Food Polysaccharides, Starch, and Protein: Processing, Characterization, and Health Benefits

Food Polysaccharides, Starch, and Protein: Processing, Characterization, and Health Benefits

Guest Editors

Jianhua Xie
Yanjun Zhang
Hansong Yu
Mingyue Shen

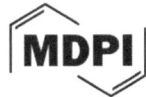

Basel • Beijing • Wuhan • Barcelona • Belgrade • Novi Sad • Cluj • Manchester

Guest Editors

Jianhua Xie
Nanchang University
Nanchang
China

Yanjun Zhang
Chinese Academy of Tropical
Agricultural Sciences
Wanning
China

Hansong Yu
Jilin Agricultural University
Changchun
China

Mingyue Shen
Nanchang University
Nanchang
China

Editorial Office
MDPI AG
Grosspeteranlage 5
4052 Basel, Switzerland

This is a reprint of the Special Issue, published open access by the journal *Foods* (ISSN 2304-8158), freely accessible at: https://www.mdpi.com/journal/foods/special_issues/2PEO4SMAM5.

For citation purposes, cite each article independently as indicated on the article page online and as indicated below:

Lastname, A.A.; Lastname, B.B. Article Title. *Journal Name* **Year**, *Volume Number*, Page Range.

ISBN 978-3-7258-3071-8 (Hbk)
ISBN 978-3-7258-3072-5 (PDF)
https://doi.org/10.3390/books978-3-7258-3072-5

© 2025 by the authors. Articles in this book are Open Access and distributed under the Creative Commons Attribution (CC BY) license. The book as a whole is distributed by MDPI under the terms and conditions of the Creative Commons Attribution-NonCommercial-NoDerivs (CC BY-NC-ND) license (https://creativecommons.org/licenses/by-nc-nd/4.0/).

Contents

About the Editors vii

Preface ix

Liyuan Rong, Mingyue Shen, Yanjun Zhang, Hansong Yu and Jianhua Xie
Food Polysaccharides and Proteins: Processing, Characterization, and Health Benefits
Reprinted from: *Foods* **2024**, *13*, 1113, https://doi.org/10.3390/foods13071113 1

Huaiwen Yang, Liang-Yu Chou and Chi-Chung Hua
Effects of Calcium and pH on Rheological Thermal Resistance of Composite Xanthan Gum and High-Methoxyl Apple Pectin Matrices Featuring Dysphagia-Friendly Consistency
Reprinted from: *Foods* **2023**, *13*, 90, https://doi.org/10.3390/foods13010090 5

Yihang Xing, Dingwen Zhang, Li Fang, Ji Wang, Chunlei Liu, Dan Wu, et al.
Complement in Human Brain Health: Potential of Dietary Food in Relation to Neurodegenerative Diseases
Reprinted from: *Foods* **2023**, *12*, 3580, https://doi.org/10.3390/foods12193580 29

Junyao Wang, Jiarui Zhang, Sainan Wang, Wenhao Liu, Wendan Jing and Hansong Yu
Isolation and Extraction of Monomers from Insoluble Dietary Fiber
Reprinted from: *Foods* **2023**, *12*, 2473, https://doi.org/10.3390/foods12132473 54

Xin Wang, Liyuan Rong, Mingyue Shen, Qiang Yu, Yi Chen, Jinwang Li and Jianhua Xie
Rheology, Texture and Swallowing Characteristics of a Texture-Modified Dysphagia Food Prepared Using Common Supplementary Materials
Reprinted from: *Foods* **2023**, *12*, 2287, https://doi.org/10.3390/foods12122287 74

Jiarui Zhang, Sainan Wang, Junyao Wang, Wenhao Liu, Hao Gong, Zhao Zhang, et al.
Insoluble Dietary Fiber from Soybean Residue (Okara) Exerts Anti-Obesity Effects by Promoting Hepatic Mitochondrial Fatty Acid Oxidation
Reprinted from: *Foods* **2023**, *12*, 2081, https://doi.org/10.3390/foods12102081 93

Anqi Xie, Hao Wan, Lei Feng, Boyun Yang and Yiqun Wan
Protective Effect of *Anoectochilus formosanus* Polysaccharide against Cyclophosphamide-Induced Immunosuppression in BALB/c Mice
Reprinted from: *Foods* **2023**, *12*, 1910, https://doi.org/10.3390/foods12091910 107

Fan Li, Tingting Li, Jiajia Zhao, Mingcong Fan, Haifeng Qian, Yan Li and Li Wang
Entanglement between Water Un-Extractable Arabinoxylan and Gliadin or Glutenins Induced a More Fragile and Soft Gluten Network Structure
Reprinted from: *Foods* **2023**, *12*, 1800, https://doi.org/10.3390/foods12091800 122

Shihua Wu, Xianxiang Chen, Ruixin Cai, Xiaodie Chen, Jian Zhang, Jianhua Xie and Mingyue Shen
Sulfated Chinese Yam Polysaccharides Alleviate LPS-Induced Acute Inflammation in Mice through Modulating Intestinal Microbiota
Reprinted from: *Foods* **2023**, *12*, 1772, https://doi.org/10.3390/foods12091772 136

Chunmei Gu, Qiuping Yang, Shujun Li, Linlin Zhao, Bo Lyu, Yingnan Wang and Hansong Yu
Effects of Soybean Trypsin Inhibitor on Pancreatic Oxidative Damage of Mice at Different Growth Periods
Reprinted from: *Foods* **2023**, *12*, 1691, https://doi.org/10.3390/foods12081691 151

Yanan Guo, Caihua Liu, Yichang Wang, Shuanghe Ren, Xueting Zheng, Jiayu Zhang, et al.
Impact of Cavitation Jet on the Structural, Emulsifying Features and Interfacial Features of Soluble Soybean Protein Oxidized Aggregates
Reprinted from: *Foods* **2023**, *12*, 909, https://doi.org/10.3390/foods12050909 . . . . **164**

Mingyue Shen, Ruixin Cai, Zhedong Li, Xiaodie Chen and Jianhua Xie
The Molecular Mechanism of Yam Polysaccharide Protected H_2O_2-Induced Oxidative Damage in IEC-6 Cells
Reprinted from: *Foods* **2023**, *12*, 262, https://doi.org/10.3390/foods12020262 . . . . **188**

Kaiying Jia, Min Wei, Yao He, Yujie Wang, Hua Wei and Xueying Tao
Characterization of Novel Exopolysaccharides from *Enterococcus hirae* WEHI01 and Its Immunomodulatory Activity
Reprinted from: *Foods* **2022**, *11*, 3538, https://doi.org/10.3390/foods11213538 . . . . **202**

Xingfen He, Bin Wang, Baotang Zhao, Yuecheng Meng, Jie Chen and Fumin Yang
Effect of Hydrothermal Treatment on the Structure and Functional Properties of Quinoa Protein Isolate
Reprinted from: *Foods* **2022**, *11*, 2954, https://doi.org/10.3390/foods11192954 . . . . **217**

About the Editors

Jianhua Xie

Jianhua Xie is a Professor of Nanchang University. He received his B.S., M.S., and Ph.D. degrees in Food Science and Engineering, Food Science and Nutrition from Nanchang University in July 2005, January 2008, and January 2015, respectively. He joined the Department of Food Science, Purdue University, as a Postdoctoral Fellow from 2016 to 2017 with a government scholarship from the China Scholarship Council. He is an Executive Council Member of the Society of Processing and Storage of Agro-products of the China Agricultural Society, a Council Member of the Food Science and Technology of Jiangxi Province, a Member of the Editorial Board of Journal of Food Nutrition and Dietetics, a Member of Institute of Food Technologist, a Member of the Institute of Food Technologist, and a Member of the American Chemical Society. His research mainly focuses on the structure and bioactivities of food carbohydrate polymers (dietary fiber and polysaccharides), and the structure–function relationships of polysaccharides. He has published more than 200 research papers and has played a leading role in many scientific and technological projects sponsored by the National Natural Science Foundation of China, the Science and Technology Support Project, sponsored by the Ministry of Science and Technology, Jiangxi Province, and so on.

Yanjun Zhang

Yanjun Zhang is a Professor at the Spice and Beverage Research Institute, the Chinese Academy of Tropical Agricultural Sciences. He graduated from Nanchang University with a major in Food Science and Engineering in 2012. He is engaged in scientific research on starch. Taking tropical grain crops and jackfruit starch as representative material, research has been carried out on the basic theory and application of technology with ideas including the relationship between starch functional characteristics and molecular structure, the pasting and retrogradation properties of starch controlled by the molecular weight of amylopectin, and starch digestion improved through innovative methods. The special functional properties and molecular structure of jackfruit starch have been clarified. The control theory of starch pasting and retrogradation has been enriched based on the knowledge of starch structure and function. An efficient preparation method has also been established for improving the digestibility and utilization rate of jackfruit starch. His previous research has led to 64 publications, 7 national invention patents, and the Hainan Provincial Science and Technology Progress Award in 2017. He has demonstrated national-level talents: Shennong Talents, Jiangxi Province Double Thousand Plan leading talents, Hainan Province South Sea famous, 515 talent project second level, hot science excellent youth, and others.

Hansong Yu

Hansong Yu is a Professor and Doctoral Supervisor at the College of Food Science and Engineering, Jilin Agricultural University. Professor Yu graduated from Jilin University's Department of Biochemistry and Molecular Biology, receiving his doctorate degree in 2008. From 2013 to 2014, he collaborated on the intensive processing of soybean products as a Fellow of the American Academy of Food Sciences (SAM K.C. CHANG, IFT Fellow, ACS Fellow) at North Dakota State University and Mississippi State University in the United States. He has presided over 13 projects of the National Agricultural Industry Technology System, the National Natural Science Foundation of China, the Major National Science and Technology Support Project, the National Ministry of Agriculture 948 Project, and other national and Jilin major projects. He won the first prize of the Jilin Provincial

Science and Technology Progress Award, first prize of the National Harvest Award for agriculture, animal husbandry, and fishery, two first prizes of the Jilin Provincial Natural Science Achievement Award, four second prizes of the Science and Technology Progress Award, and one third prize. He has published more than 300 papers (90 papers included in SCI and EI) and two monographs and textbooks. Moreover, he has applied for and obtained 25 patents and participated in the formulation of four national and industry standards.

Mingyue Shen

Mingyue Shen is a Professor and Doctoral Supervisor at the State Key Laboratory of Food Science and Resources, Nanchang University. She received her B.S., M.S., and Ph.D. degrees in Food Science and Engineering from Nanchang University in July 2005, January 2008, and June 2016, respectively. She joined the University of California, Davi, as a Postdoctoral Fellow from 2020 to 2022 with a government scholarship from the China Scholarship Council. She has presided over 10 projects of the National Natural Science Foundation of China, the Major National Science and Technology Support Project of Jiangxi Provincial. She won the second prize of the Jiangxi Provincial Science and Technology Progress Award and has published more than 120 papers (90 papers included in SCI and EI), two monographs and textbooks, and 20 invention patents.

Preface

Polysaccharides, starch, and protein are naturally occurring polymers with efficient, safe and green characteristics. These food components show different physico-chemical properties, functional properties and biological activity. The structural characteristics and functional activity of these natural components are gradually being recognized, and they are widely applied in the food industry as important raw materials. Nowadays, the unsatisfactory characteristics of natural components including their insolubility at lower temperatures, instability under certain conditions, viscosity change, and lack of functional properties still limit their specialized mass production and downstream processing with high added value. Therefore, research studies on the modification and application of polysaccharides, starch, and protein are needed. Our Special Issue, "Food Polysaccharides and Proteins: Processing, Characterization, and Health Benefits", with two reviews and eleven articles, offers a broad perspective on recent in-depth studies of these components. The Guest Editors are very grateful to all the authors for their contributions and the entire MDPI team for their professional support.

Jianhua Xie, Yanjun Zhang, Hansong Yu, and Mingyue Shen
Guest Editors

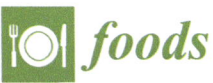

Editorial

Food Polysaccharides and Proteins: Processing, Characterization, and Health Benefits

Liyuan Rong [1], Mingyue Shen [1], Yanjun Zhang [2], Hansong Yu [3] and Jianhua Xie [1,*]

[1] State Key Laboratory of Food Science and Resources, Nanchang University, Nanchang 330047, China; rongliyuan01@163.com (L.R.); shenmingyue1107@163.com (M.S.)
[2] Spice and Beverage Research Institute, Chinese Academy of Tropical Agricultural Sciences, Wanning 571533, China; zhangyanjun0305@163.com
[3] College of Food Science and Engineering, Jilin Agricultural University, Changchun 130118, China; yuhansong@163.com
* Correspondence: xiejianhua7879@163.com; Tel./Fax: +86-791-8830-4347

Natural macromolecular substances are prevalent in the organs of plants and animals, such as polysaccharides, resins, proteins, etc. With the progress of modern isolation technology as well as the development of enzyme engineering and modification technologies, the structural characteristics and functional activity of these natural components are gradually recognized, and they are widely applied in the food industry as important raw materials. Nowadays, the unsatisfactory characteristics of natural components, including their insolubility at lower temperatures, instability under certain conditions, viscosity change, and lack of functional properties, still limit their specialized mass production and downstream processing with high added value. Researchers in specific subjects from around the world devote themselves to further investigating the critical properties and mechanisms during the process, and a Special Issue titled "Food Polysaccharides, Starch, and Protein: Processing, Characterization, and Health Benefits" was launched for peers in related fields to exchange recent research progress on the modification of natural active substances and their functional activities.

Among these accepted manuscripts, various critical properties and mechanisms of natural macromolecular substances had been put forward, many focusing on the separation and purification of new protein and polysaccharide resources, as well as their changes in structure and nutritional function during processing. Polysaccharides are biomacromolecule carbohydrates wildly found in nature, consisting of multiple monosaccharide units connected by glycosidic bonds [1]. The advancement in isolation and identification techniques has led to a significant surge of interest and research in polysaccharides. The polysaccharides discovered in recent years have exhibited diverse biological activities, including anti-tumor, antioxidant, antibacterial, anti-inflammatory, and immunomodulatory effects [2,3]. Lu et al. [4] revealed that the Iljinskaja polysaccharide and Chinese yam polysaccharide (CYP) improved colitis symptoms in dextran sulfate sodium-induced mice by enhancing the production of IL-10, inhibiting cytokines (IL-1β and TNF), and reducing myeloperoxidase (MBO) activity. They also reduced the contents of lipopolysaccharide-binding protein (LBP) and endotoxin (ET) in serum and oxidative stress in the liver, promoting the expression of mucin MUC-2, ZO-1, and occluding to maintain the integrity of the intestine. The pretreatment of CYP relieved excessive oxidative stress by modulating the MAPK signaling pathway, with a corresponding preventive role against injury to the intestinal barrier [5].

Polysaccharides are applied to the development of special foods and packing materials due to their special composition and structure, such as dysphagia diet [6], 3D printing foods [7], and biodegradable food packaging [8]. The biological activities of natural polysaccharides extracted from various sources may not always meet satisfactory requirements

---

Citation: Rong, L.; Shen, M.; Zhang, Y.; Yu, H.; Xie, J. Food Polysaccharides and Proteins: Processing, Characterization, and Health Benefits. *Foods* **2024**, *13*, 1113. https://doi.org/10.3390/foods13071113

Received: 17 March 2024
Revised: 28 March 2024
Accepted: 2 April 2024
Published: 5 April 2024

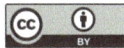

Copyright: © 2024 by the authors. Licensee MDPI, Basel, Switzerland. This article is an open access article distributed under the terms and conditions of the Creative Commons Attribution (CC BY) license (https://creativecommons.org/licenses/by/4.0/).

and can even demonstrate suboptimal performance. The exploration and molecular modification of polysaccharide resources play a crucial role in promoting the utilization of polysaccharides in both the food and non-food industries [9,10]. Among the manuscripts accepted by the Special Issue, the exopolysaccharide (EPS) was successfully isolated and purified from probiotic *Enterococcus hirae* WEHI01. EPS was composed of I01-1, I01-2, I01-3, and I01-4, while I01-2 and I01-4 raised the viability and phagocytic function of macrophage cells, boosted NO generation, and encouraged the release of cytokines including TNF-α and IL-6 in RAW 264.7 macrophages. The main components of *Anoectochilus formosanus* polysaccharide (AFP) were galacturonic acid, glucose, and galactose, and AFP alleviated cyclophosphamide-induced immunosuppression and significantly improved the immunity of mice via stimulating the production of cytokines (IgA, IgG, SIgA, IL-2, IL-6, and IFN-γ). Obesity has become a global public health matter; it always causes a series of severe chronic diseases, such as metabolic syndrome, cardiovascular disease, type 2 diabetes, and neurodegenerative diseases [11]. In this Special Issue, the potential regulatory mechanisms of high-purity insoluble dietary fiber from soybean residue (HPSIDF) on hepatic fatty acid oxidation were investigated. The medium- and long-chain fatty acid oxidation in hepatic mitochondria was accelerated because HPSIDF effectively increased the levels of acyl-coenzyme A oxidase 1, malonyl coenzyme A, acetyl coenzyme A synthase, acetyl coenzyme A carboxylase, and carnitine palmitoyl transferase-1. HPSIDF supplementation significantly ameliorated co-occurring symptoms in high-fat diet-induced mice, including body weight gain, fat accumulation, dyslipidemia, and hepatic steatosis. As an important part of the innate immune system, the complement pathway is critical for identifying and clearing pathogens that rapidly react to defend the body against external pathogens. Xing et al. [12] reviewed the function and immunomodulatory mechanisms of complement component 1q (C1q), and they summarized the foods, including polysaccharides, with beneficial effects in neurodegenerative diseases via C1q and the complement pathway. For instance, *Artemisia annua* polysaccharides exhibited noteworthy efficacy in anticomplement activities through the classical pathway and alternative pathway, and *Prunella vulgaris* polysaccharides exhibited a potential value in addressing ailments correlated with the excessive activation of the complement system, while they could interact with C1q, exerting an influence on the C2, C3, C5, and C9 constituents of the complement system.

The physicochemical properties of natural polysaccharides always need to be modified to meet the development of food science and technology, and there are considerable differences between the natural and modified polysaccharides [13]. This Special Issue highlighted that CYP and sulfated Chinese yam polysaccharides (SCYP) both promoted the proliferation of polysaccharide-degrading bacteria and facilitated the intestinal de-utilization of polysaccharides by producing more biomarkers of the gut microbiome. Differently, CYP regulated the gut microbiota by decreasing *Desulfovibrio* and *Sutterella* and increasing *Prevotella*, while SCYP changed the gut microbiota by decreasing *Desulfovibrio* and increasing *Coprococcus*, which reversed the microbiota dysbiosis caused by lipopolysaccharide. SCYP was more effective than CYP in reducing hepatic TNF-α, IL-6, and IL-1β secretion. Special dietary foods are specifically formulated to meet the nutritional needs of individuals with unique requirements. The dysphagia diet is a special eating plan for dysphagia patients, such as newborns, the elderly, and patients with postoperative muscle loss, neurological impairment, and Alzheimer's disease [14]. In this Special Issue, high-methoxyl apple pectin was employed as the main component to improve the rheological behaviors for developing dysphagia-friendly fluidized alimentary matrices. The researchers prepared dysphagia foods using rice starch, perilla seed oil, and whey isolate protein and evaluated the positive effects of food supplements (vitamins, minerals, salt, and sugar) on the swallowing characteristics and rheological and textural properties of the prepared products. The work revealed that polysaccharides hold great potential for the special diet's application, and the combination of the nutritional functional activity and the sensory physical properties could be the research priorities in the following research work [15,16]. As a macromolecular polysaccharide aggregate, insoluble dietary fiber will also be focused on in the Special Issue, and the developing status of technologies for the separation and extraction of single components in insoluble dietary fiber will be reviewed, aiming to expand their application in the food and non-food fields.

Proteins play a major role in human life, serving as the basic structural material of the body as well as biochemical catalysts and regulators of genes [17,18]. The soybean trypsin inhibitors caused structural damage and secretory dysfunction of the pancreas, increasing lipid peroxidation and injuring the enzymatic and non-enzymatic antioxidant defenses in the soybean trypsin inhibitor diet-fed mice. Proteins could be denatured, altering their physiochemical properties and functions during thermal or non-thermal treatment. The denaturation of proteins is a prevalent occurrence in processing, and comprehending and harnessing the principles and mechanisms behind protein denaturation holds immense significance [19,20]. Among the papers published in the Special Issue, suitable cavitation jet treatment (CJT) improved the food proteins' functionalities by adjusting the structural and functional features of solvable oxidized soybean protein accumulations. The CJT at a short treatment time destroyed the core aggregation skeleton of soybean protein insoluble aggregates and transferred the insoluble aggregates into soluble aggregates. The prolonged CJT reaggregated the soluble oxidized aggregates through an anti-parallel intermolecular β-sheet, resulting in a lower emulsification activity index (EAI) and emulsification stability index (ESI) and a higher interfacial tension. The effects of hydrothermal treatment on the structure and functional properties of quinoa protein isolate (QPI) were studied. The secondary and tertiary structures of QPI were significantly changed after hydrothermal treatment, which accounted for the hydrothermal treatment. QPI exhibited a better functional property, while the suitable hydrothermal treatment improved its water-holding and oil-holding capacity, emulsifying activity, emulsion stability, and solubility [21]. As the main macromolecules concerned in this Special Issue, proteins and polysaccharides were also studied in innovative combinations. Water-unextractable arabinoxylan (WUAX) improved the textural property of flour by interacting with starch or gluten and investigating its structure-activity relationship [22]. WUAX increased the free sulfhydryl of gliadins and glutenins, inhibiting the formation of covalent bonds. WUAX decreased the β-sheet content and increased the β-turn prevalence of gliadins and glutenins. Differently, the WUAX decreased the contents of α-helixes and β-sheets for glutenins, and it did not significantly change these values of gliadins [22]. Consequently, WUAX could cause a quality deterioration of gluten by weakening the structure of the gliadins and glutenins.

In summary, the manuscripts published in this Special Issue have explored various innovative bioactive macromolecular resources and studied their structural characteristics, bioactivity, and nutritional function properties, as well as their application potential in the food industry. These results are helpful for colleagues to understand the health benefits of homologous resources in medicine and food and the characterization methods in the discovery process. The information presented in this Special Issue will promote the widespread use of macromolecules such as polysaccharides and proteins in the food industry.

Author Contributions: L.R. and J.X. conceived and wrote this editorial L.R., M.S., Y.Z., H.Y. and J.X. Did writing—review and editing of this editorial. All authors have read and agreed to the published version of the manuscript.

Funding: The authors gratefully acknowledge the financial support provided by the National Key Research and Development Program of China (2023YFF1104001-3) and the Jiangxi Provincial Natural Science Foundation, China (20232BCD44003).

Conflicts of Interest: The authors declare no conflicts of interest.

References

1. Gao, Y.; Tan, J.; Sang, Y.; Tang, J.; Cai, X.; Xue, H. Preparation, structure, and biological activities of the polysaccharides from fruits and vegetables: A review. *Food Biosci.* **2023**, *54*, 102909. [CrossRef]
2. Subhash, A.; Bamigbade, G.; al-Ramadi, B.; Kamal-Eldin, A.; Gan, R.; Ranadheera, C.; Ayyash, M. Characterizing date seed polysaccharides: A comprehensive study on extraction, biological activities, prebiotic potential, gut microbiota modulation, and rheology using microwave-assisted deep eutectic solvent. *Food Chem.* **2024**, *444*, 138618. [CrossRef] [PubMed]

3. Geng, X.; Guo, D.; Wu, B.; Wang, W.; Zhang, D.; Hou, S.; Bau, T.; Lei, J.; Xu, L.; Cheng, Y.; et al. Effects of different extraction methods on the physico-chemical characteristics and biological activities of polysaccharides from Clitocybe squamulose. *Int. J. Biol. Macromol.* **2024**, *259 Pt 2*, 2024129234. [CrossRef] [PubMed]
4. Lu, H.; Shen, M.; Chen, Y.; Yu, Q.; Chen, T.; Xie, J. Alleviative effects of natural plant polysaccharides against DSS-induced ulcerative colitis via inhibiting inflammation and modulating gut microbiota. *Food Res. Int.* **2023**, *167*, 112630. [CrossRef]
5. Shen, M.; Cai, R.; Li, Z.; Chen, X.; Xie, J. The Molecular Mechanism of Yam Polysaccharide Protected H_2O_2-Induced Oxidative Damage in IEC-6 Cells. *Foods* **2023**, *12*, 262. [CrossRef]
6. Zhang, C.; Wang, C.; Girard, M.; Therriault, D.; Heuzey, M. 3D printed protein/polysaccharide food simulant for dysphagia diet: Impact of cellulose nanocrystals. *Food Hydrocol.* **2024**, *148*, 109455. [CrossRef]
7. Wang, J.; Jiang, Q.; Huang, Z.; Muhammad, A.; Gharsallaoui, A.; Cai, M.; Yang, K.; Sun, P. Rheological and mechanical behavior of soy protein-polysaccharide composite paste for extrusion-based 3D food printing: Effects of type and concentration of polysaccharides. *Food Hydrocol.* **2024**, *153*, 109942. [CrossRef]
8. Deng, J.; Zhu, E.-Q.; Xu, G.-F.; Naik, N.; Murugadoss, V.; Ma, M.-G.; Guo, Z.; Shi, Z.-J. Overview of renewable polysaccharide-based composites for biodegradable food packaging applications. *Green Chem.* **2022**, *24*, 480–492. [CrossRef]
9. Guan, X.; Wang, F.; Zhou, B.; Sang, X.; Zhao, Q. The nutritional function of active polysaccharides from marine animals: A review. *Food Biosci.* **2024**, *58*, 103693. [CrossRef]
10. Qin, Z.; Huang, M.; Zhang, X.; Hua, Y.; Zhang, X.; Li, X.; Fan, C.; Li, R.; Yang, J. Structural and in vivo-in vitro myocardial injury protection features of two novel polysaccharides from *Allium macrostemon* Bunge and *Allium chinense* G. Don. *Int. J. Biol. Macromol.* **2024**, *264 Pt 1*, 130537. [CrossRef]
11. Kolsi, R.; Jardak, N.; Hajkacem, F.; Chaaben, R.; Jribi, I.; Feki, A.; Rebai, T.; Jamoussi, K.; Fki, L.; Belghith, H.; et al. Anti-obesity effect and protection of liver-kidney functions by Codium fragile sulphated polysaccharide on high fat diet induced obese rats. *Int. J. Biol. Macromol.* **2017**, *102*, 119–129. [CrossRef] [PubMed]
12. Xing, Y.; Zhang, D.; Fang, L.; Wang, J.; Liu, C.; Wu, D.; Liu, X.; Wang, X.; Min, W. Complement in Human Brain Health: Potential of Dietary Food in Relation to Neurodegenerative Diseases. *Foods* **2023**, *12*, 3580. [CrossRef]
13. Uzeme, P.; Aluta, Z.; Aderolu, O.; Ishola, A.; Gordon, A.; Olumayokun, A. Chemical characterisation of sulfated polysaccharides from the red seaweed *Centroceras clavulatum* and their in vitro immunostimulatory and antioxidant properties. *Food Hydrocoll. Health* **2023**, *3*, 100135.
14. Min, C.; Zhang, C.; Cao, Y.; Li, H.; Pu, H.; Huang, J.; Xiong, Y. Rheological, textural, and water-immobilizing properties of mung bean starch and flaxseed protein composite gels as potential dysphagia food: The effect of Astragalus polysaccharide. *Int. J. Biol. Macromol.* **2023**, *239*, 124236. [CrossRef]
15. Funami, T.; Nakauma, M. Cation-responsive food polysaccharides and their usage in food and pharmaceutical products for improved quality of life. *Food Hydrocol.* **2023**, *141*, 108675. [CrossRef]
16. Yong, H.; Liu, J. Polysaccharide-catechin conjugates: Synthesis methods, structural characteristics, physicochemical properties, bioactivities and potential applications in food industry. *Trends Food Sci. Technol.* **2024**, *145*, 104353. [CrossRef]
17. Qi, X.; Li, Y.; Li, J.; Rong, L.; Pan, W.; Shen, M.; Xie, J. Fibrillation modification to improve the viscosity, emulsifying, and foaming properties of rice protein. *Food Res. Int.* **2023**, *166*, 112609. [CrossRef]
18. Liu, S.; Li, Z.; Yu, B.; Wang, S.; Shen, Y.; Cong, H. Recent advances on protein separation and purification methods. *Adv. Colloid Interface Sci.* **2020**, *284*, 102254. [CrossRef] [PubMed]
19. Cheng, S.; Langrish, A. Fluidized bed drying of chickpeas: Developing a new drying schedule to reduce protein denaturation and remove trypsin inhibitors. *J. Food Eng.* **2023**, *351*, 111515. [CrossRef]
20. Ren, C.; Hong, S.; Qi, L.; Wang, Z.; Sun, L.; Xu, X.; Du, M.; Wu, C. Heat-induced gelation of SAM myofibrillar proteins as affected by ionic strength, heating time and temperature: With emphasis on protein denaturation and conformational changes. *Food Biosci.* **2023**, *56*, 103320. [CrossRef]
21. Lu, X.; Zhan, J.; Ma, R.; Tian, Y. Structure, thermal stability, and in vitro digestibility of rice starch–protein hydrolysate complexes prepared using different hydrothermal treatments. *Int. J. Biol. Macromol.* **2023**, *230*, 123130. [CrossRef] [PubMed]
22. Li, F.; Li, T.; Zhao, J.; Fan, M.; Qian, H.; Li, Y.; Wang, L. Entanglement between Water Un-Extractable Arabinoxylan and Gliadin or Glutenins Induced a More Fragile and Soft Gluten Network Structure. *Foods* **2023**, *12*, 1800. [CrossRef] [PubMed]

Disclaimer/Publisher's Note: The statements, opinions and data contained in all publications are solely those of the individual author(s) and contributor(s) and not of MDPI and/or the editor(s). MDPI and/or the editor(s) disclaim responsibility for any injury to people or property resulting from any ideas, methods, instructions or products referred to in the content.

Article

Effects of Calcium and pH on Rheological Thermal Resistance of Composite Xanthan Gum and High-Methoxyl Apple Pectin Matrices Featuring Dysphagia-Friendly Consistency

Huaiwen Yang [1,*], Liang-Yu Chou [1] and Chi-Chung Hua [2,*]

1. Department of Food Science, National Chiayi University, Chiayi City 60004, Taiwan
2. Department of Chemical Engineering, National Chung Cheng University, Chiayi City 621301, Taiwan
* Correspondence: calyang@g.ncyu.edu.tw (H.Y.); chmcch@ccu.edu.tw (C.-C.H.); Tel.: +886-52717620 (C.-C.H.)

Abstract: High-methoxyl apple pectin (AP) derived from apple was employed as the main ingredient facilitating rheological modification features in developing dysphagia-friendly fluidized alimentary matrices. Xanthan gum (XG) was also included as a composite counterpart to modify the viscoelastic properties of the thickened system under different thermal processes. The results indicate that AP is extremely sensitive to thermal processing, and the viscosity is greatly depleted under a neutral pH level. Moreover, the inclusion of calcium ions echoed the modification effect on the rheological properties of AP, and both the elastic property and viscosity value were promoted after thermal processing. The modification effect of viscoelastic properties (G' and G'') was observed whne XG was incorporated into the composite formula. Increasing the XG ratio from 7:3 to 6:4 (AP:XG) triggers the rheological transformation from a liquid-like form to a solid-like state, and the viscosity value shows that the AP-XG composite system exhibits better thermal stability after thermal processing. The ambient modifiers of pH (pH < 4) and calcium chloride concentration (7.5%) with an optimal AP-XG ratio of 7:3 led to weak-gel-like behavior ($G'' < G'$), helping to maintain the texture properties of dysphagia-friendly features similar to those prior to the thermal processing.

Keywords: high-methoxyl pectin; thermal processing; xanthan gum; rheological properties; texture profile analysis; dysphagia

1. Introduction

Aging can lead to dysphagia, a condition characterized by the degradation of swallowing function involving the oropharyngeal muscles and nerves [1–3]. The prevalence of dysphagia among the elderly in the Midwest of the United States ranges from 6% to 9%, but it is estimated to be 15–22% in community residents over 50 years old and as high as 40–60% among those in assisted living facilities and nursing homes [3]. Diseases such as stroke, Parkinson's disease, multiple sclerosis, and neoplasms can also cause dysphagia [4,5]. To ensure the safe swallowing of flowable foods for individuals with dysphagia, thickeners are often used to modify the consistency of thin liquids, creating a safe-progressive alimentary bolus that can pass through the esophagus safely [6]. Consequently, thickeners serve as the foundation for creating dysphagia-friendly matrices for consistency adjustment [1,4–6].

A multi-disciplinary volunteer committee organized by the International Dysphagia Diet Standardisation Initiative (IDDSI) developed a general diet framework for with dysphagia [7]. The framework categorizes the consistency of food fluids into several levels by assessing a designated 10 mL syringe without a needle within a period of 10 s in contrast to a fork drip test [7,8]. The IDDSI framework is developed as per the guidelines issued by the most recognized organizations, such as the National Dysphagia Diet (NDD) proposed by the American Dietetic Association in 2002 [9], the Dysphagia Diet Committee of the Japanese Society of Dysphagia Rehabilitation [10,11] and the Australian Standardised Labels and Definitions [12]. These organizations also indicate that a fluidized food matrix bearing a viscosity greater than 50 mPa.s at a designated shear rate of 50 1/s is generally considered dysphagia-friendly [7–12].

The IDDSI framework, despite not including viscosity measurement, emphasizes the importance of food matrices having consistent apparent viscosity (thickness) at the specified test shear rate (50 1/s) to influence flow behavior and rheological characteristics [13–16]. While the IDDSI guideline is straightforward and accessible, it predominantly provides qualitative descriptions of food texture and liquid consistency. It lacks quantitative information on the textural and rheological characteristics of food and liquids. This gap makes it challenging for industry partners to ensure the quality of their modified diet products consistently [8]. The lack of quantitative data hinders researchers from exploring how food texture and liquid rheology affect swallowing [17]. Relying solely on qualitative assessments cannot capture the nuanced variations in food or liquids categorized within the same IDDSI level [18]. Consequently, there is a need to create quantitative metrics for the textural and rheological properties of food and liquids to enhance and support the IDDSI guidelines [17–19]. Cichero et al. highlighted the practical and scientific challenges in accessing rheological testing equipment and expertise needed for more comprehensive studies [7]. Furthermore, understanding the non-Newtonian and elastic behaviors of thickened food matrices requires careful observation and consideration using rheological methods beyond rotary viscometers [20–23].

Starch- and gum-based thickeners are commonly used to create dysphagia-friendly formulations that yield suitable fluidized matrices [24,25]. Starch-based thickened matrices may require additional carbohydrate calories to sustain primary energy metabolism [26]. However, these matrices are susceptible to viscosity reduction within a short 10 s window due to amylase-containing saliva during oral processing, posing a risk of accidental inhalation and aspiration pneumonia for dysphagic individuals [27–29]. The molecular degradation and consistency reduction of starch-based matrices due to the enzymatic activity of saliva alpha-amylase presents a significant concern. These changes can compromise the safety of the food bolus, increasing the risk of accidental inhalation and, consequently, aspiration pneumonia. Acknowledging these risks, it is clear that choosing non-starch-based (gum-based) matrices is a preferable approach. These alternatives are inherently more resistant to enzymatic breakdown, offering a more stable and predictable consistency. This stability is crucial in reducing the risk of aspiration and ensuring the safety and efficacy of dysphagia diets. Hydrocolloid gums are often added to stabilize the consistency of commercially available dysphagia-friendly products. Among these, xanthan gum is highly versatile, capable of forming networks, resistant to acidity, and can serve as an excipient when used alone or in combination with other polymers [30]. Yoon and Yoo studied the rheological behaviors of xanthan gum-based thickened formulas with 8 g of carbohydrate per 100 mL and found significant differences in shear-thinning behavior [31]. Ortega et al. reported that matrices with a consistency between 250 and 1000 mPa·s, achieved with a mixed starch and xanthan gum product, resulted in safe swallowing [32]. However, starch-based thickened matrices may face texture depletion during thermal processing, with significant viscosity reduction reported after simulated pasteurization [33]. Considering these challenges, gum-based matrices, such as pectin materials, have gained attention as thickeners, particularly when calorie supplementation is not a primary concern.

Pectin materials, found in plant cell walls, are chemically complex polysaccharides composed of various components, including homogalacturonans, rhamnogalacturonans-I, rhamnogalacturonans-II, xylogalacturonan, and apio-galacturonan moieties [34–37]. Their primary structure consists of repeating units of α-D-galacturonic acid linked with 1,4-glucosidic bonds and esterified with methyl residues at C-6 [36]. Commercial pectin products are classified as high- (>50%) or low- (<50%) methoxyl pectin based on their degree of methyl esterification (DE), with the European regulation requiring at least 65% α-D-galacturonic acid [36]. Pectin molecules can form three-dimensional aggregates, allowing them to create hydrocolloidal matrices with thickening properties [37]. These properties make them suitable as texture modifiers to meet dysphagia-friendly requirements [38].

Additionally, pectin materials offer health benefits beyond their rheological and mechanical properties, including antioxidant activities [34], anti-diabetic effects [39,40], and reductions in low-density lipoprotein [41]. They also serve as dietary fiber sources that function as prebiotics for intestinal fermentation [42–44]. We previously reported on the rheological and texture properties of a low-degree-of-esterification (DE = 45.4%) apple pectin-based composite formula with xanthan gum as a modifier, showing potential for dysphagia-friendly applications [33]. However, the effects of thermal processes on xanthan gum–apple pectin (XG–AP) composite formulas with varying DE levels of pectin materials remain unexplored and warrant investigation.

In this study, we used high-methoxyl apple pectin (AP) as the base thickener to develop thickened model matrices intended for commercial distribution within a sterilized logistics chain involving thermal processing that causes variations in rheological behavior. Therefore, the aims of this study are: (1) to investigate how blending xanthan gum (XG) and AP in varying proportions modifies rheological properties and determines the optimal thermal stability ratio; (2) to explore the modification effects and identify the optimal thermal stability formula by introducing calcium ions and adjusting pH in the XG–AP system; and (3) to assess the suitability of the XG–AP system as a thickening formula for dysphagia-friendly fluidized matrices.

2. Materials and Methods

2.1. Materials and Chemicals

The XG thickener used in this study was generously provided by a local food additive agency (Gemfont Co. Ltd., Taipei, Taiwan). XG is a long-chain polysaccharide (circa 2000 kDa) with d-glucose, d-mannose, and d-glucuronic acid as the main building skeleton in a nearly equal ratio in terms of quantitative molecule amounts with a high number of trisaccharide side chains associated with cations of sodium, potassium, and calcium [45,46]. The powdered apple pectin (AP) (Solgar, Inc., Leonia, NJ, USA) was purchased. Its degree of esterification was subjected to our in-house titration evaluation and reported in Section 3; we deemed it as presumably a high-methoxy AP. Calcium chloride anhydrous (CCA) as a divalent calcium source was obtained from Sigma-Aldrich Co. (St. Louis, MO, USA). A commercial powder, Neo-high Toromeal III® (TRM, Food-care, Inc., Tokyo, Japan), was obtained as the control sample for the texture examination. Unless stated otherwise, all other chemicals in this study were of chemical grade, such as powdered citric acid and sodium bicarbonate.

2.2. Degree of Esterification (DE)

The DE of apple pectin (AP) was estimated as described previously [47] with minor modifications. Briefly, 0.2 g of powdered apple pectin was thoroughly dissolved in 200 mL of deionized water by stirring under ambient temperature for 2 h. Upon complete mixing, 3–5 drops of phenolphthalein indicator solution ($C_{20}H_{14}O_4$, Sigma-Aldrich Co., St. Louis, MO, USA) were employed, and the dissolved AP solution was thereafter subjected to titration with 0.1 M NaOH until the mixture turned pink, and this lasted for 30 s; the depletion volume of NaOH (mL) was recorded as V_1. Another 10 mL of NaOH was added and underwent stirring for 30 min. Subsequently, 10 mL of 0.1 M HCl was thoroughly mixed with the pink solution to neutralize the solution until it turned transparent, followed by a second titration of 0.1 M NaOH until the solution turned pink again for another 30 s. The second depletion volume of NaOH was recorded as V_2. The DE was calculated according to Equation (1):

$$\text{DE\%} = \frac{V_1}{V_1 + V_2} \times 100 \tag{1}$$

2.3. Sample Preparation

To measure the basic characteristics of AP and to evaluate its optimal formula with possible modifications, sample matrices were prepared according to the formulae listed in

Table 1. Sample powders were weighed and dispersed evenly in reverse osmosis water; to adjust the designated pH of the sample matrices, a small amount of reverse osmosis water was taken to dissolve the hydrocolloid completely, and then the pH was adjusted with a citric acid solution and sodium bicarbonate solution. The mixed matrix was stirred with an electronic stirrer at ambient temperature for complete dissolution, and the sample was poured into a 15 mL centrifuge tube and stored at 4 °C for future usage.

Table 1. List of formulating parameters and groups of hydrocolloidal matrices with their corresponding codes.

Group		Matrix Code	Concentrations/pH or Ca^{+2}
Preliminary			
	Control	--	AP = 2 wt%
	pH adjusted	pH3, pH4, pH 5, and pH6	AP = 2 wt%/Acid or alkaline
	Ca^{+2} addition	Ca2.5, Ca5, Ca7.5, and Ca10	AP = 2 wt%/calcium chloride anhydrous (CCA)
Composite			
	Composite ratio	XG0.6AP1.4	XG = 0.6 wt% and AP = 1.4 wt%
		XG0.8AP1.2	XG = 0.8 wt% and AP = 1.2 wt%
Solitary XG		XG0.6	XG = 0.6 wt%
		XG0.8	XG = 0.8 wt%
Modifier			
	Ca^{+2}	XG0.6AP1.4-Ca2.5	XG = 0.6 wt% and AP = 1.4 wt% with 2.5 wt% CCA
		XG0.6AP1.4-Ca7.5	XG = 0.6 wt% and AP = 1.4 wt% with 7.5 wt% CCA
	pH	[pH5, XG0.6AP1.4-Ca2.5] [pH6, XG0.6AP1.4-Ca2.5] [pH5, XG0.6AP1.4-Ca7.5] [pH6, XG0.6AP1.4-Ca7.5]	Corresponding CCA level with pH adjustment

2.4. Thermal Processes

We employed a retort autoclave (SS-325, Tomy Seiko Co., Ltd., Tokyo, Japan) in simulating thermal processing. Control sample matrices (2 wt% AP) were sealed in designated centrifuge tubes equipped with temperature data loggers (MadgeTech, Inc., Warner, NH, USA). They were subjected to programmed treatments, including 5 or 10 min at 95 °C, 5 min at 105 °C, and 1 min at 115 °C. Appendix A illustrates the sample matrices' actual temperature profiles over time, showing slight variations from the programmed temperature patterns due to thermal penetration delays. We selected 95 °C and 105 °C for 5 min as our thermal treatment settings, as these temperatures are commonly used for sterilizing high-acid foods. Pectin-based matrices typically have a pH below 4.6, categorizing them as high-acid (acidified) food matrices.

2.5. Rheological Measurements and Flow Behavior Characterization

A stress-controlled rheometer (DHR-2, TA Instruments, New Castle, DE, USA) equipped with a plate-and-plate stainless fixture (diameter = 40 mm, gap distance = 1000 μm) or a cylindrical double-gap fixture (inner cup diameter = 30.2 mm, inner motor diameter = 31.97 mm and outer diameter = 34.98 mm) was used. A Peltier temperature controller was used to maintain the temperature measurement at 25 °C. A solvent trap was employed to prevent moisture loss. The rheological measurements in chronological order are: (1) dynamic oscillatory strain sweeps to identify the linear viscoelastic region (LVR), (2) frequency sweeps with 2 min of rest duration after strain sweeps, (3) shear rate-dependent viscosities with 2 min rest duration after frequency sweep. The measurement parameters are listed in Table 2.

Table 2. Experimental parameters for the employed rheometer.

Experiment	Temperature (°C)	Strain (%)	Frequency (rad/s)	Shear Rate (1/s)
Strain sweep	25	0.01-100	50	-
Frequency sweep	25	1	0.1-100	-
Shear-rate-dependent viscosity	25	-	-	0.1, 0.3, 1, 3, 10, 30, 50, 70, and 100

2.6. Texture Profile Analysis (TPA)

The authorized method of TPA issued in 2009 by the Japanese Ministry of Consumers, "Food for patients with swallowing difficulty", under the regulation of "Food for special dietary uses", was adopted for the characterization of model food matrices [35].

2.7. Data Manipulation and Statistical Analysis

The experimental data of this study were plotted and presented by Sigmaplot® version 10.0. One-way ANOVA for LVR and loss tangent (tan δ) and two-way ANOVA for shear rate dependent viscosity were performed to determine significant differences using Duncan's multiple range tests based on three replications; paired sample t-tests were utilized to justify the significance of differences among the mean values of textural properties based on nine replications. SPSS (Statistical Package for the Social Science) version 19.0 was used for the statistical analysis, and difference comparisons were made within the confidence interval of 95%, unless otherwise specified.

3. Results and Discussion

3.1. DE Evaluation of Apple Pectin Sample Powder

The AP sample used in this study exhibited a degree of esterification of 73.9 ± 1.00%, indicating its high-methoxyl form. However, achieving a weak-gel-like texture solely with high-methoxyl pectin is challenging due to its strict gel-forming conditions (requiring soluble solids >55% and pH < 3.5). Thus, the study explores composite formulas to create food matrices with the desired texture, with xanthan gum (XG) assistance. XG matrices generally exhibit elastic characteristics and contribute to the formation of thickened composite matrices (TCMs). Building on our previous study [35], we prepared two types of 2 wt% TCMs with different XG-to-AP ratios (4:6 and 3:7) to assess their rheological properties. Additionally, we prepared solitary (standalone) XG matrices using the same formula as a reference to evaluate the improvement in thermal stability brought about by TCMs.

3.2. Thermal Stability Analysis of Thickened Composite Matrices (TCM)

3.2.1. Effects of Xanthan Gum (XG) and High-Methoxy Apple Pectin (AP) Composite Ratio on Rheological Behavior

Figure 1A(a) displays the strain sweep profiles (50 rad/s) of the composite XG–AP and standalone XG thickened matrices without thermal processing, both constrained to 2% weight. The 2% AP matrix exhibits liquid-like behavior (Appendix B), while standalone XG matrices (0.6% or 0.8%) exhibit solid-like behavior within the linear viscoelastic region (LVR), as summarized in Table 3. Increasing the XG ratio from XG0.6AP1.4 to XG0.8AP1.2 shifts the viscoelastic characteristics from liquid-like to solid-like. Figure 1A(b) presents frequency sweep profiles at 1% strain for the samples without thermal processing. The results indicate that the qualitative features, as exhibited by the slopes of G′ for standalone XG (XG0.6 and XG0.8) and composite XG–AP (XG0.6AP1.4 and XG0.8AP1.2) matrices, are similar, while the slopes of the G″ curve vary significantly. The overall trends suggest that the addition of AP to the composite XG–AP group imparts viscous characteristics to the samples, while XG primarily contributes to the elastic characteristics of the composite

XG–AP matrices. Table 4 provides the viscosity values at different shear rates for all samples. The viscosity of each sample decreases as the shear rate increases, with the standalone XG group (XG0.6, XG0.8) exhibiting a larger degree of shear thinning compared to the composite groups XG0.6AP1.4 and XG0.8AP1.2.

To evaluate the modification effect of the XG composite ratio on the thermal stability of thickened matrices with the AP base, the set thermal processes for 5 min at 95 °C and 105 °C were imposed, and the results are presented in Figures 1B and 1C, respectively. Comparing the results of solitary (standalone) XG samples (XG0.6 and XG0.8) in terms of strain sweep and frequency sweep, both G' and G'' values decreased significantly after the thermal processing, and the increase in thermal processing temperature resulted in a more significant decrease. For composite matrices, the strain sweep profile of the 95 °C processing shows that the decreases in G' and G'' in the XG0.6AP1.4 sample are less than those in the XG0.8AP1.2 sample. The viscoelastic characteristics of the former (XG0.6AP1.4) indicate good thermal stability at 95 °C for 5 min. However, the matrices treated at 105 °C (Figure 1C) show very different trends.

Table 3. Linear viscoelastic region data resulted from the strain sweep due to different thermal processes. Storage modulus (G'_{LVR}); loss modulus (G''_{LVR}); loss tangent (tan δ_{LVR}) [†].

Treatment	Sample	G'_{LVR} (Pa)	G''_{LVR} (Pa)	tan δ_{LVR}
Prior	XG0.6	25.63 ± 0.12 [c]	6.94 ± 0.14 [d]	0.27 ± 0.01 [c]
	XG0.6AP1.4	19.91 ± 0.70 [d]	22.55 ± 0.35 [b]	1.13 ± 0.05 [a]
	XG0.8	71.06 ± 0.31 [a]	13.77 ± 0.11 [c]	0.19 ± 0.00 [d]
	XG0.8AP1.2	40.69 ± 0.64 [b]	27.33 ± 0.16 [a]	0.67 ± 0.0145 [b]
95 °C	XG0.6	19.55 ± 0.08 [c]	5.78 ± 0.11 [d]	0.30 ± 0.01 [c]
	XG0.6AP1.4	17.67 ± 0.76 [d]	19.55 ± 0.16 [b]	1.11 ± 0.06 [a]
	XG0.8	39.63 ± 0.05 [a]	9.20 ± 0.02 [c]	0.23 ± 0.00 [d]
	XG0.8AP1.2	29.36 ± 0.12 [b]	20.55 ± 0.06 [a]	0.70 ± 0.00 [b]
105 °C	XG0.6	14.49 ± 0.06 [d]	4.88 ± 0.04 [d]	0.34 ± 0.00 [c]
	XG0.6AP1.4	23.97 ± 0.38 [c]	17.53 ± 0.10 [a]	0.73 ± 0.01 [a]
	XG0.8	25.25 ± 0.06 [b]	7.97 ± 0.05 [c]	0.32 ± 0.00 [d]
	XG0.8AP1.2	26.84 ± 0.05 [a]	13.42 ± 0.06 [b]	0.50 ± 0.00 [b]
Prior	XG0.6AP1.4	19.91 ± 0.70 [c]	22.55 ± 0.35 [c]	1.13 ± 0.05 [a]
	XG0.6AP1.4Ca2.5	34.49 ± 0.46 [b]	24.26 ± 0.13 [a]	0.70 ± 0.01 [b]
	XG0.6AP1.4Ca7.5	40.25 ± 0.30 [a]	23.74 ± 0.22 [b]	0.59 ± 0.01 [c]
95 °C	XG0.6AP1.4	17.67 ± 0.76 [c]	19.55 ± 0.16 [c]	1.11 ± 0.06 [a]
	XG0.6AP1.4Ca2.5	39.35 ± 0.41 [a]	19.73 ± 0.17 [b]	0.50 ± 0.01 [c]
	XG0.6AP1.4Ca7.5	30.21 ± 0.49 [b]	20.75 ± 0.17 [a]	0.69 ± 0.02 [b]
105 °C	XG0.6AP1.4	23.97 ± 0.38 [c]	17.53 ± 0.10 [a]	0.73 ± 0.01 [a]
	XG0.6AP1.4Ca2.5	35.47 ± 0.53 [a]	16.00 ± 0.10 [c]	0.45 ± 0.01 [c]
	XG0.6AP1.4Ca7.5	34.24 ± 0.19 [b]	17.37 ± 0.12 [b]	0.51 ± 0.00 [b]
Prior	XG0.6AP1.4Ca7.5	40.25 ± 0.298 [a]	23.74 ± 0.22 [a]	0.59 ± 0.01 [c]
	XG0.6AP1.4Ca7.5 (pH 5)	19.04 ± 0.42 [b]	17.92 ± 0.15 [b]	0.94 ± 0.03 [a]
	XG0.6AP1.4Ca7.5 (pH 6)	15.72 ± 0.46 [c]	13.79 ± 0.33 [c]	0.88 ± 0.04 [b]
95 °C	XG0.6AP1.4Ca7.5	30.21 ± 0.49 [a]	20.75 ± 0.17 [a]	0.69 ± 0.02 [a]
	XG0.6AP1.4Ca7.5 (pH 5)	15.31 ± 0.45 [c]	6.37 ± 0.10 [b]	0.42 ± 0.02 [b]
	XG0.6AP1.4Ca7.5 (pH 6)	19.38 ± 0.23 [b]	5.74 ± 0.03 [c]	0.30 ± 0.00 [c]
105 °C	XG0.6AP1.4Ca7.5	34.24 ± 0.19 [a]	17.37 ± 0.12 [a]	0.51 ± 0.00 [a]
	XG0.6AP1.4Ca7.5 (pH 5)	19.54 ± 0.22 [b]	5.56 ± 0.03 [b]	0.28 ± 0.00 [b]
	XG0.6AP1.4Ca7.5 (pH 6)	18.07 ± 0.33 [c]	5.26 ± 0.16 [c]	0.29 ± 0.01 [b]

[†] Means ± SD of triplicate analyses are given. [a–d] Means with different lowercase superscripts within an individual thermal treatment (sub-column) differ significantly.

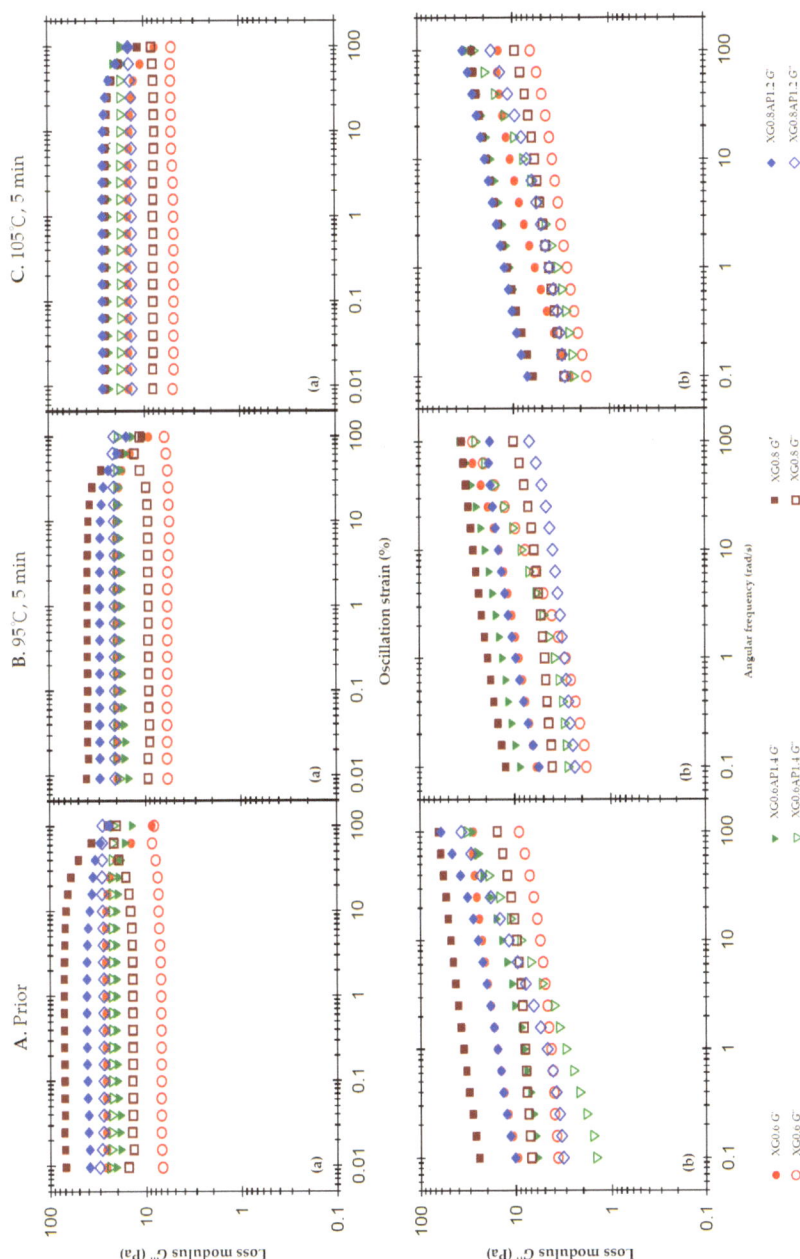

Figure 1. Storage modulus (G') and loss modulus (G'') of composite xanthan gum and high-methoxy apple pectin (XG-AP) formula and the corresponding standalone XG thickened matrices based on a 2% weight constraint experiencing different thermal processing conditions: (**A**). prior to thermal processes, (**B**). after a 95 °C for 5 min process and (**C**). after a 105 °C for 5 min. (**a**) oscillatory strain sweeps at the frequency of 50 rad./s, and (**b**) angular frequency sweeps at 1% strain.

Table 4. Shear-rate-dependent (10–100 1/s) viscosity (mPa·s) due to the thermal processing for different composite formulations with dysphagia-friendly potential [†].

Formula [†]	Processing	Modifier	Shear Rate (1/s)				
			10	30	50	70	100
XG0.6	Prior	--	1036.8 ± 0.76 [3, a]	411.9 ± 0.63 [3, a]	280.4 ± 0.67 [3, a]	222.0 ± 1.41 [3, a]	178.7 ± 0.78 [4, a]
	95 °C, 5 min	--	755.8 ± 0.60 [b]	272.1 ± 0.14 [b]	174.8 ± 0.18 [b]	129.9 ± 0.09 [b]	95.1 ± 0.09 [b]
	105 °C, 5 min	--	615.3 ± 0.23 [c]	228.6 ± 0.05 [c]	142.0 ± 0.03 [c]	103.9 ± 0.01 [c]	74.8 ± 0.01 [c]
XG0.6AP1.4	Prior	--	1327.7 ± 3.91 [2, b]	808.3 ± 1.55 [1, a]	638.7 ± 0.51 [1, a]	549.4 ± 0.59 [1, a]	465.6 ± 0.43 [1, a]
	95 °C, 5 min	--	1299.2 ± 4.09 [c]	754.7 ± 1.50 [b]	584.6 ± 0.61 [b]	496.5 ± 0.81 [b]	416.2 ± 0.71 [b]
	105 °C, 5 min	--	1376.0 ± 4.89 [a]	753.7 ± 1.58 [c]	568.9 ± 0.73 [c]	476.7 ± 0.72 [c]	394.0 ± 0.74 [c]
XG0.8	Prior	--	2542.4 ± 3.84 [1, a]	1060.1 ± 2.00 [2, a]	732.9 ± 0.85 [2, a]	576.6 ± 1.21 [2, a]	450.2 ± 0.94 [3, a]
	95 °C, 5 min	--	1145.7 ± 1.96 [b]	430.2 ± 0.40 [b]	281.2 ± 0.55 [b]	217.2 ± 0.46 [b]	162.2 ± 0.48 [b]
	105 °C, 5 min	--	860.1 ± 0.22 [c]	319.6 ± 0.10 [c]	200.7 ± 0.04 [c]	147.1 ± 0.04 [c]	105.6 ± 0.02 [c]
XG0.8AP1.2	Prior	--	2180.0 ± 4.92 [1, a]	1167.3 ± 1.88 [1, a]	870.1 ± 0.80 [1, a]	719.1 ± 0.83 [1, a]	583.8 ± 0.71 [2, a]
	95 °C, 5 min	--	1376.9 ± 3.87 [b]	718.4 ± 1.38 [b]	528.8 ± 0.70 [b]	433.8 ± 0.67 [b]	349.6 ± 0.64 [b]
	105 °C, 5 min	--	1204.3 ± 2.48 [c]	555.4 ± 0.95 [c]	385.1 ± 0.48 [c]	305.6 ± 0.46 [c]	239.4 ± 0.43 [c]
AP2.0	Prior	control	290.8 ± 0.27 [β, A, a]	270.3 ± 0.14 [β, A, a]	258.1 ± 0.12 [β, A, a]	249.2 ± 0.10 [β, A, a]	238.5 ± 0.06 [β, A, a]
	95 °C, 5 min	control	123.4 ± 0.21 [b]	120.4 ± 0.13 [b]	118.5 ± 0.12 [b]	116.5 ± 0.08 [b]	113.8 ± 0.09 [b]
	105 °C, 5 min	control	55.0 ± 0.14 [c]	53.6 ± 0.11 [c]	53.3 ± 0.09 [c]	53.0 ± 0.06 [c]	52.6 ± 0.04 [c]
	Prior	pH = 3	270.6 ± 1.04 [A, a]	253.4 ± 0.33 [A, a]	243.2 ± 0.21 [A, a]	235.3 ± 0.14 [A, a]	225.5 ± 0.08 [A, a]
	95 °C, 5 min	pH = 3	116.1 ± 0.22 [b]	112.6 ± 0.20 [b]	110.6 ± 0.18 [b]	108.8 ± 0.16 [b]	106.4 ± 0.00 [b]
	105 °C, 5 min	pH = 3	48.8 ± 0.11 [c]	47.1 ± 0.03 [c]	46.6 ± 0.03 [c]	46.3 ± 0.02 [c]	46.0 ± 0.01 [c]
	Prior	pH = 4	247.9 ± 0.70 [A, a]	233.6 ± 0.25 [A, a]	223.7 ± 0.11 [A, a]	216.0 ± 0.12 [A, a]	206.7 ± 0.07 [A, a]
	95 °C, 5 min	pH = 4	119.2 ± 0.17 [b]	115.6 ± 0.10 [b]	113.1 ± 0.08 [b]	111.0 ± 0.04 [b]	108.1 ± 0.05 [b]
	105 °C, 5 min	pH = 4	61.9 ± 0.18 [c]	60.9 ± 0.09 [c]	60.4 ± 0.09 [c]	60.0 ± 0.07 [c]	59.4 ± 0.05 [c]
	Prior	pH = 5	257.2 ± 0.53 [B, a]	237.5 ± 0.42 [B, a]	224.8 ± 0.38 [B, a]	214.8 ± 0.12 [B, a]	203.0 ± 0.28 [B, a]
	95 °C, 5 min	pH = 5	60.8 ± 0.18 [b]	60.1 ± 0.09 [b]	59.8 ± 0.08 [b]	59.5 ± 0.07 [b]	59.0 ± 0.02 [b]
	105 °C, 5 min	pH = 5	17.4 ± 0.13 [c]	17.3 ± 0.05 [c]	17.2 ± 0.04 [c]	17.2 ± 0.01 [c]	17.2 ± 0.02 [c]

Table 4. Cont.

Formula [†]	Processing	Modifier	Shear Rate (1/s)				
			10	30	50	70	100
	Prior	pH = 6	240.5 ± 0.16 [B,a]	225.6 ± 0.08 [B,a]	215.5 ± 0.07 [B,a]	207.2 ± 0.05 [B,a]	197.0 ± 0.03 [B,a]
	95 °C, 5 min	pH = 6	11.4 ± 0.10 [b]	11.1 ± 0.03 [b]	11.0 ± 0.02 [b]	10.9 ± 0.00 [b]	10.9 ± 0.02 [b]
	105 °C, 5 min	pH = 6	5.91 ± 0.05 [c]	5.49 ± 0.01 [c]	5.39 ± 0.00 [c]	5.3 ± 0.00 [c]	5.2 ± 0.00 [c]
	Prior	Ca2.5	721.9 ± 0.64 [α,a]	563.4 ± 0.26 [α,a]	496.5 ± 0.22 [α,a]	454.6 ± 0.21 [α,a]	411.4 ± 0.20 [α,a]
	95 °C, 5 min	Ca2.5	260.1 ± 0.40 [b]	214.7 ± 0.27 [b]	195.2 ± 0.26 [b]	182.7 ± 0.11 [b]	169.6 ± 0.24 [b]
	105 °C, 5 min	Ca2.5	79.2 ± 0.20 [c]	69.5 ± 0.14 [c]	65.6 ± 0.12 [c]	63.2 ± 0.06 [c]	60.6 ± 0.08 [c]
	Prior	Ca5	578.1 ± 1.16 [α,a]	459.2 ± 0.39 [α,a]	408.9 ± 0.27 [α,a]	376.9 ± 0.20 [α,a]	343.8 ± 0.18 [α,a]
	95 °C, 5 min	Ca5	232.0 ± 0.14 [b]	192.4 ± 0.06 [b]	175.4 ± 0.05 [b]	164.6 ± 0.05 [b]	153.3 ± 0.05 [b]
AP2.0	105 °C, 5 min	Ca5	73.3 ± 73.3 [c]	64.6 ± 0.11 [c]	60.8 ± 0.08 [c]	58.5 ± 0.06 [c]	55.9 ± 0.03 [c]
	Prior	Ca7.5	577.0 ± 0.86 [α,a]	461.9 ± 0.31 [α,a]	412.5 ± 0.17 [α,a]	380.6 ± 0.16 [α,a]	366.8 ± 0.16 [α,a]
	95 °C, 5 min	Ca7.5	272.8 ± 0.23 [b]	225.0 ± 0.16 [b]	204.9 ± 0.14 [b]	191.7 ± 0.13 [b]	177.7 ± 0.12 [b]
	105 °C, 5 min	Ca7.5	91.3 ± 0.18 [c]	78.5 ± 0.11 [c]	73.4 ± 0.08 [c]	70.3 ± 0.05 [c]	67.0 ± 0.04 [c]
	Prior	Ca10	555.5 ± 0.88 [α,a]	444.4 ± 0.30 [α,a]	397.0 ± 0.25 [α,a]	347.4 ± 0.11 [α,a]	335.6 ± 0.10 [α,a]
	95 °C, 5 min	Ca10	259.3 ± 0.31 [b]	215.0 ± 0.25 [b]	195.7 ± 0.23 [b]	183.3 ± 0.19 [b]	170.1 ± 0.11 [b]
	105 °C, 5 min	Ca10	76.5 ± 0.17 [c]	67.3 ± 0.10 [c]	63.6 ± 0.08 [c]	61.3 ± 0.06 [c]	58.8 ± 0.05 [c]
	Prior *	Ca40	482.0 ± 0.76	391.2 ± 0.43	348.9 ± 0.32	322.4 ± 0.33	295.3 ± 0.27
	Prior	Ca2.5	2129.3 ± 7.94 [a]	1039.3 ± 2.83 [a]	757.6 ± 1.26 [a]	625.4 ± 1.27 [a]	511.6 ± 1.02 [a]
	95 °C, 5 min	Ca2.5	1958.4 ± 6.89 [b]	934.2 ± 2.51 [b]	674.8 ± 1.05 [b]	554.7 ± 1.04 [b]	452.2 ± 0.88 [b]
XG0.6AP1.4	105 °C, 5 min	Ca2.5	1698.0 ± 4.90 [c]	806.5 ± 1.82 [c]	579.9 ± 0.84 [c]	474.4 ± 0.87 [c]	384.9 ± 0.72 [c]
	Prior	Ca7.5	2245.7 ± 7.63 [a]	1109.7 ± 3.49 [a]	807.7 ± 1.54 [a]	666.3 ± 1.49 [a]	544.6 ± 1.29 [a]
	95 °C, 5 min	Ca7.5	1883.6 ± 5.68 [b]	930.0 ± 2.31 [b]	676.5 ± 1.24 [b]	557.8 ± 1.15 [b]	455.8 ± 0.98 [b]
	105 °C, 5 min	Ca7.5	1746.8 ± 5.19 [c]	841.5 ± 2.13 [c]	606.2 ± 1.11 [c]	496.7 ± 1.10 [c]	403.5 ± 0.98 [c]

* Control without statistical comparison. [†] Means ± SD of triplicate analyses are given. [a–c] Means with different lowercase superscripts within an individual thermal treatment at a specific shear rate (sub-column) differ significantly. [A–B] Means with different lowercase superscripts indicate significant differences due to pH values for AP2.0 matrices; [α–β] Means due to Ca (CCA) concentrations for AP2.0 matrices; [1–4] Means due to composite ratio of formula.

Compared with the results in Figure 1B(a) for the 95 °C processing, the sample XG0.8AP1.2 in Figure 1C(a) does not show a significant decrease in G', but shows a substantial decrease in G''. Presumably, the G'' of the aforementioned composite matrices (0.8/1.2) is mainly dominated by apple pectin molecules, so the rise in temperature aggravates the degradation of apple pectin. It leads to the decline of composite matrices, which can also be observed from the results of the XG0.6AP1.4 sample. In the strain sweep profile, the XG0.6AP1.4 matrix shows liquid-like characteristics ($G' < G''$) after thermal processing at 95 °C; however, the temperature rise would promote pectin degradation. As a result, the XG0.6AP1.4 sample shifted to a solid-like behavior ($G'' < G'$) shown in the strain sweep profile after the thermal processing at 105 °C. The frequency sweep results of thermal processing at 105 °C also indicate that the viscoelastic moduli of XG (control) group samples are lower than those of samples subjected to thermal processing at 95 °C due to the increase in temperature. In the composite group, because pectin is the main component contributing to the viscous characteristics, the slope of the G'' curve of XG0.6AP1.4 is significantly greater than that of XG0.8AP1.2, and both samples demonstrate more remarkable elastic characteristics with the increase in pectin degradation after the thermal processing.

Table 4 exhibits the shear-rate-dependent viscosity of the composite matrices and their corresponding controls prior to and after the designated thermal processing. All samples show a similar trend of shear thinning, while the standalone XG sample matrices show the most significant degree of shear thinning. For the XG0.8AP1.2 composite matrix, the degree of shear thinning is close to that of the standalone XG group due to its higher XG ratio.

Following a 5 min exposure to a 95 °C thermal load, the viscosity at a shear rate of 50 1/s decreased by varying amounts: 37.6% for XG0.6 (i.e., 280 → 174 mPa.s), 61.6% for XG0.6AP1.4, 8.5% for XG0.8, 39.2% for XG0.8AP1.2, and 54.1% for AP2.0. These results indicate that higher concentrations of standalone XG matrices correspond to more substantial viscosity reductions after thermal processing. Notably, XG itself does not provide resistance to thermal processing, aligning with findings reported by Naji et al. [48].

While the viscosity of AP matrices also decreased significantly post-thermal processing, composite matrices experienced only slight reductions. Notably, the XG0.6AP1.4 matrix exhibited the least viscosity reduction, at 8.5%. The composite XG–AP matrices present stronger thermal stability than the standalone XG or AP, and XG0.6AP1.4 (or 3:7 in ratio) is the best among them. This may be due to certain co-structures formed by XG and AP that impart the composite matrices' excellent thermal stability. Therefore, the ideal modification effect can be achieved by exploring the optimized mixing ratio of XG and AP.

Deducing from the observations above, the remarkable rheological behavior provided by XG can be utilized to modify the viscoelastic characteristics of the AP matrices, which are dominated by viscous characteristics at low concentrations. In addition, the composite matrices can provide the corresponding hydrocolloidal matrices with a polymer system possessing more robust thermal stability. Therefore, including composite matrices into thickened edible fluid matrices for seniors is quite exploitable, and provides products featuring thermal stability after high-temperature processing.

3.2.2. Modification Effects of pH and CCA on the Rheological Behavior of Thickened XG–AP Matrices

- Preliminary tests

The pH of the 2% AP is approximately 3.3 (control), and Appendix B provides insights into the rheological behavior of the 2% AP matrices under varying pH and thermal conditions. Thahur et al. [49] have reported that carboxyl dissociation in AP matrices can be hindered under low-pH conditions. Following thermal processing at 95 °C and 105 °C, it is evident that the G'' for matrices at pH 5 and 6 are significantly lower compared to those at pH 3 and 4. This observation suggests that β-elimination reactions may occur most rapidly at pH levels near neutrality during the thermal pyrolysis of pectin, aligning with the findings of Fraeye et al. [50]. Additionally, high-methoxy pectin is generally considered resistant to acid hydrolysis. In summary, AP matrices subjected to 5 min thermal loading at 95 °C exhibit higher apparent viscosity compared to those at 105 °C. Furthermore, it can be inferred that maintaining a low pH can help mitigate thermal degradation in terms of consistency.

Appendix C illustrates the impact of calcium ions (Ca2.5 through 10) on standalone 2% AP matrices. The addition of CCA as the calcium ion source was expected to hydrate the water in the matrices, resulting in a denser intermolecular pectin structure. A prior study by Noriah et al. [51] noted that the addition of calcium ions to low-concentration pectin matrices led to an increase in G', consistent with the findings in this study. While the loss tangent value for samples with added calcium ions is slightly higher, ~1 (Table 3), compared to the control samples, it can be inferred that incorporating CCA as the calcium ion source predominantly enhances the elastic properties of pectin m matrices rather than the viscosity properties, making the samples closer to a solid-like state. The experimental results, both before and after thermal processing, indicate that the formulations containing Ca2.5 and 7.5 exhibit more favorable modification effects, and are therefore selected for further formulation evaluation.

- Effects of CCA Concentration

Previous experiments indicate that adding CCA as a calcium ion source can modify the viscoelastic characteristics of the 2% standalone AP matrices, and the samples added with calcium ions show higher viscosity (thickening effect) after thermal processing. Therefore, this section aims to explore the effect of calcium ion (CCA) dosage on the rheological properties of the samples. The groups with the highest viscosity after thermal processing (added with 2.5% and 7.5% CCA) in the previous experiment and the XG0.6AP1.4 matrix base without CCA addition were employed for the investigation.

Figure 2A displays the rheological profiles of the three samples before thermal processing. The strain sweep (at a high frequency of 50 rad/s) reveals that the liquid-like state of XG0.6AP1.4 transitions to a solid-like state when calcium ions are added (XG0.6AP1.4-Ca2.5 and XG0.6AP1.4-Ca7.5), consistent with previous experimental findings that the addition of CCA enhances the elasticity of the matrices. The influence of CCA on XG–AP composite matrices is evident, maintaining the desirable weak-gel-like state pursued in this study. Notably, in the absence of CCA, the G'' of composite matrices exhibits significant changes after thermal processing (Figure 2A(a)). Furthermore, in frequency sweep tests, the samples with added CCA (Ca2.5 and Ca7.5) consistently exhibit significantly higher values of G' and G'' compared to matrices in the absence of CCA.

It is hypothesized that calcium ions may enhance the molecular structure of composite matrices, making them more robust. When examining the frequency sweep profile, particularly in the high-frequency region, samples lacking CCA exhibit characteristics that are more viscous than elastic. Notably, a crossover point is observable in this context. However, the sample's molecular structure is more stable after the addition of calcium ions, as the sample's elasticity becomes dominant and there is no crossover point within the same range of frequencies. Therefore, the dominance of viscosity would occur only at still higher frequencies. In examining the impact of CCA addition, the results before thermal processing reveal that the XG0.6AP1.4-Ca2.5 and XG0.6AP1.4-Ca7.5 curves closely coincide in both strain and frequency sweep profiles. This suggests that calcium ions from CCA exert a limited modifying effect on the samples prior to heating. Therefore, a further investigation was conducted to assess whether calcium ion concentration would affect the rheological properties of the samples after thermal processing.

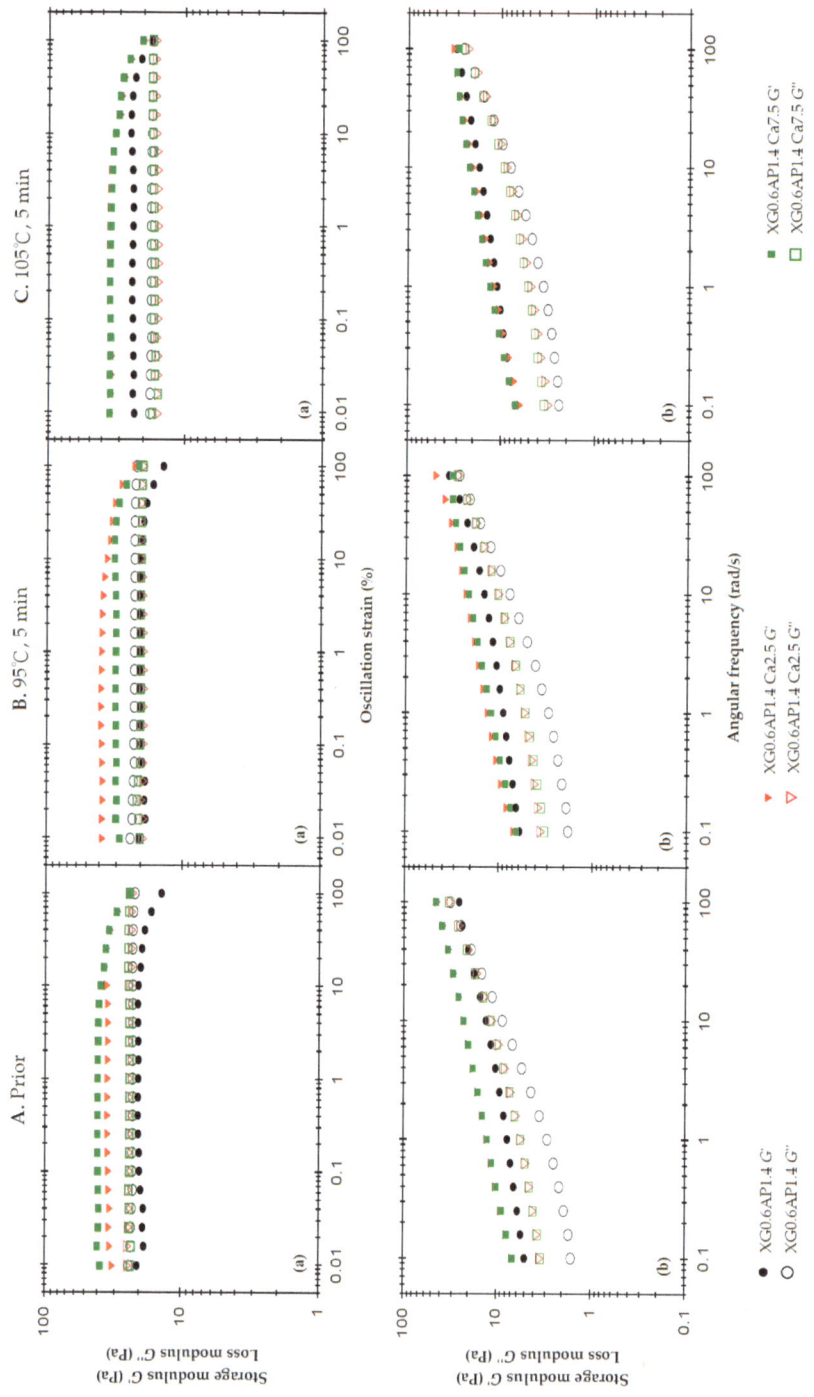

Figure 2. The effects of 2.5% and 7.5% calcium chloride anhydrous on storage modulus (G') and loss modulus (G'') of the composite XG–AP (XG0.6AP1.4) thickened matrix experiencing different thermal processing conditions: (**A**) prior to thermal process, (**B**) after a 95 °C for 5 min process and (**C**) after a 105 °C for 5 min process with (**a**) oscillatory strain sweeps at the frequency of 50 rad/s, and (**b**) angular frequency sweeps at 1% strain.

Figure 2B displays the rheological profiles of the samples subjected to a 5 min thermal treatment at 95 °C. In the strain sweep profile, it is observed that the G' of XG0.6AP1.4-Ca2.5 is higher than that of XG0.6AP1.4-Ca7.5. However, the G'' of XG0.6AP1.4-Ca2.5 is slightly lower than that of XG0.6AP1.4-Ca7.5. This outcome aligns with previous experimental findings when comparing the impact of CCA addition on standalone 2% AP matrices, where Ca2.5 and Ca7.5 exhibited the most favorable modification effects prior to thermal processing.

However, after undergoing thermal processing at 95 °C for 5 min, it becomes evident that XG0.6AP1.4-Ca7.5 exhibits superior thermal stability compared to XG0.6AP1.4-Ca2.5. The latter, XG0.6AP1.4-Ca2.5, displays reduced thermal stability due to a decrease in G'', indicating a weakening of the pectin structure. This results in the XG–AP composite matrices leaning more towards a viscoelastic profile biased towards XG, and consequently experiencing an increase in elastic characteristics. A notable difference in the frequency sweep profile compared to the pre-thermal group is in the absence of the original crossover point in the high-frequency region for XG0.6AP1.4. This absence is attributed to the partial degradation of the pectin structure. The results obtained from the 5 min thermal processing at 95 °C highlight that a higher calcium ion concentration is effective.

Figure 2C shows the rheological profiles of the samples affected by a 5 min thermal load at 105 °C. Due to the increase in temperature compared to the temperature of 95 °C, XG0.6AP1.4-Ca7.5 presents almost the same rheological characteristics as XG0.6AP1.4-Ca2.5 in its strain sweep and frequency sweep results. As the temperature rises to 105 °C, the increase in calcium ion concentration ceases to enhance the thermal stability. It has been reported that the addition of calcium ions can enhance the associative strength of high-methoxyl pectins [52,53], diverging from the "egg-box" model seen in low-methoxyl pectins and more closely resembling alginate gelation [54]. Yang et al. [55] have noted that a calcium-concentrating process, brought about by water evaporation, enables high-methoxyl pectin molecules to improve their hydrophobic interactions, which is crucial for gel formation. However, the specific molecular interactions between high-methoxyl pectin and calcium ions require further investigation to be fully understood. Therefore, the addition of CCA can improve the thermal stability of composite matrices only at a lower temperature (95 °C) under the same processing duration.

The viscosities (Table 4) measured at a shear rate of 50 Hz (1/s) were used to investigate the effect of CCA addition on the sample viscosity. The viscosity values of XG0.6AP1.4, XG0.6AP1.4-Ca2.5, and XG0.6AP1.4-Ca7.5 prior to thermal processing are 638.8, 757.6, and 807.7 mPa.s, respectively. They become lower after thermal processing at 95 °C, and even lower after thermal processing at 105 °C. The existence of calcium ions can promote the viscosity of the sample with or without thermal processing. According to the above results, the viscosity of XG0.6AP1.4-Ca7.5 is comparatively higher in all three conditions, although the disparity is small in general. We also observed that the inclusion of calcium ions into XG0.6AP1.4 composite matrices has a modification effect on both the viscoelastic characteristics and viscosities. Especially with Ca7.5, the viscoelastic characteristics after thermal processing at 95 °C are closer to the weak-gel-like state, and the viscosities are also the highest in all cases at a shear rate of 50 Hz (1/s). Therefore, XG0.6AP1.4-Ca7.5 is considered a better choice for the dysphagia-friendly fluid model system for use in the following evaluation.

- Effects of pH

For the evaluation of the pH effect, an XG–AP composite ratio of 3:7 with 7.5% CCA was employed (i.e., XG0.6AP1.4-Ca7.5). The measured pH is 2.92 prior to any adjustment, which is in line with the low-pH environment. Therefore, samples with pH 5 and 6 are additionally prepared to investigate the influence of pH on the rheological properties and matrix stability after thermal processing.

Figure 3 presents the results of the rheological analysis concerning the pH effect. In Figure 3A, we observe the rheological profiles of the samples before thermal processing. The previous strain sweep results indicate that the incorporation of CCA substantially enhances the elasticity of XG0.6AP1.4 composite matrices, which originally exhibited liquid-like characteristics, to the extent that G' surpasses G'' and demonstrates a weak-gel-like behavior. Notably, the samples with pH adjusted to 5 and 6 also exhibit a weak-gel-like pattern, but with both G' and G'' values higher than those of the original XG0.6AP1.4-Ca7.5.

The frequency sweep also shows results similar to the strain sweep, and additionally, the viscosities of the three samples exhibit shear-thinning characteristics. At a shear rate of 50 1/s, the measured viscosity follows the trend: control, XG0.6AP1.4-Ca7.5 (807.7 mPa.s) > pH 5, XG0.6AP1.4-Ca7.5 (565.0 mPa.s) > pH 6, XG0.6AP1.4-Ca7.5 (393.0 mPa.s).

Figure 3B shows the rheology profile of the same set of samples subjected to a 5 min thermal load at 95 °C. The strain sweep and frequency sweep profiles show that the G' of the XG0.6AP1.4-Ca7.5 sample with unadjusted pH value (pH = 2.92, control) did not decrease significantly, and the sample still exhibited weak-gel-like characteristics. Thus, the composite matrices can maintain properties similar to those prior to thermal processing with good stability. In contrast, the other two samples with pH values adjusted to be close to the neutral one (pH = 7) showed quite different trends. The G' and G'' pH 5, XG0.6AP1.4-Ca7.5 sample decreased, and especially the G''; the G'' of the pH 6, XG0.6AP1.4-Ca7.5 sample also decreased, while the G' increased.

Therefore, the above and previous experimental findings (as detailed in Appendix B) offer mutual support. When subjected to heating under pH 5 and 6 conditions, pectin undergoes more pronounced degradation compared to lower pH levels. This degradation similarly affects XG–AP composite matrices. The degradation of apple pectin, primarily responsible for imparting viscosity to the samples, results in a significant reduction in G'' for the pH 5 and 6 samples. It is speculated that the degree of AP degradation in the pH 6 environment exceeds that in the pH 5 environment, causing a weaker modification effect on XG–AP composite matrices in the latter. Consequently, both samples exhibit increased G', resembling the viscoelastic traits of XG.

In Figure 3C, which showcases the rheological profiles of the samples after thermal processing at 105 °C for 5 min, the overall trend remains largely consistent with that observed after thermal processing at 95 °C. As a higher temperature will accelerate pectin degradation, a decrease in G'' can be seen from the strain sweep profile of the XG0.6AP1.4-Ca7.5 sample (Figure 3C(a)). For comparison, the pH 5, XG0.6AP1.4-Ca7.5 sample exhibited a similar increase in the elastic characteristics as the pH 6, XG0.6AP1.4-Ca7.5 sample when the thermal processing temperature was increased to 105 °C.

The changes in viscosity due to thermal processing are calculated from the reported data shown in Table 4. For the measured viscosity at a shear rate of 50 1/s, the viscosity of all samples decreased after thermal processing. However, it can be seen that the two samples with pH close to the neutral state exhibited more pronounced viscosity reductions than those of lower pH values. After being heated at 95 °C and 105 °C for 5 min, the viscosity of the control, XG0.6AP1.4-Ca7.5 sample decreased by 16.24% and 24.9% (807.7 → 676.5 and 807.7 → 606.3 mPa.s), respectively; the pH 5, XG0.6AP1.4-Ca7.5 sample decreased by 57.8% and 62.1% (565.0 → 238.3 and 565.0 → 214.1 mPa.s), respectively; the pH 6, XG0.6AP1.4-0Ca7.5 sample decreased by 45.8% and 52.4% (393.0 → 213.1 and 393.0 → 186.9 mPa.s), respectively.

As per the previous discussions on the effects of the pH values of the matrix systems, the viscoelasticity and viscosity of the XG–AP composite matrices can be observed to decrease more significantly after thermal processing, with pH closer to the neutral state (pH 5 or 6). The degradation of apple pectin in these samples leads to decreased viscous characteristics, resulting in promoted elastic characteristics (similar to the rheological characteristics of XG). The viscosity, which currently serves as the primary standard [9,10,13,56] of dysphagia-friendly edible fluids, decreased significantly and most notably. Therefore, it can be deduced that the pH value is crucial when preparing edible fluid models. When high-methoxy pectin is used as the major thickener base, better thermal stability can be ensured with acid-base ones.

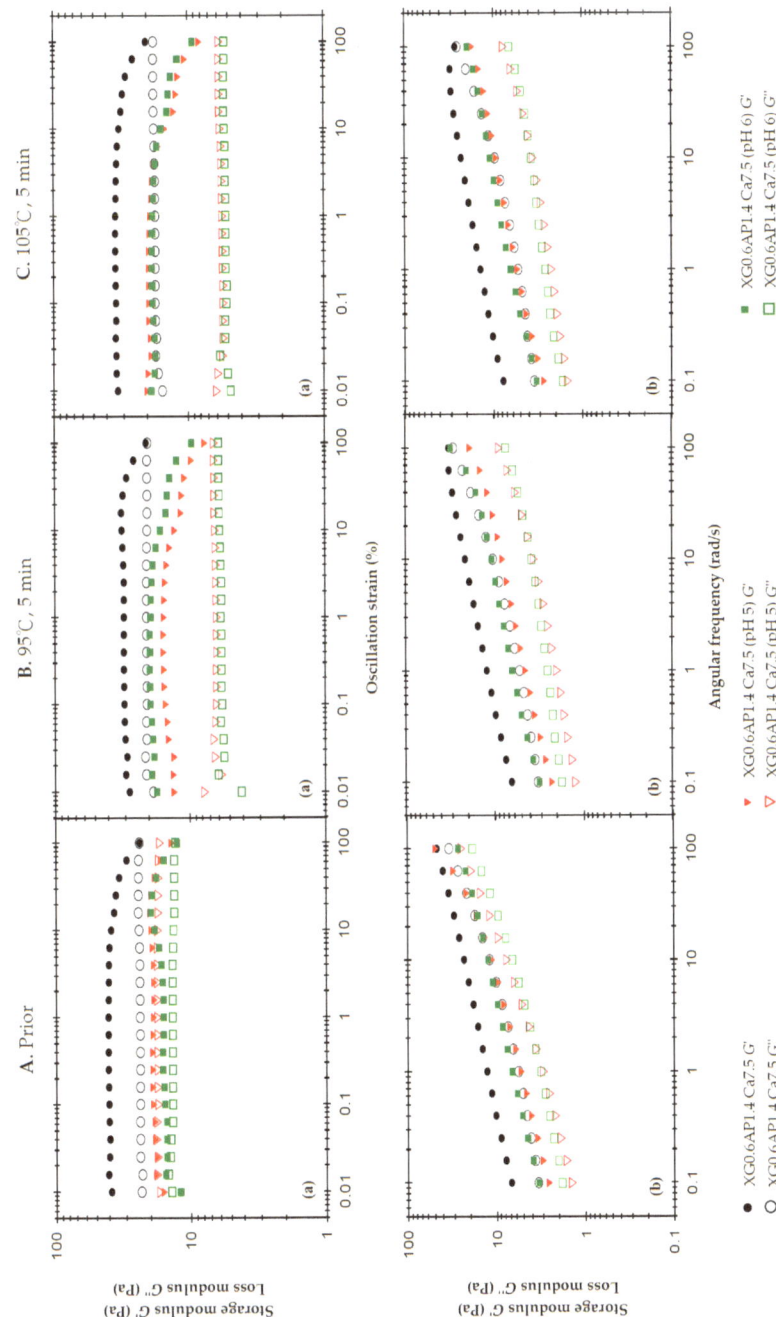

Figure 3. The effects of the pH of 2.5% and 7.5% calcium chloride anhydrous on storage modulus (G′) and loss modulus (G″) of the composite XG0.6AP1.4 thickened matrix with 7.5% calcium chloride anhydrous addition (XG0.6AP1.4-Ca7.5) experiencing different thermal processing conditions: (**A**) prior to thermal process, (**B**) after a 95 °C for 5 min process and (**C**) after a 105 °C for 5 min process with (**a**) oscillatory strain sweeps at the frequency of 50 rad/s, and (**b**) angular frequency sweeps at 1% strain.

3.3. Summary of Rheological Behavior of Sample Matrices

Cichero [56] and Burning [57] highlighted a shift from starch-based dysphagia products to gum-based ones, citing improved palatability, stable thickness, and patient preference for serving temperature. Leonard et al. conducted a clinical trial with 118 enrolled dysphagia patients, comparing gum-thickened matrices to thin water and starch-thickened ones, all designated as having the consistency of nectar [58]. They found that gum-based administration resulted in reduced aspiration difficulty and lower PAS ratings [55]. Additional studies explored gum-based thickeners, focusing on amylase-resistance properties [27,28]. A study on 120 post-stroke patients with dysphagia showed that gum-based thickeners with a viscosity range of 150 to 800 mPa.s significantly improved swallowing safety [59]. Burnip [57] and Cichero [56] noted that applying these recommendations clinically may be limited due to the viscosity labeling system's requirement of laboratory-grade rheometers and engineering expertise.

Chemical β-elimination, a major nonenzymatic degradation in pectin, involves hydrogen and glycosidic residue removal due to heating [60]. Other known pectin degradation methods include acid hydrolysis and demethylation [60,61]. Studies indicate that alkalized pectin allows β-elimination [62] and demethylation [63]. Diaz et al. found that β-elimination increases with higher temperatures, with an activation energy of 136 kJ/mol at pH 4.5, suggesting temperature dependency [60]. Higher temperatures promote β-elimination, while increased pH promotes demethylation [64,65]. Our results in the previous section align with these findings, especially at higher pH values (5 and 6) and with thermal treatment.

Calcium chloride, designated as E-509 [66], is an approved food additive in the European Union, authorized for its sequestrant and firming agent properties. When fortifying food matrices with various calcium sources, moisture absorption during storage is a concern. To ensure experimental precision, we opted for calcium chloride anhydrous (CCA) as the calcium ion source due to its resistance to moisture absorption during storage. According to the manufacturer's specifications, CCA exhibits a solubility of up to 74.5 g/100 mL in water at ambient temperature. We utilized a 40 g/100 mL solution for shear-rate-dependent viscosity measurements as another control. Notably, the calcium ion concentrations range from Ca2.5 to Ca40 and span from 0.91% to 14.55% (wt).

Table 3 gathers the results of G', G'', and tan δ of different TCMs; a high versatility of these systems can be observed. The as-prepared matrices vary in behavior, and range from an almost creamy matrix (G' or G'' lower than 20 Pa; tan δ > 0.7) to a weak-gel-like system (tan δ < 0.25), comparable to a previously reported multiple-layered w/o/w emulsion system [67]. Liu et al. [68] investigated the rheological and structural properties of different acidified (pH 4.8–6.2) and rennet-treated milk gels and reported that no data were obtained from their milk gel samples, which gave high tan δ values >1.0 and low G' < 1. They highlight that the tan δ values of milk gel samples with renneting extents of 55% and 74% at pH 6.2 were identical (0.27); as the pH progressively reduced and became as low as 4.8 due to acidification, the tan δ values were promoted to 0.72 and 0.92, respectively.

Based on the frequency sweep spectra, Ross-Murphy [69] demonstrated that the viscoelasticity of flowable matrices is generally classified into dilute and concentrated solutions and real gels. We noted that the standalone 2% apple pectin-based (AP2.0) matrices present a dilute solution pattern regardless of the thermal treatments, pH, and CCA fortification (Figure A2B(b) and Figure A3C(b)). In contrast, the composite XG–AP matrices present gel behavior (Figure 1(b), Figure 2(b) and Figure 3(b)) regardless of the thermal conditions, pH, and CCA fortification, indicating the modification effect of XG.

XG-based thickeners like ThickenUP Clear® (Nestlé Health Science, Vevey, Switzerland) are commonly used for individuals with dysphagia. Rofes et al. [28] found that adding 2.4 g of this commercial XG-based thickening formula to 100 mL of mineral water can create a honey-like viscosity. Our XG matrices, at 0.8 g/100 mL before thermal treatment, have a honey-like viscosity (351–1750 mPa.s). This similarity highlights the need for the careful consideration of source variations in dysphagia oral administration. Additionally, the frequency-dependent rheological moduli of XG0.6AP1.4-Ca7.5 following thermal treatments under controlled pH (Figure 3(b)) converge at 100 1/s due to a G' dip. This behavior may result from β-elimination in the pectin and the negatively charged nature of XG, while 1 mg/mL XG, with or without 1 mg/mL Na-caseinate, was prepared within the pH 2.7–6.6 range, after incubation at 37 °C for 60 min [70]. In addition to interpreting the rheological behavior, we conducted a comprehensive statistical analysis of shear-rate-dependent viscosities, as presented in Table 4. Generally, a more rigorous thermal treatment (indicated by lowercase letters) resulted in higher viscosity levels ($p < 0.05$), except for the case of XG0.6AP1.4 at a shear rate of 10 1/s. It is worth emphasizing that at the composite ratio of 3/7, these matrices exhibited the best thermal stability, or, equivalently, the least variation in viscosity. The influence of pH values on the AP2.0 matrices is indicated by uppercase letters. Specifically, pH 5 and 6 led to significantly lower viscosity levels ($p < 0.05$) compared to the control at pH 3. In contrast, at pH 4, intensive thermal treatment also resulted in a significant viscosity reduction, rendering it unsuitable for claiming dysphagia-friendly status. With the incorporation of CCA into AP2.0, viscosity also experienced a significant increase ($p < 0.05$), although its overall impact remained statistically insignificant ($p > 0.05$). When varying the composite ratio of thickeners, changes in viscosity were found to be shear-rate-dependent, with no clear trends across the entire range (indicated as numbers). However, considering that the typical shear rate associated with human swallowing is approximately 50 1/s, it is noteworthy that viscosity within the range of 30 to 70 1/s consistently followed the trend of XG0.8AP1.2 = XG0.6AP1.4 > XG0.8 > XG0.6 ($p < 0.05$). Hence, it is deducible that pectin not only efficiently modulates the viscosity of XG-based hydrocolloids, but also acts as a beneficial dietary fiber source.

Our previous study [33] reported on the rheological behavior of distilled water and acidic orange juice, each individually thickened with tapioca starch and xanthan gum (XG) to achieve a nectar-like consistency. These beverages exhibited distinct rheological responses following a 6 min thermal treatment at 80 °C. Specifically, the tapioca-thickened distilled water consistently exhibited a viscous behavior after the thermal treatment, while the tapioca-thickened orange juice initially displayed an elastic behavior before transitioning to a viscous behavior after treatment. Furthermore, we observed that the XG-thickened samples consistently exhibited an elastic behavior in an aqueous base (distilled water or orange juice) before or after the thermal treatment. Our current study subjected the XG–AP composite matrices to more severe thermal loads of 95 °C and 105 °C. This further confirmed that XG allows the XG–AP composite matrices to consistently exhibit elastic dominance features, regardless of the pH condition and calcium content, even though the standalone AP matrices at 2% concentration exhibited viscous dominance features.

3.4. Texture Analysis

Under various thermal processing conditions, prior rheological measurements showed that the thickened XG–AP model matrix has good thermal stability under the processing condition of 95 °C for 5 min. The texture analysis results of samples prior to and after heating under the processing condition of 95 °C for 5 min were further compared, as shown in Table 5. The hardness of the XG0.6AP1.4-Ca7.5 sample prior to thermal processing was higher than that of other samples. However, after thermal processing, the hardness decreased significantly ($p < 0.01$). It can be deduced that the strength of the network structure of the samples significantly decreased after thermal processing. The adhesiveness of XG0.6AP1.4-Ca7.5 prior to and after the thermal processing shows only a slight decrease. Overall, it seems that thermal processing had little effect on the adhesiveness of the samples investigated.

Table 5. Texture profile analysis (TPA) of the [XG0.6AP1.4-Ca7.5] of hydrocolloidal matrix prior to and after a 95 °C-5 min thermal processing.

Processing	Hardness (N/m^2)	Adhesiveness (J/m^3)	Cohesiveness	Gumminess (N/m^2)
Prior	583.14 ± 25.60	19.74 ± 1.42	0.73 ± 0.03	423.84 ± 14.54
95 °C-5 min	487.65 ± 7.26 **	18.46 ± 2.66	0.70 ± 0.02 *	340.76 ± 13.27 **

n = 9 represent the standard deviations based on nine replicates, *, ** t-test for ($p < 0.05$) or ($p < 0.01$).

The cohesiveness of all samples decreased after thermal processing, and there were significant differences. It can be inferred that after thermal processing, the bonding strength of the internal structure of the samples will decrease. According to the Japanese Society of Dysphagia Rehabilitation, foods are designated from 0.2 to 0.9; the measured results of the samples (prior to or after thermal processing) in this study are all within the standard range. The gumminess values prior to and after thermal processing for the XG0.6AP1.4-Ca7.5 sample show a very significant difference ($p < 0.01$). However, both gumminess values are greater than those with the same XG–AP ratio as the thickeners and a low-methoxy AP (DE = 45.2%) [35]. However, in our previous study, we measured a commercial powder product, Neo-high Toromeal III® (TRM, Food-care, Inc., Tokyo, Japan), with the recommended concentration of 1.5% [35], as the control sample for texture profile analysis. The gumminess observed in this case (282 N/m^2) was similar to that found in the current study. The measured gumminess after thermal processing was reasonable because the Japanese Society of Dysphagia Rehabilitation Foods standard [10] recommends that hardness to fall in the range of 300–10,000 N/m^2, and that the maximum adhesiveness be less than 1500 J/m^3. The current results show that the composite formula of XG0.6AP1.4-Ca7.5 meets these standards. Therefore, the proposed approach of adding pectin as the thickener seems reasonable for the matrix required for further thermal processing.

In this study, we found that the AP sample had a DE value of 73.9%, while in previous reports, the DE value of the AP sample was noted as 45.2%. In both instances, XG effectively functioned as a texture modifier. To mitigate the issues arising from material variations or complexity, adherence to existing standardization measures is recommended. For instance, the texture analysis standards provided by the Japanese Society of Dysphagia Rehabilitation Foods [10] are a reliable indicator of product specification and acceptance. To manage this complexity and ensure a robust and standardized formulation, we have conducted preliminary studies focusing on crucial formulation parameters, notably the calcium concentration and the ambient pH. These studies are essential for optimizing the pectin's viscoelastic characteristics. Additionally, we have investigated the formulation ratio of xanthan gum, a known consistency modifier, to complement the pectin matrix. This approach allows us to fine-tune the texture and viscosity of the preparation, thereby addressing potentially acceptable consistency. By systematically studying these parameters and their interactions, we have developed a formulation: the ambient modifiers of pH (pH < 4) and calcium chloride concentration (7.5%) with an optimal AP–XG ratio of 7:3 led to weak-gel-like behavior ($G'' < G'$) that helps to maintain the texture properties of dysphagia-friendly features similar to those prior to the thermal processing. The IDDSI framework does not include a direct measurement of viscosity because it is an empirical method. The framework is designed to be a guideline for nursing professionals preparing food bolus with a dysphagia-friendly consistency to serve individuals with dysphagia over the duration of a certain meal. However, formulae and standards such as the Japanese Society of Dysphagia Rehabilitation Foods are available [10]. The flowable matrices still need to be defined and classified by specified shear-rate-dependent (10–100 1/s) viscosities [13], as we listed in Table 4. Our motivation for assessing rheology is related to the pursuit of scale-up potential, including extended shelf life with possible thermal processing for microbial/sanitation control and possible unit operation dissolving, mixing, or aseptic heat exchanging in terms of the viscoelastic characteristics. Chemical β-elimination, and other degradation processes such as acid hydrolysis and demethylation, affect pectin, especially under conditions of higher temperature and pH. Our studies align with previous findings, showing that these conditions promote pectin's degradation. However, our composite XG–AP matrices, particularly XG0.6AP1.4, demonstrated superior thermal stability with minimal viscosity reduction, likely due to the presence of stabilizing co-structures between XG and AP. Optimizing the XG and AP composite ratio is key to enhancing the thermal stability of pectin-based matrices. We have previously reported on the co-structure of XG–AP composite matrices [35]. The composite thickener (AP1.8XG0.2) demonstrated smoother surfaces compared to the calcium ion sample (AP2Ca5) and other single thickener formulas through scanning electron microscopic image observations; additional research is needed to gain deeper insights. Starch-based matrices, often used in formulations for individuals with dysphagia, tend to decrease in viscosity when exposed to amylase in saliva. This reduction can increase the risk of accidental inhalation and aspiration pneumonia. Addressing this concern aligns with our research goals. We experimented with composite XG–AP matrices, selected for their unique structures. These matrices lack the alpha-1,4 glucosidic bonds usually present in starch, which are key to ensuring they do not pose inhalation or aspiration risks for those with dysphagia. Generally, significant viscosity depletion highlights the limitations of starch-based matrices. Therefore, our non-starch-based composite XG–AP formula could offer a more reliable alternative, given its better stability and alpha-amylase resistance for developing dysphagia-friendly matrices.

4. Conclusions

This study demonstrated that the inclusion of XG can effectively modify the original AP matrices' rheological properties, and substantially extend the accessible range of viscoelastic properties, resulting in ubiquitous weak-gel-like characteristics, as with commercially available geriatric foods. Furthermore, regarding thermal stability, the change in viscosity of the composite matrices after thermal processing is smaller than that of the standalone AP or XG matrices, and the group with AP:XG = 7:3 showed the best performance. The formula with 7.5% CCA showed the optimal viscoelastic characteristics after thermal processing. Especially with the addition of calcium ions, the viscoelastic characteristics of the XG0.6AP1.4 matrices were shown to change from liquid-like to solid-like for the full range of frequencies investigated—an ideal rheological feature for the further fortification of the minor nutrients required for individuals with dysphagia.

Author Contributions: Conceptualization, H.Y., L.-Y.C. and C.-C.H.; methodology, H.Y., L.-Y.C. and C.-C.H.; software, H.Y. and L.-Y.C.; validation, H.Y., L.-Y.C. and C.-C.H.; formal analysis, H.Y. and L.-Y.C.; investigation, H.Y. and L.-Y.C.; resources, H.Y. and C.-C.H.; data curation, H.Y. and L.-Y.C.; writing—original draft preparation, H.Y. and L.-Y.C.; writing—review and editing, H.Y. and L.-Y.C.; visualization, H.Y., L.-Y.C. and C.-C.H.; supervision, H.Y. and C.-C.H.; project administration, H.Y. and C.-C.H.; funding acquisition, H.Y. All authors have read and agreed to the published version of the manuscript.

Funding: This study was sponsored by the TAIWAN MINISTRY OF AGRICULTURE, grant number 107-3.5.2-Z1(1).

Institutional Review Board Statement: Not applicable.

Informed Consent Statement: Not applicable.

Data Availability Statement: Data is contained within the article or appendix material.

Acknowledgments: The authors acknowledge the administrative help provided by the Department of Food Science, National Chiayi University, and the Department of Chemical Engineering, National Chung Cheng University Taiwan, China.

Conflicts of Interest: The authors declare no conflicts of interest.

Appendix A

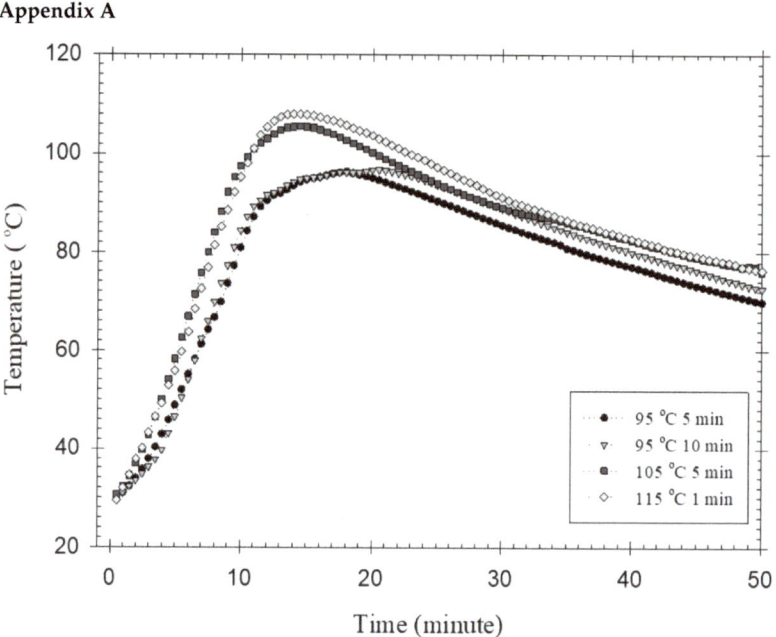

Figure A1. The measured center temperature profile of the 2 wt% high-methoxy AP matrix experienced the preset thermal processes with different time-temperature combinations.

Appendix B

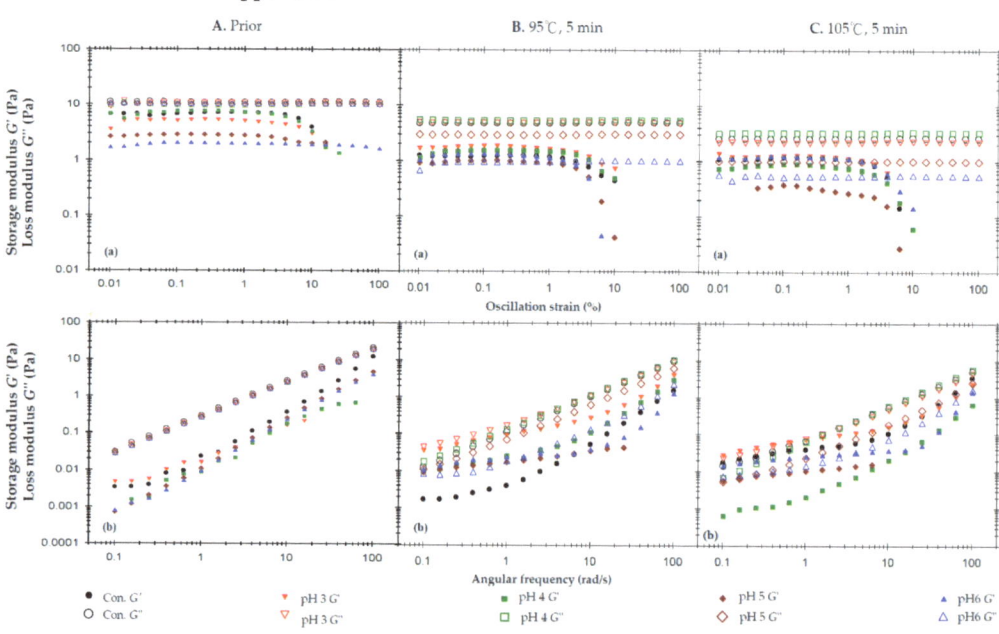

Figure A2. The effects of pH on storage modulus (G') and loss modulus (G'') of the 2% AP matrices experiencing different thermal processing conditions: (**A**) prior to thermal process, (**B**) after a 95 °C for 5 min process and (**C**) after a 105 °C for 5 min process; (**a**) oscillatory strain sweeps at the frequency of 50 rad/s, and (**b**) angular frequency sweeps at 1% strain.

Appendix C

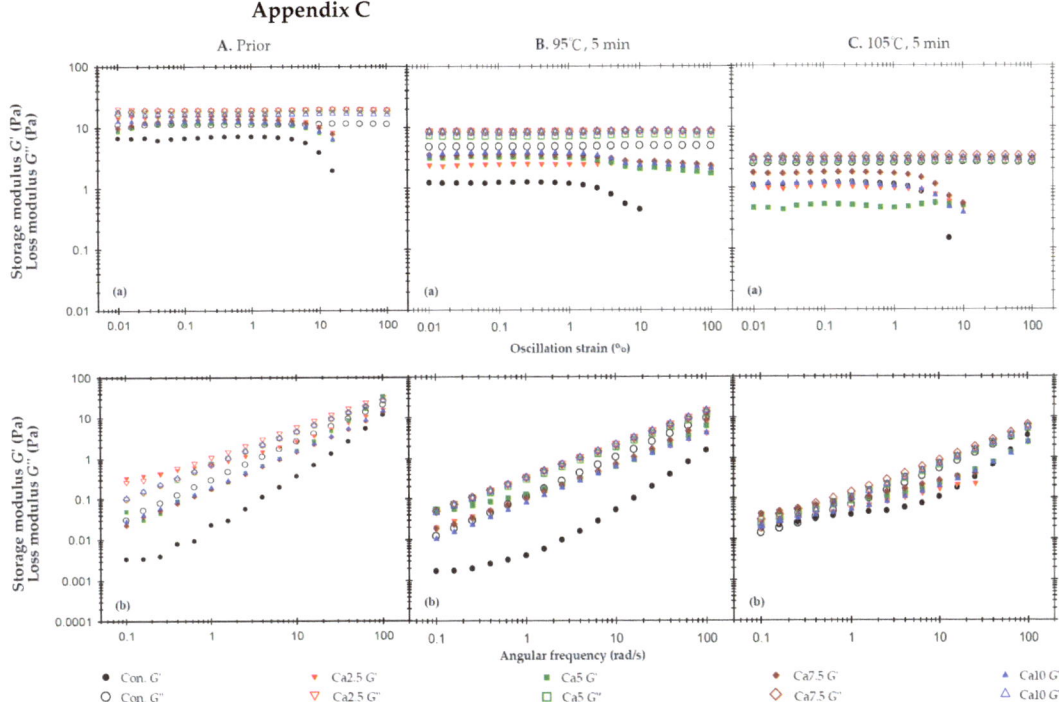

Figure A3. The effects of added calcium chloride anhydrous on storage modulus (G') and loss modulus (G'') of the 2% AP experiencing a 95 °C thermal process for 5 min: (**a**) oscillatory strain sweeps at the frequency of 50 rad/s, and (**b**) angular frequency sweeps at 1% strain.

References

1. Methacanon, P.; Gamonpilas, C.; Kongjaroen, A.; Buathongjan, C. Food polysaccharides and roles of rheology and tribology in the rational design of thickened liquids for oropharyngeal dysphagia: A review. *Compr. Rev. Food Sci. Food Saf.* **2021**, *20*, 4101–4119. [CrossRef] [PubMed]
2. Dodds, W.J. The physiology of swallowing. *Dysphagia* **1989**, *3*, 171–178. [CrossRef] [PubMed]
3. Aslam, M.; Vaezi, M.F. Dysphagia in the elderly. *Gastroenterol. Hepatol.* **2013**, *9*, 784. [CrossRef]
4. Hudson, H.M.; Daubert, C.R.; Mills, R.H. The interdependency of protein-energy malnutrition, aging, and dysphagia. *Dysphagia* **2000**, *15*, 31–38. [CrossRef] [PubMed]
5. Newman, R.; Vilardell, N.; Clavé, P.; Speyer, R. Effect of bolus viscosity on the safety and efficacy of swallowing and the kinematics of the swallow response in patients with oropharyngeal dysphagia: White paper by the European Society for Swallowing Disorders (ESSD). *Dysphagia* **2016**, *31*, 232–249. [CrossRef] [PubMed]
6. Funami, T. Next target for food hydrocolloid studies: Texture design of foods using hydrocolloid technology. *Food Hydrocoll.* **2011**, *25*, 1904–1914. [CrossRef]
7. Cichero, J.A.; Lam, P.; Steele, C.M.; Hanson, B.; Chen, J.; Dantas, R.O.; Duivestein, J.; Kayashita, J.; Lecko, C.; Murray, J.; et al. Development of international terminology and definitions for texture-modified foods and thickened fluids used in dysphagia management: The IDDSI framework. *Dysphagia* **2017**, *32*, 293–314. [CrossRef]
8. Hadde, E.K.; Prakash, S.; Chen, W.; Chen, J. Instrumental texture assessment of IDDSI texture levels for dysphagia management. Part 1: Thickened fluids. *J. Texture Stud.* **2022**, *53*, 609–616. [CrossRef]
9. National Dysphagia Diet Task Force. In *National Dysphagia Diet: Standardization for Optimal Care*; American Dietetic Association: Chicago, IL, USA, 2002.
10. The Dysphagia Diet Committee of the Japanese Society of Dysphagia Rehabilitation. The Japanese Dysphagia diet 2013. *Jpn. J. Dysphagia Rehabil.* **2013**, *17*, 255–267. (In Japanses)
11. Watanabe, E.; Yamagata, Y.; Fujitani, J.; Fujishima, I.; Takahashi, K.; Uyama, R.; Ogoshi, H.; Kojo, A.; Maeda, H.; Ueda, K.; et al. The criteria of thickened liquid for dysphagia management in Japan. *Dysphagia* **2018**, *33*, 26–32. [CrossRef]
12. Dietitians Association of Australia, and Speech Pathology Association of Australia Limited. Texture-modified foods and thickened fluids as used for individuals with dysphagia: Australian standardised labels and definitions. *Nutr. Diet.* **2007**, *64*, S53–S76. [CrossRef]

13. Steele, C.M.; Alsanei, W.A.; Ayanikalath, S.; Barbon, C.E.A.; Chen, J.; Cichero, J.A.Y.; Coutts, K.; Dantas, R.O.; Duivestein, J.; Giosa, L.; et al. The Influence of Food Texture and Liquid Consistency Modification on Swallowing Physiology and Function: A Systematic Review. *Dysphagia* **2015**, *30*, 2–26. [CrossRef] [PubMed]
14. Vickers, Z.; Damodhar, H.; Grummer, C.; Mendenhall, H.; Banaszynski, K.; Hartel, R.; Hind, J.; Joyce, A.; Kaufman, A.; Robbins, J. Relationships among rheological, sensory texture, and swallowing pressure measurements of hydrocolloid-thickened fluids. *Dysphagia* **2015**, *30*, 702–713. [CrossRef]
15. Funami, T.; Ishihara, S.; Nakauma, M.; Kohyama, K.; Nishinari, K. Texture design for products using food hydrocolloids. *Food Hydrocoll.* **2012**, *26*, 412–420. [CrossRef]
16. Garcia, J.M.; Chambers, E.; Matta, Z.; Clark, M. Viscosity measurements of nectar-and honey-thick liquids: Product, liquid, and time comparisons. *Dysphagia* **2005**, *20*, 325–335. [CrossRef] [PubMed]
17. Hadde, E.K.; Chen, J. Texture and texture assessment of thickened fluids and texture-modified food for dysphagia management. *J. Texture Stud.* **2021**, *52*, 4–15. [CrossRef] [PubMed]
18. Kunimaru, W.; Ito, S.; Motohashi, R.; Arai, E. Ease of swallowing potato paste in people with dysphagia: Effect of potato variety. *Int. J. Food Prop.* **2021**, *24*, 615–626. [CrossRef]
19. Wong, M.C.; Chan, K.M.K.; Wong, T.T.; Tang, H.W.; Chung, H.Y.; Kwan, H.S. Quantitative Textural and Rheological Data on Different Levels of Texture-Modified Food and Thickened Liquids Classified Using the International Dysphagia Diet Standardisation Initiative (IDDSI) Guideline. *Foods* **2023**, *12*, 3765. [CrossRef]
20. Sopade, P.; Halley, P.; Cichero, J.; Ward, L. Rheological characterisation of food thickeners marketed in Australia in various media for the management of dysphagia. I: Water and cordial. *J. Food Eng.* **2007**, *79*, 69–82. [CrossRef]
21. Sopade, P.; Halley, P.; Cichero, J.; Ward, L.; Hui, L.; Teo, K. Rheological characterisation of food thickeners marketed in Australia in various media for the management of dysphagia. II. Milk as a dispersing medium. *J. Food Eng.* **2008**, *84*, 553–562. [CrossRef]
22. Sopade, P.; Halley, P.; Cichero, J.; Ward, L.; Liu, J.; Varliveli, S. Rheological characterization of food thickeners marketed in Australia in various media for the management of dysphagia. III. Fruit juice as a dispersing medium. *J. Food Eng.* **2008**, *86*, 604–615. [CrossRef]
23. Hadde, E.K.; Nicholson, T.M.; Cichero, J.A.Y. Rheological characterisation of thickened fluids under different temperature, pH and fat contents. *Nutr. Food Sci.* **2015**, *45*, 270–285. [CrossRef]
24. Mackley, M.; Tock, C.; Anthony, R.; Butler, S.; Chapman, G.; Vadillo, D. The rheology and processing behavior of starch and gum-based dysphagia thickeners. *J. Rheol.* **2013**, *57*, 1533–1553. [CrossRef]
25. Payne, C.; Methven, L.; Fairfield, C.; Gosney, M.; Bell, A.E. Variability of starch-based thickened drinks for patients with dysphagia in the hospital setting. *J. Texture Stud.* **2012**, *43*, 95–105. [CrossRef]
26. Yang, H.-W.; Dai, H.-D.; Huang, W.-C.; Sombatngamwilai, T. Formulations of dysphagia-friendly food matrices with calorie-dense starchy thickeners and their stability assessments. *J. Food Meas. Charact.* **2020**, *14*, 3089–3102. [CrossRef]
27. Hanson, B.; O'Leary, M.T.; Smith, C.H. The effect of saliva on the viscosity of thickened drinks. *Dysphagia* **2012**, *27*, 10–19. [CrossRef] [PubMed]
28. Rofes, L.; Arreola, V.; Mukherjee, R.; Swanson, J.; Clavé, P. The effects of a xanthan gum-based thickener on the swallowing function of patients with dysphagia. *Aliment. Pharmacol. Ther.* **2014**, *39*, 1169–1179. [CrossRef] [PubMed]
29. Marik, P.E.; Kaplan, D. Aspiration pneumonia and dysphagia in the elderly. *Chest* **2003**, *124*, 328–336. [CrossRef]
30. Petri, D.F. Xanthan gum: A versatile biopolymer for biomedical and technological applications. *J. Appl. Polym. Sci.* **2015**, *132*, 42035. [CrossRef]
31. Yoon, S.-N.; Yoo, B. Rheological behaviors of thickened infant formula prepared with xanthan gum-based food thickeners for dysphagic infants. *Dysphagia* **2017**, *32*, 454–462. [CrossRef]
32. Ortega, O.; Bolívar-Prados, M.; Arreola, V.; Nascimento, W.V.; Tomsen, N.; Gallegos, C.; Brito-de La Fuente, E.; Clavé, P. Therapeutic effect, rheological properties and α-amylase resistance of a new mixed starch and xanthan gum thickener on four different phenotypes of patients with oropharyngeal dysphagia. *Nutrients* **2020**, *12*, 1873. [CrossRef] [PubMed]
33. Yang, H.; Lin, Y.J.P. Effect of thermal processing on flow properties and stability of thickened fluid matrices formulated by tapioca starch, hydroxyl distarch phosphate (E-1442), and xanthan gum associating dysphagia-friendly potential. *Polymers* **2021**, *13*, 162. [CrossRef] [PubMed]
34. Alexandri, M.; Kachrimanidou, V.; Papapostolou, H.; Papadaki, A.; Kopsahelis, N. Sustainable Food Systems: The Case of Functional Compounds towards the Development of Clean Label Food Products. *Foods* **2022**, *11*, 2796. [CrossRef] [PubMed]
35. Zhang, S.; Waterhouse, G.I.; Xu, F.; He, Z.; Du, Y.; Lian, Y.; Wu, P.; Sun-Waterhouse, D. Recent advances in utilization of pectins in biomedical applications: A review focusing on molecular structure-directing health-promoting properties. *Crit. Rev. Food Sci. Nutr.* **2021**, *63*, 3386–3419. [CrossRef] [PubMed]
36. Cui, J.; Zhao, C.; Feng, L.; Han, Y.; Du, H.; Xiao, H.; Zheng, J. Pectins from fruits: Relationships between extraction methods, structural characteristics, and functional properties. *Trends Food Sci. Technol.* **2021**, *110*, 39–54. [CrossRef]
37. Thibault, J.-F.; Ralet, M.-C. Physico-chemical properties of pectins in the cell walls and after extraction. In *Advances in Pectin and Pectinase Research*; Springer: Berlin/Heidelberg, Germany, 2003; pp. 91–105.
38. Yang, H.; Tsai, C.-C.; Jiang, J.-S.; Hua, C.-C. Rheological and textural properties of apple pectin-based composite formula with xanthan gum modification for preparation of thickened matrices with dysphagia-friendly potential. *Polymers* **2021**, *13*, 873. [CrossRef] [PubMed]

39. Wicker, L.; Kim, Y.; Kim, M.-J.; Thirkield, B.; Lin, Z.; Jung, J. Pectin as a bioactive polysaccharide–Extracting tailored function from less. *Food Hydrocoll.* **2014**, *42*, 251–259. [CrossRef]
40. Makarova, E.; Górnaś, P.; Konrade, I.; Tirzite, D.; Cirule, H.; Gulbe, A.; Pugajeva, I.; Seglina, D.; Dambrova, M. Acute antihyperglycaemic effects of an unripe apple preparation containing phlorizin in healthy volunteers: A preliminary study. *J. Sci. Food Agric.* **2015**, *95*, 560–568. [CrossRef]
41. Gunness, P.; Gidley, M.J. Mechanisms underlying the cholesterol-lowering properties of soluble dietary fibre polysaccharides. *Food Funct.* **2010**, *1*, 149–155. [CrossRef]
42. Gómez, B.; Gullon, B.; Remoroza, C.; Schols, H.A.; Parajo, J.C.; Alonso, J.L. Purification, characterization, and prebiotic properties of pectic oligosaccharides from orange peel wastes. *J. Agric. Food Chem.* **2014**, *62*, 9769–9782. [CrossRef]
43. Gómez, B.; Gullón, B.; Yáñez, R.; Schols, H.; Alonso, J.L. Prebiotic potential of pectins and pectic oligosaccharides derived from lemon peel wastes and sugar beet pulp: A comparative evaluation. *J. Funct. Foods.* **2016**, *20*, 108–121. [CrossRef]
44. Chung, W.S.F.; Meijerink, M.; Zeuner, B.; Holck, J.; Louis, P.; Meyer, A.S.; Wells, J.M.; Flint, H.J.; Duncan, S.H. Prebiotic potential of pectin and pectic oligosaccharides to promote anti-inflammatory commensal bacteria in the human colon. *FEMS Microbiol. Ecol.* **2017**, *93*, fix127. [CrossRef] [PubMed]
45. Patel, J.; Maji, B.; Moorthy, N.H.N.; Maiti, S. Xanthan gum derivatives: Review of synthesis, properties and diverse applications. *RSC Adv.* **2020**, *10*, 27103–27136. [CrossRef] [PubMed]
46. Kumar, A.; Rao, K.M.; Han, S.S. Application of xanthan gum as polysaccharide in tissue engineering: A review. *Carbohydr. Polym.* **2018**, *180*, 128–144. [CrossRef] [PubMed]
47. Singthong, J.; Cui, S.W.; Ningsanond, S.; Goff, H.D. Structural characterization, degree of esterification and some gelling properties of Krueo Ma Noy (*Cissampelos pareira*) pectin. *Carbohydr. Polym.* **2004**, *58*, 391–400. [CrossRef]
48. Naji, S.; Razavi, S.M.; Karazhiyan, H. Effect of thermal treatments on functional properties of cress seed (*Lepidium sativum*) and xanthan gums: A comparative study. *Food Hydrocoll.* **2012**, *28*, 75–81. [CrossRef]
49. Thakur, B.R.; Singh, R.K.; Handa, A.K.; Rao, M. Chemistry and uses of pectin—A review. *Crit. Rev. Food Sci. Nutr.* **1997**, *37*, 47–73. [CrossRef]
50. Fraeye, I.; De Roeck, A.; Duvetter, T.; Verlent, I.; Hendrickx, M.; Van Loey, A. Influence of pectin properties and processing conditions on thermal pectin degradation. *Food Chem.* **2007**, *105*, 555–563. [CrossRef]
51. Norziah, M.; Kong, S.; Abd Karim, A.; Seow, C. Pectin–sucrose–Ca^{2+} interactions: Effects on rheological properties. *Food Hydrocoll.* **2001**, *15*, 491–498. [CrossRef]
52. Löfgren, C.; Guillotin, S.; Evenbratt, H.; Schols, H.; Hermansson, A.-M. Effects of calcium, pH, and blockiness on kinetic rheological behavior and microstructure of HM pectin gels. *Biomacromolecules* **2005**, *6*, 646–652. [CrossRef]
53. Neidhart, S.; Hannak, C.; Gierschner, K. Investigations of the influence of various cations on the rheological properties of high-esterified pectin gels. *Prog. Biotechnol.* **1996**, *14*, 583–590. [CrossRef]
54. Morris, E.R.; Powell, D.A.; Gidley, M.J.; Rees, D.A. Conformations and interactions of pectins: I. Polymorphism between gel and solid states of calcium polygalacturonate. *J. Mol. Biol.* **1982**, *155*, 507–516. [CrossRef] [PubMed]
55. Yang, Y.; Zhang, G.; Hong, Y.; Gu, Z.; Fang, F. Calcium cation triggers and accelerates the gelation of high methoxy pectin. *Food Hydrocoll.* **2013**, *32*, 228–234. [CrossRef]
56. Cichero, J.A.; Steele, C.; Duivestein, J.; Clavé, P.; Chen, J.; Kayashita, J.; Dantas, R.; Lecko, C.; Speyer, R.; Lam, P. The need for international terminology and definitions for texture-modified foods and thickened liquids used in dysphagia management: Foundations of a global initiative. *Curr. Phys. Med. Rehabil. Rep.* **2013**, *1*, 280–291. [CrossRef] [PubMed]
57. Burnip, E.; Cichero, J.A.Y. Review of the effect of amylase-resistant dysphagia products on swallowing safety. *Curr. Opin. Otolaryngol. Head Neck Surg.* **2022**, *30*, 169–176. [CrossRef] [PubMed]
58. Leonard, R.J.; White, C.; McKenzie, S.; Belafsky, P.C. Effects of bolus rheology on aspiration in patients with dysphagia. *J. Acad. Nutr. Diet.* **2014**, *114*, 590–594. [CrossRef] [PubMed]
59. Bolivar-Prados, M.; Rofes, L.; Arreola, V.; Guida, S.; Nascimento, W.V.; Martin, A.; Vilardell, N.; Ortega Fernandez, O.; Ripken, D.; Lansink, M.J.N. Effect of a gum-based thickener on the safety of swallowing in patients with poststroke oropharyngeal dysphagia. *Neurogastroenterol. Motil.* **2019**, *31*, e13695. [CrossRef]
60. Diaz, J.V.; Anthon, G.E.; Barrett, D.M. Nonenzymatic degradation of citrus pectin and pectate during prolonged heating: Effects of pH, temperature, and degree of methyl esterification. *J. Agric. Food Chem.* **2007**, *55*, 5131–5136. [CrossRef]
61. Krall, S.M.; McFeeters, R.F. Pectin hydrolysis: Effect of temperature, degree of methylation, pH, and calcium on hydrolysis rates. *J. Agric. Food Chem.* **1998**, *46*, 1311–1315. [CrossRef]
62. Kiss, J. β-Eliminative degradation of carbohydrates containing uronic acid residues. In *Advances in Carbohydrate Chemistry and Biochemistry*; Elsevier: Amsterdam, The Netherlands, 1974; Volume 29, pp. 229–303. [CrossRef]
63. Renard, C.M.; Thibault, J.F. Degradation of pectins in alkaline conditions: Kinetics of demethylation. *Carbohydr. Res.* **1996**, *286*, 139–150. [CrossRef]
64. Albersheim, P.; Neukom, H.; Deuel, H. Splitting of pectin chain molecules in neutral solutions. *Arch. Biochem. Biophys.* **1960**, *90*, 46–51. [CrossRef] [PubMed]
65. Sila, D.N.; Smout, C.; Elliot, F.; Loey, A.V.; Hendrickx, M.J. Non-enzymatic depolymerization of carrot pectin: Toward a better understanding of carrot texture during thermal processing. *J. Food Sci.* **2006**, *71*, E1–E9. [CrossRef]

66. Tiwari, P.; Joshi, A.; Varghese, E.; Thakur, M. Process standardization and storability of calcium fortified potato chips through vacuum impregnation. *J. Food Sci. Technol.* **2018**, *55*, 3221–3231. [CrossRef] [PubMed]
67. Márquez, A.L.; Wagner, J.R. Rheology of double (W/O/W) emulsions prepared with soybean milk and fortified with calcium. *J. Texture Stud.* **2010**, *41*, 651–671. [CrossRef]
68. Liu, X.T.; Zhang, H.; Wang, F.; Luo, J.; Guo, H.Y.; Ren, F.Z. Rheological and structural properties of differently acidified and renneted milk gels. *J. Dairy Sci.* **2014**, *97*, 3292–3299. [CrossRef]
69. Ross-Murphy, S.B. Small deformation measurements. In *Food Sturcture—Its Creation and Evaluation*; Blanshard, J.M.V., Mitchel, J.R., Eds.; Butterworths Ltd.: London, UK, 1992; pp. 387–400.
70. Kobori, T.; Matsumoto, A.; Sugiyama, S. PH-dependent interaction between sodium caseinate and xanthan gum. *Carbohydr. Polym.* **2009**, *75*, 719–723. [CrossRef]

Disclaimer/Publisher's Note: The statements, opinions and data contained in all publications are solely those of the individual author(s) and contributor(s) and not of MDPI and/or the editor(s). MDPI and/or the editor(s) disclaim responsibility for any injury to people or property resulting from any ideas, methods, instructions or products referred to in the content.

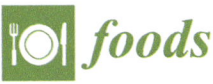

Review

Complement in Human Brain Health: Potential of Dietary Food in Relation to Neurodegenerative Diseases

Yihang Xing [1], Dingwen Zhang [1], Li Fang [1], Ji Wang [1], Chunlei Liu [1], Dan Wu [1], Xiaoting Liu [1], Xiyan Wang [1,*] and Weihong Min [2,*]

[1] College of Food Science and Engineering, Jilin Agricultural University, Changchun 130118, China; xyh15943188342@163.com (Y.X.); 15104353149@163.com (D.Z.); fangli1014@126.com (L.F.); wangji198644@163.com (J.W.); liuchunlei0709@jlau.edu.cn (C.L.); wudan@jlau.edu.cn (D.W.); liuxiaoting@jlau.edu.cn (X.L.)

[2] College of Food and Health, Zhejiang A&F University, Hangzhou 311300, China

* Correspondence: wangxiyan199294@163.com (X.W.); minwh2000@zafu.edu.cn (W.M.)

Abstract: The complement pathway is a major component of the innate immune system, which is critical for recognizing and clearing pathogens that rapidly react to defend the body against external pathogens. Many components of this pathway are expressed throughout the brain and play a beneficial role in synaptic pruning in the developing central nervous system (CNS). However, excessive complement-mediated synaptic pruning in the aging or injured brain may play a contributing role in a wide range of neurodegenerative diseases. Complement Component 1q (C1q), an initiating recognition molecule of the classical complement pathway, can interact with a variety of ligands and perform a range of functions in physiological and pathophysiological conditions of the CNS. This review considers the function and immunomodulatory mechanisms of C1q; the emerging role of C1q on synaptic pruning in developing, aging, or pathological CNS; the relevance of C1q; the complement pathway to neurodegenerative diseases; and, finally, it summarizes the foods with beneficial effects in neurodegenerative diseases via C1q and complement pathway and highlights the need for further research to clarify these roles. This paper aims to provide references for the subsequent study of food functions related to C1q, complement, neurodegenerative diseases, and human health.

Keywords: C1q; complement pathway; synaptic pruning; microglia; neurodegenerative diseases; dietary food

1. Introduction

In 1894, Jules Bordet discovered the presence of a thermally unstable component or group of components of serum that acted as a complement to antibodies and interacted with bacteria. Based on its function as an antibody supplement, Paul Ehrlich named the new substance "complement" (Figure 1a). Complement is a multimolecular self-assembling biologically active system consisting of nearly 20 plasma proteins with different physico-chemical and immunological properties. When activated, the precursor molecules react in a chained enzymatic reaction in a particular order. In this process, C1q acts as a promoter of the complement pathway and participates in the body's defense by binding to antigen–antibody complexes to activate the classical complement pathway. However, in addition to the traditional role of complement activation, C1q plays other important roles in a complement-independent manner. Recent investigations have unveiled that the complement molecule C1q is involved in both neuroprotection and neurodegenerative diseases. It has been shown that C1q levels in the brains of Alzheimer's disease (AD) mouse models are significantly higher than in normal rats [1]. C1q plays a role in neurodegenerative diseases by inducing microglia to phagocytose synapses, which ultimately results in cognitive–behavioral deficits caused by synaptic loss. The inhibition of C1q activity resulted in a diminution of microglial count, a mitigation of initial synaptic attrition, and a notable amelioration in cognitive memory impairments [2]. Suggesting that the induction of microglia phagocytosis of synapses by C1q plays an important role in neurodegenerative diseases.

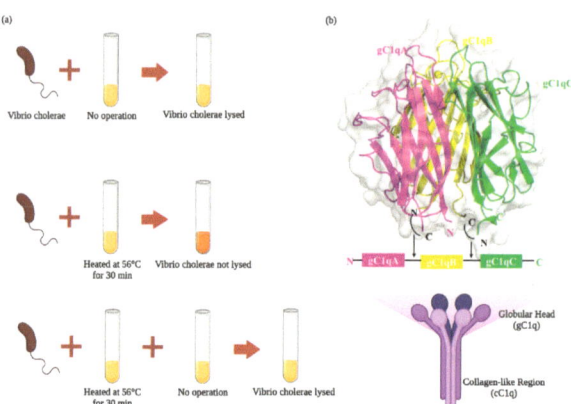

Figure 1. (**a**) Complementation findings. Sheep anti-cholera serum was able to lyse Vibrio cholera, while sheep anti-cholera serum lost the ability to lyse Vibrio cholera when heated at 56 °C for 30 min, and Vibrio cholera was again lyzed when fresh non-immune-serum was added to the heated serum again. (**b**) The structure of C1q (Created with BioRender.com accessed on 28 April 2023).

Synapses are the fundamental structures of neural networks that translate information into various brain regions and cell types. Throughout the developmental journey, the establishment of fully fledged neural networks necessitates the judicious eradication of unsuitable synaptic bonds, an intricate choreography wherein microglia and astrocytes partake, orchestrating synaptic honing under the tutelage of C1q [3]. C1q is neuroprotective during the initial stages of CNS injury, where it can hold a pivotal position in avoiding the release of cell-damaging factors by enhancing the phagocytosis of microglia and macrophages and regulating inflammation [4]. However, when excessive activation of C1q occurs, it may lead to direct synaptic damage. C1q induces localized activation of microglia and astrocytes, which, by acting synergistically with other proinflammatory pathways, ultimately leads to memory-related neurodegenerative disorders such as AD, Huntington's disease (HD), and traumatic brain injury (TBI) [5,6]. The clinical hallmark of Parkinson's disease (PD) is a motor syndrome characterized by bradykinesia, rest tremor, and rigidity, as well as changes in posture and gait [7]. In PD cases, neurons seemed to be opsonized by C1q [8]. In contrast, blocking C1q activation using C1q knockdown or antibodies has been shown to significantly reduce synaptic phagocytosis and cognitive dysfunction [1].

With today's rapid advances in medicine and the increasing emphasis on the prevention of diseases before they develop, there is a growing interest in utilizing bioactive substances in food to maintain health and combat chronic human diseases, in addition to the nutritional supply of food. A number of functional food factors have been shown to delay the development of neurodegenerative diseases by modulating C1q levels. In this article, we present a review of the recent advances in the role of C1q in neurodegenerative diseases, focusing on the specific mechanisms of synaptic elimination of C1q through the classical complement pathway in CNS development, aging, and disease, as well as the targeting of C1q by food components to slow down the progression of neurodegenerative diseases. The aim of this study is to provide a new theoretical basis to further explore the role of functional food factors in the development of neurodegenerative diseases and to hypothesize that C1q can be an effective target and marker for delaying the development of neurodegenerative diseases, such as AD.

2. C1q Structure and Biological Function

2.1. C1q Structure

C1, the inaugural sentinel within the precincts of the classical pathway inherent to the innate immune system, comprises the trinity of C1q, C1r, and C1s. The self-initiation of C1r, a serine protease, ensues, cascading into the enzymatic cleavage and activation of another akin serine protease, C1s. This orchestration is precipitated upon the embrace of antibodies or the surfaces of pathogens by C1q, serving as the harbinger of this sequence. Thus, a symphony of elements coalesces, culminating in the creation of a C1 complex, wherein one C1q molecule interlaces with twin counterparts of C1r and C1s. The unveiling of this assembly activates the classical complement pathway, precipitating a transformative shift in the collagenic domain [9].

The intact C1q molecule is a complex of 18 chains: 6A, 6B, and 6C, which are connected by covalent and noncovalent bonds to form ABC-CBA triple-helical structural units [10–12]. Each chain of C1q has its ligand, and each region mediates different physiological functions by binding to different ligands and receptors, such as regulation of various immune cells (e.g., dendritic cells, platelets, microglia, and lymphocytes), clearance of apoptotic cells, a range of cellular processes such as differentiation, chemotaxis, aggregation, and adhesion, and neurodegenerative diseases and pathogenesis of SLE [13,14]. Interestingly, studies have observed that the B and C chains of C1q are highly conserved, and little ligands were recognized by B and C chains. Deoxy-D-ribose and heparan sulfate were recognized specifically by the globular domain of C1q involving interactions with ArgC98, ArgC111, AsnC113 and LysC129, TyrC155, TrpC190, respectively. Helena et al. reported that phosphatidylserine is one of the C1q ligands on apoptotic cells and interacts with subunit C of C1q, which unfolds during the nascent phases of apoptosis [15]. Moreover, plausible 3D models of the C1q globular domain in complex with C-reactive protein (CRP) and IgG were proposed; ArgB114, ArgB129, and ArgB163 were involved in the interaction with IgG, while LysA200, TyrB175, and LysC170 at the top of the C1q head directed toward CRP [16]. Furthermore, the A chain is the exact opposite, with a collagen region containing a major binding site for nonimmunoglobulin substances that can bind Adiponectin [17], Von Willebrand factor [18], C-reactive protein [19,20], Serum amyloid P [21], DNA [22], Aβ [22], and Heme [23]. Among them, IgM [24,25], LPS [26], GAPDH [27], Blood platelets [28], Fibronectin [29], Adiponectin [17], C-reactive protein [19,20], Serum amyloid P [21], and Aβ [22] can activate the classical complement pathway by binding C1q, whose binding sites are the cationic regions 14–26 and 76–92 of the C1q A chain, and the use of the same peptide as residues 14–26 can regulate ligand binding to C1q to activate the classical complement pathway [22]. In accordance, one may posit the conjecture that the preponderance of C1q's functionalities seems to derive primarily from the A chain. The target ligands and versatile recognition properties of C1q are summarized in Table 1.

Some studies have also shown that the B-chain of C1q plays a crucial role in tumorigenesis binding of multiple tumors. Yamada and colleagues have laid bare that elevated C1qB expression exhibited a marked correlation with unfavorable prognostication within the context of renal cell carcinoma. In contrast, the work of Linnartz-Gerlach and collaborators uncovered the downregulation of C1qB in the cerebral milieu of triggering receptors expressed on myeloid cell-2 (TREM2) knock-out mice. Intriguingly, it merits noting that TREM2 has been brought to the forefront as a conduit for intracellular messaging, effectuated via its partnered transmembrane adapter, TYROBP [30]. Demonstrations have borne witness to a robust linkage existing between TYROBP and C1qB expression amidst individuals afflicted by gastric carcinoma [31]. Analogously, investigations have illuminated that a disruption within this signaling conduit engenders an array of perturbations in physiological equilibrium and confers susceptibility to an array of maladies encompassing the likes of senescence and age-linked neuronal attrition [32,33]. Concurrently, evidence has surfaced elucidating that C1q within the realm of IgG-mediated acquired immunity underscores the centrality of Arg114 and Arg129 within the B chain, marking them as pivotal residues in the tapestry of IgG binding. This discourse further accentuates the role of Arg162 in the A chain, along with Arg163 in the B chain and Arg156 in the C chain, as integral participants in the orchestration of C1q-IgG interplay [34,35]. Although there are fewer studies on the C1qC chain, it is clear that each of the three C1q chains may be functionally independent and capable of differentially splicing ligands.

The globular "head" of each ABC chain is connected to a fibrillar central region by six collagen-like "stalks" that form two distinct structural and functional domains: the collagen-like region (cC1q) and a spherical "head" structure (gC1q) [36]. The ultimate configuration of the C1q molecule mirrors the semblance of a cluster of tulip blossoms (Figure 1b). Interestingly, these two domains acted as separate parts from each other and interacted with diverse biological structures, including pathogen- and cell-associated molecules. The collagen-like regions of C1q are engaged in immune response effector mechanisms through their interaction with a tetramer of complement C1r and C1s proteases (C1r2s2) or receptors on immune cell surfaces [37,38]. More prominently, the globular regions support the recognition properties of C1q with the striking ability to sense a wide variety of ligands [39,40]. (As shown in Table 1) In general, gC1q was performed to investigate the location binding interactions and recognition specificity of C1q-ligands complexes, as well as in the regulation of C1 activation, such as the lipopolysaccharides (LPS) inside Table 1. LPS interacts specifically with the gC1q domain in a calcium-dependent manner. LPS and IgG-binding sites on the gC1q domain appear to be overlapping, and this interaction can be inhibited by a synthetic C1q inhibitor, suggesting common interacting mechanisms [26]. However, it does not work when only the C1q tail or C1q globules are present; in other words, the complete C1q is required to affect the organism [4].

Table 1. The versatile recognition properties of C1q.

C1q Ligand	C1q Binding Region/Binding Site	Function	Ref.
IgM	C1q globular domain	Activate the classical complement pathway	[24,25]
IgG	C1q globular domain	Activate the classical complement pathway	[16]
LPS	C1q globular domain	Activate the classical complement pathway	[26]
GAPDH	C1q globular domain	Activate the classical complement pathway	[27]
Blood platelets	C1q globular domain	Activate the classical complement pathway	[28]
CRP	C1q globular domain	Activate the classical complement pathway	[5,19,20]
Pentraxin 3	C1q globular domain	Interacts with C1q and inhibits the classical complement pathway	[41]
Fibronectin	C1q globular domain	Activate the classical complement pathway	[29]
Calreticulin	C1q globular domain	recognize apoptotic cells	[42,43]
Heparin	C1q globular domain	Inhibit the classical complement pathway	[44]
ApoE	C1q stalk	Inhibit the classical complement pathway	[45]
Adiponectin	Globular domain of the C1q A chain	Activate the classical complement pathway	[17]
Von Willebrand factor	N-terminal of the C1q A chain	Inhibit the classical complement pathway	[18]
Serum amyloid P	Residues 14–26 and 76–92 of the C1q A chain	Activate the classical complement pathway	[21]
DNA	Residues 14–26 of the C1q A chain	Activate the classical complement pathway	[22]
Aβ	Residues 14–26 of the C1q A chain	Activate the classical complement pathway	[22]
Heme	TyrA122 of the C1q A chain	Inhibit the classical complement pathway	[23]
Deoxy-D-ribose	Residues Arg98, Arg111, Asn113 of the C1q C chain	Inhibit C1 activation	[44]
Heparan sulfate	Residues Lys129, Tyr155, Trp190 of the C1q C chain	Inhibit C1 activation	[44]
PS	Globular domain of the C1q C chain	Efficient apoptotic cell removal determined synaptic vulnerability	[15,46,47]

2.2. C1q Biological Functions

C1q serves as the herald of the complement pathway, adroitly bridging the realms of innate and adaptive immunity. In the context of innate defense, the dearth of C1q is intimately tied to the constellation of systemic lupus erythematosus (SLE) [48]. Within this intricate framework, one of the conjectured mechanisms, aptly denominated the waste disposal paradigm [49], propounds that C1q assumes an indispensable role in the expunction of deceased cells. In the unfortunate absence of C1q, this regulatory function falters, impeding the efficient clearance of expired cellular constituents [50]. The cascading result is the exposure of intracellular moieties, inciting an immune retort against these very (self) entities [51]. In addition to its influence within the realm of innate immunity, C1q unfurls a diverse spectrum of roles within adaptive immunity. Human T cells bear the imprint of C1q receptors, bestowing upon C1q the capacity to navigate the complex terrain of T-cell responses. Recent investigations in mouse models have cast light upon the intriguing prospect that C1q might indeed wield a discernible influence on T-cell immunity. Within mouse models emblematic of SLE, a striking phenomenon emerges: C1q assumes the role of an inhibitor, quelling the vigor of CD8 T-cell responses [52]. The authors propose a mechanism in which C1q is internalized and impacts mitochondrial function via C1q receptors. In emphysema, the absence of C1q leads to a shift from suppressive regulatory T-cell responses to pro-inflammatory Th17 responses [53]. The synergy between human observational studies and mouse models showed that C1q acts on the T-cell suppressor [3]. From these studies, it is clear that C1q stands as a regulator, dictating the amplitude and caliber of T-cell responses, reflecting the important role of C1q in adaptive immunity. In contradistinction to the diminished levels of C1q noted across various autoimmune conditions, an augmentation in C1q levels has been documented within the annals of numerous infectious and neurodegenerative maladies, including AD and PD. Hence, increasing awareness of the distinct roles of C1q, as well as the relationship between C1q level with autoimmune diseases and neurodegenerative diseases, highlights the need for a thorough understanding of C1q in innate immunity and adaptive immunity.

3. Complement in the Brain

The complement cascade is a key effector mechanism of the innate immune system that contributes to the rapid clearance of pathogens and dead or dying cells and increases the extent and limits of the inflammatory immune response. C1q, the promoter of the classical complement pathway in the complement cascade, has been clearly shown to play a beneficial role in synaptic elimination during neurological development, but excessive C1q-mediated synaptic pruning in the adult or injured brain may be detrimental in a variety of neurodegenerative diseases.

3.1. C1q and the Complement Pathway

The complement pathway stands as a crucial constituent nestled within the precincts of the innate immune system that can participate in host defense by rapidly recognizing and eliminating pathogens, cellular debris, and misfolded proteins, facilitating the clearance of dead cells or antibody–antigen complexes [54]. In response to multiple endogenous or exogenous substances, the components of the complement body are activated sequentially in a chain reaction to produce various biological effects.

The classical complement pathway, lectin pathway, and alternate pathway are three commonly accepted pathways of complement system activation. The complement pathways share commonalities but also have their characteristics. The three complement pathways are mainly initiated by promoters, mediated by C3 converting enzyme and C5 converting enzyme, and activated by a series of pathway amplification reactions to activate the complement system and form membrane attack complex (MAC), resulting in the lysis and rupture of the plasma membrane of the antigen-bearing cells, and the outflow of the cellular contents, which triggers the inflammatory response [55]. The details are shown in Figure 2.

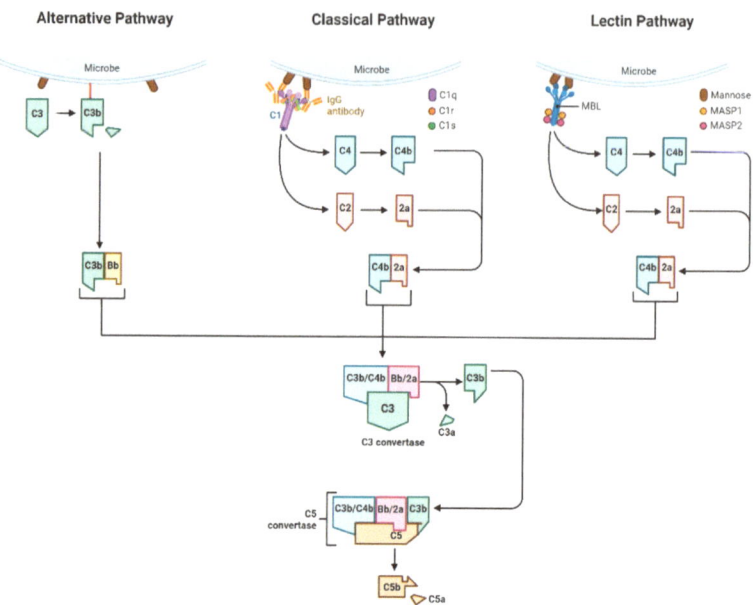

Figure 2. Complement pathways (created with BioRender.com accessed on 12 October 2022).

Similarly, the lectin pathway's activation mirrors that of the classical pathway, albeit with a distinct initiator—mannose-binding lectin (MBL). MBL undertakes the task of forming multimeric lectin complexes upon engaging ficolin. This intricate association ushers in the activation of MBL-associated serine protease (MASP), heralding the initiation of the complement pathway. MASP-1 and MASP-2 bear semblance to C1r and C1s, respectively. Their counterparts in this realm, MASP-1 and MASP-2, wield the power to usher in the complete activation of the complement system by cleaving C4 and C2, thus assembling the C3 convertase.

Diverging from the trajectory of classical activation, the alternative pathway circumvents the involvement of C1, C4, and C2. Instead, it forges a direct path towards the activation of C3, thereby igniting a cascading sequence that propels the components from C5 through C9 to fulfillment. Meanwhile, the lectin pathway and the classical pathway formation of C3 convertase from C4b and 2a, whereas the alternative pathway is via C3b and Bb. The alternative pathway can play a significant anti-inflammatory role as a low-level sustained activation of nonspecific immunity by acting directly on invading microorganisms and other foreign bodies at the early stage of pathogen infection before specific antibodies are produced.

Given that the initiation of the classical complement pathway hinges upon the genesis of antigen–antibody complexes before their binding with C1q, and the birth of antibodies necessitates a specific immune retort, it follows that the classical complement pathway predominantly exerts its influence during the latter phases of infection.

3.2. C1q through Classical Pathway Activation Mediated Synapse Pruning

Within the complement pathways, it is the classical complement pathway that predominantly takes on a significant role within the CNS, in which C1q acts as a recognition protein and plays different roles at different stages of the CNS.

3.2.1. C1q in Developing CNS

During the development of the CNS, precise neural circuits are vital for the development and functional maturation of the brain. Complement pathway activation products are crucial to modulate synapse formation to avoid redundant, spider web-like neural network growth. A subset of synapses in neurons is pruned while other presynaptic or postsynaptic axons from the parent neuron are positively stabilized and strengthened [56]. C1q activates the downstream complement component C3 by labeling abnormal synapses or inappropriate synaptic connections, and C3 binds to the receptor CR3 on microglia, initiating the complement pathway and the exercise of synaptic pruning by microglia (Figure 3). In this way, it participates in beneficial synaptic elimination and promotes neuronal development and functional maturation.

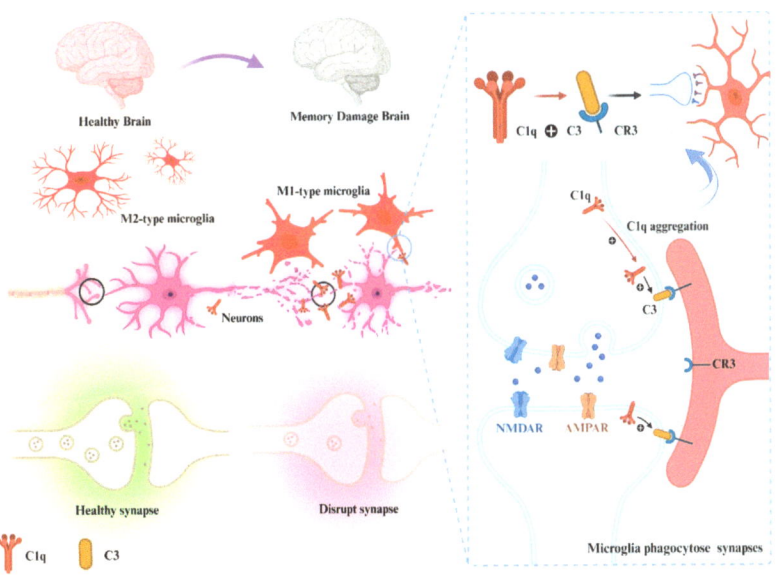

Figure 3. Microglia phagocytose synapses. C1q is expressed in microglia or neurons and localizes at synapses by recognizing ligands, leading to downstream deposition of complement protein C3, which binds to C3 receptors on microglia and activates phagocytosis of microglia to directly trigger synaptic loss (Created with BioRender.com accessed on 11 August 2023).

Synaptic pruning removes less active or "weak" synapses, strengthens synaptic connections appropriately, and promotes neuronal maturation, meaning that C1q can "detect" morphofunctional changes in synapses [57]. As long as the "weak" synapses are labeled by C1q and subsequently removed by phagocytic microglia via synaptic pruning [55,58]. To what kind of synapses are "weak" that contribute to labeling by C1q during the synaptic pruning remains unclear.

Györffy et al. divulged the existence of processes akin to apoptosis within synapses adorned with C1q, as unveiled through a proteomic exploration and pathway analysis of synaptosomes labeled with C1q [58]. The presence of apoptosis-like processes in C1q-labeled synapses and the fact that synaptic apoptosis induces increased C1q levels suggest that synaptic pruning based on C1q labeling may be triggered by synaptic apoptosis, which can be inhibited by increased synaptic activity. In conditions of normalcy, the proclivity for C1q to bind surfaces leans toward late apoptotic cells in comparison to their early apoptotic counterparts [59]. It has also been shown that microglia preferentially phagocytose apoptotic cells, whereas in the absence of C1q, the level of phagocytosis by microglia is reduced [60]. Bioinformatics analysis showed that C1q-labeled synapses contained higher levels of caspase 3 and caspase 5, both markers of apoptosis, compared with C1q-negative synapses [58], suggesting that synaptic pruning and clearance of apoptotic cells are similar in the mechanism. Phosphatidylserine (PS) is one of the C1q ligands on apoptotic cells [15].

An apoptosis-like process exists in C1q-labeled synapses, and the synaptic apoptotic mechanism induces elevated C1q levels, while synaptic pruning based on C1q labeling may be triggered by gC1q-PS binding effects [44]. During normal growth and development, synapses may be induced by increased apoptotic signaling while C1q levels are increased and aggregated toward them, while C1q stimulation also causes apoptotic cells and cell debris clearance. In contrast, in neurodegenerative diseases, synapses may be triggered to apoptosis by increased levels of C1q, leading to their "misrecognition" by microglia and their engulfment.

The perturbation of C1q's equilibrium precipitates anomalies in synaptic pruning, culminating in compromised synaptic transmission, diminished cerebral connectivity, impairments in social engagement, and heightened instances of repetitive behavioral traits. This intricate web of repercussions interweaves with the realms of epilepsy, as well as a spectrum of neurodevelopmental and neuropsychiatric afflictions [61]. Concurrently, mice lacking in the complement protein C1q or its downstream counterpart, complement protein C3, manifest pronounced and enduring deficiencies in the process of CNS synapse elimination. This is starkly evidenced through the thwarting of anatomical refinement within retinogeniculate connections, along with the retention of superfluous retinal innervation amongst lateral geniculate neurons [62]. In a study involving a mouse model of the CNS, C1q was upregulated after birth and peaked within two weeks [3]. Increased synaptic connectivity and epileptic activity were shown in C1q knockout mice that were unable to establish proper synaptic connections [63].

3.2.2. C1q in Aging

The wane of cognitive prowess has surfaced as a formidable health menace during the later stages of life. Within this purview, the decline in cognitive function is intrinsically linked to the perturbed neuronal circuitry that comes with advancing age. Unlike the rise in C1q levels during development, neuronal C1q is normally downregulated in the adult CNS. Certain inquiries have unearthed a notable resurgence in C1q protein levels within the confines of the aging mouse and human brain [64,65]. In harmony with the rise in serum C1q concentrations that accompany the passage of time, a commensurate augmentation in C1q levels within the cerebrospinal fluid (CSF) has been duly noted [66]. Significant disparages in the C1q protein abundance within mouse and human brain tissue emerged palpably through the lens of immunohistochemistry, particularly when juxtaposing brain specimens from the early stages of life to those in advanced age [67]. This escalation predominantly manifested near synapses, materializing at the nascent stages and with remarkable intensity in specific cerebral domains. Among these locales, a subset—but not the entirety—comprising regions acknowledged for their predisposition to neurodegenerative disorders underwent this surge, i.e., the hippocampus, substantia nigra, and piriform cortex [67]. C1q-deficient mice exhibited enhanced synaptic plasticity in the aging and reorganization of the circuitry in the aging hippocampal dentate gyrus [10].

3.2.3. C1q in Diseases

Changes in the expression level of C1q in different diseases have different effects on the disease process or pathological changes. Diminished levels of C1q have surfaced within the context of autoimmune disorders, select inflammatory ailments, and numerous tumor types. Notably, an elevation in anti-C1q antibodies has been unveiled to precede renal flares in lupus. Furthermore, autoantibodies targeting C1q have also been documented in the annals of diverse spontaneous mouse models of systemic lupus erythematosus (SLE) [68]. C1q deficiencies have been correlated with heightened vulnerability to infections triggered by encapsulated bacteria, particularly cases of pneumonia and meningitis. Additionally, recurrent respiratory infections are known to afflict individuals with such deficiencies [69]. The conceptualization of C1q's role in the genesis of cancer remains in a state of continuous evolution. Evidence has emerged indicating that elevated C1q levels bear a favorable prognostic implication for disease-free survival in basal-like breast cancer, as well as for overall survival in HER2-positive breast cancer. However, a converse narrative unfolds when exploring its influence within the landscape of lung adenocarcinoma and clear cell renal cell carcinoma, where C1q appears to assume a pro-tumorigenic role [70]. C1q seems to encompass a binary function within the realm of cancer, manifesting itself as both a catalyst for tumor advancement and a guardian against tumors, its stance oscillating in tandem with the intricate context of the disease at hand. Elevated C1q levels have been detected across a spectrum of domains, including aging, infectious diseases, assorted inflammatory disorders, and cardiac and cerebral ailments. In the context of infectious diseases, the surge in circulating C1q levels is likely attributed to an escalated production of C1q as a countermeasure against pathogens. However, the localized surges noted in conditions such as neuroborreliosis and meningitis could potentially stem from augmented leakage from the circulation. C1q can regulate cytokine expression, and when cells are injured or encounter trauma, the concentration of free C1q becomes high, which can stimulate neutrophils to move toward the lesion [71]. Also, neutrophils are recruited to the site of cell injury accompanied by the accumulation of C1q, IgM, and albumin; among others, accumulation of C1q, IgM, and albumin is accompanied by the accumulation of these proteins [4]. Also, in neurodegenerative diseases, increased C1q levels are a consequence of increased (local) C1q production. C1q engages in a deleterious interaction with anomalous protein aggregates, thus embroiling itself in the genesis of neurodegenerative afflictions like AD alongside other neuropsychiatric disorders [71]. Mouse models lacking C1q, although showing the "plaque" structure characteristic of AD, those mice lacking C1q have significantly less inflammation around these plaques and significantly more neuronal integrity compared with transgenic mice with an intact complement system [72]. Studies have shown that ANX005 is a potent anti-C1q-targeting antibody that binds to C1q, inhibits its interaction with multiple substrates, and prevents classical complement pathway activation while leaving the lectin and alternative complement pathways intact [73].

3.3. The Role of C1q in the Complement-Independent Manner

Indeed, C1q is widely acknowledged for its role as an initiator within the classical complement pathway, culminating in the activation of the complement system. This activation intricately aids in the swift elimination of pathogens and dead cells. It is of significance to note that C1q assumes roles that extend beyond its involvement in the complement pathway, encompassing the maintenance of homeostasis and regulatory functions in a manner distinct from its engagement within the complement system. There is some evidence that C1q can be synthesized in peripheral tissue bone marrow cells in the absence of C1q-associated C1 serine proteases C1r and C1s [74]. Within the CNS, the synthesis of C1q experiences an augmentation as an initial retort to injury in numerous instances, yet this response occurs independently from the simultaneous synthesis of the C1 serine proteases, indicating C1q-mediated activities individually without a complement pathway. Demonstrations have illuminated that C1q possesses the ability to induce a gene expression program that champions neuroprotection. In doing so, it potentially furnishes a shield against the menace posed by Aβ, particularly in the preclinical phase of AD and other neurodegenerative pathways [75]. Moreover, C1q presents a protective impact on primary neuronal viability in rodents from Aβ and serum amyloid P (SAP)-induced neurotoxicity in the absence of other downstream factors of the complement pathway [4]. C1q, distinct from C1, engages with myeloid cells, which encompass microglia, fostering an expedited elimination of apoptotic cells and neuronal fragments, thereby curbing the production of pro-inflammatory cytokines [76]. Another study has proved that C1q, heightened in vivo as an early rejoinder to injury, disengaged from the simultaneous upregulation of other complement constituents, has the potential to incite a genetic orchestration fostering neuroprotection [75]. In the presence of blood–brain barrier (BBB) dysfunction, C1q was accompanied by a rapid increase in proinflammatory factors such as interleukin-1β and tumor necrosis factor α but not in C1q-associated C1 serine proteases C1r and C1s [70]. This suggests that C1q can exert neuroprotective effects independently of the classical complement pathway. These results reveal a role for C1q in physiological changes and pathological changes without activating the classical complement pathway.

4. Local Synthesis of C1q in the Brain

Initially, the presence of C1q was studied as a component of the immune system in the blood, with its main site of synthesis in the liver. However, it is now recognized that under conditions of inflammation, external injury, and cellular stress in the CNS, C1q can be expressed and regulated from a variety of cell types, including neurons, microglia, and astrocytes.18 Each of these cells plays a role in regulation, homeostasis, and destruction in the CNS.

4.1. C1q and Microglia

Microglia are the resident immune cells of the brain, and their dysfunction may contribute to neurodegenerative and psychiatric disorders [77]. C1q is synthesized within the cerebral domain, primarily by microglia. In states of equilibrium, C1q is upheld at a subdued magnitude. Yet, when microglia are galvanized into action, the amplitude of C1q escalates, heralding the stimulation of pro-inflammatory cytokines such as interleukin-6 (IL-6) and TNF-α, thereby culminating in the demise of neurons [70]. Simultaneously, the affinity of C1q for apoptotic cells or neuronal fragments sets forth an augmentation in phagocytic activity within microglia. Remarkably, there are instances when heightened C1q levels yield a transient surge in reactive oxygen species (ROS), nitric oxide (NO), and calcium. Furthermore, this surge in C1q can serve to arrest the proliferation of microglia [78].

Microglia are activated in response to stimulation and accompanied by transcriptional adaptive functional changes, and microglia can generally be differentiated into two extreme states: the classical (M1) phenotype and the alternative (M2) phenotype [79]. M1-type microglia release proinflammatory factors and toxic substances, which enhance brain injury. M2 microglia, on the other hand, achieve neuroprotective effects by promoting tissue repair and regeneration [80]. Microglia are the main source of C1q in the brain [81]. This elucidates the rationale behind the presence of C1q not only within the circulatory system but also within the CNS. In states of equilibrium, the levels of C1q are deliberately maintained at a subdued magnitude; however, when microglia are overactivated, C1q levels increase rapidly [78]. M1-type microglia can play a protective role in the early stages of neurodegenerative diseases by secreting C1q involved in the clearance of protein aggregates. However, as the disease progresses, the deleterious effects of M1-type microglia outweigh their beneficial effects, and their clearance becomes less efficient. Moreover, neuronal dysfunction, injury, and degeneration result from the release of large amounts of C1q [82,83].

4.2. C1q and Astrocytes

Astrocytes are among the most numerous cells in the CNS and are critical for potassium homeostasis, neurotransmitter uptake, synapse formation, BBB regulation, and nervous system development [84]. Recent studies have found that neuroinflammation and ischemia induce two distinct phenotypes of astrocytes, control microglia "M1" and "M2" named "A1" and "A2". The A1 phenotype is close to that induced by lipid polysaccharide-induced neuroinflammation, acute CNS injury, and the underlying pathology of many neurodegenerative diseases [85]. In contrast, A2-type astrocytes strongly promote neuronal survival and repair. Moreover, activated microglia can induce neuronal death by secreting C1q to induce astrocytes to shift to the A1 phenotype [18]. In contrast, genes expressed by A1-type astrocytes were significantly downregulated in the absence of C1q, suggesting an important role of C1q in the polarization of astrocytes toward the A1 phenotype [86]. It has been shown that *Astragalus* polysaccharide inhibits the formation of A1-type astrocytes by inhibiting C1q secretion by microglia [87]. In patients with multiple sclerosis, the detection of CNS plaques is an important marker for the co-localization of C1q with reactive astrocytes [88]. A slew of contemporary investigations have unveiled the prospect that C1q originating from astrocytes might exert influence over the attenuation and deterioration of neuronal synapses amidst the trajectory of neurodegeneration [89]. The augmented expression of reactive astrocyte genes spurred by aging was notably dampened in mice devoid of microglial-secreted C1q, a stimulator recognized for inciting the formation of A1 reactive astrocytes. This observation signifies that microglia wield a role in fomenting astrocyte activation during the aging process. Simultaneously, A1 reactive astrocytes forfeit their capacity to execute customary functions. Moreover, the escalated up-regulation of reactive genes within astrocytes triggered by aging might underpin the cognitive regression witnessed within susceptible cerebral domains during normal aging. Additionally, this accentuates the heightened vulnerability of the aged brain to damage [86]. Chen and colleagues' work showcased the inhibitory prowess of Cholecystokinin octapeptide in curtailing the induction of A1-reactive astrocytes by diminishing C1q levels. This intervention concurrently stimulated the genesis of glutamatergic synapses, thus fostering neurocognitive resurgence within aged dNCR model mice [90].

4.3. C1q and Neurons

Neurons integrate thousands of synapses to process and transmit information [3,91]. Whereas neurons are another cell regulating C1q secretion in the brain in addition to astrocytes and microglia, neurons respond to neuroinflammation and other inflammatory mediators [92,93]. The complement factor C1q, sourced from cells within the central CNS, is also intrinsically linked to conferring neuroprotection against external infections [94]. C1q is deemed advantageous in the elimination of aggregated proteins after the activation of the complement factor due to the engagement of low levels of aggregates. C1q production is induced in large numbers when neurons are damaged, enhancing neuronal activity and protecting neurons from Aβ- and SAP-induced neurotoxicity [4]. Nonetheless, when the complement factor is persistently triggered, it can prove detrimental to the CNS as a result of the activation of microglia and the subsequent release of pro-inflammatory cytokines [95]. Interestingly, cholesterol distribution and levels are also influenced by C1q in neurons, which can enhance neurons indirectly by regulating cholesterol levels, and C1q affects neuronal construction by regulating lipid metabolism and membrane-associated gene expression [96].

C1q plays different roles under different cellular expressions and regulations and ultimately serves different roles in a variety of neurodegenerative diseases. In the subsequent overview, we use C1q as an entry point to systematically understand the various mechanisms of neurodegenerative diseases.

5. C1q in Neurodegenerative Diseases

Beyond its established roles in CNS growth, development, and bodily immunization, a novel facet of C1q's functionality has been freshly unveiled within the intricate tapestry of neuropathological pathways that underpin neurodegenerative disorders and TBI. This revelation has cast a spotlight on C1q as a prospective therapeutic avenue for safeguarding neuronal well-being or for retarding the progression of neurodegenerative maladies.

5.1. Alzheimer's Disease

In a series of experiments, excessive complement-mediated synapse pruning was found to be involved in the process of forgetting in AD. Region-specific loss of synaptic salience is a more potent contributor to cognitive decline in AD than the hallmark features of AD, Aβ plaques, and Tau protein hyperphosphorylation [1]. Unlike the state of synapses requiring proper pruning during growth and development, it has been shown that the number of synapses is significantly reduced in patients with early AD. The number of synapses in 75% of patients with mild cognitive impairment was lower than the average of normal individuals, and the number of synapses correlated significantly with the cognitive–behavioral status of AD patients [97–99]. Similarly, synapses in the temporal cortex are reduced by 38% and in the frontal cortex by 14% in AD patients compared with normal subjects [98]. AD mice lacking C1q display reduced synapse loss, supporting a role for C1q in mediating synapse removal [2]. At the end of AD, synapse number decreases positively with the degree of cognitive–behavioral impairment in AD patients [99]. Interestingly, C1q can be observed colocalized with either pre-synaptic or post-synaptic markers in animal models of aging-related diseases, including AD. Accordingly, the upregulation of C1q-tagged synapses is also proved in AD and other neurogenerative disorders-induced cognitive loss. Conversely, the knockdown or blockade of C1q in mouse models of AD has been shown to protect synapses and prevent cognitive impairment, suggesting the detrimental influence of C1q in synaptic loss, and even C1q-labeled synaptic loss may directly contribute to the worsening of AD.

AD is characterized by synaptic dysfunction and neurodegeneration, which are often caused by the deposition of Aβ plaques and neurofibrillary tangles [100]. The deposition of Aβ plaques triggers a series of chain reactions that lead to intracellular Tau protein misfolding and assembly, which subsequently allows the spread of the lesion throughout the neural circuit as well as the cortex, ultimately leading to neurological failure and cognitive decline. C1q plays an important role in this. It has been shown that blocking C1q activation by genetic or antibody-mediated means can attenuate the toxic effects of Aβ and hyperphosphorylated Tau on synapses [101]. This provides another direct evidence for a deleterious effect of C1q during the process of AD (Figure 4).

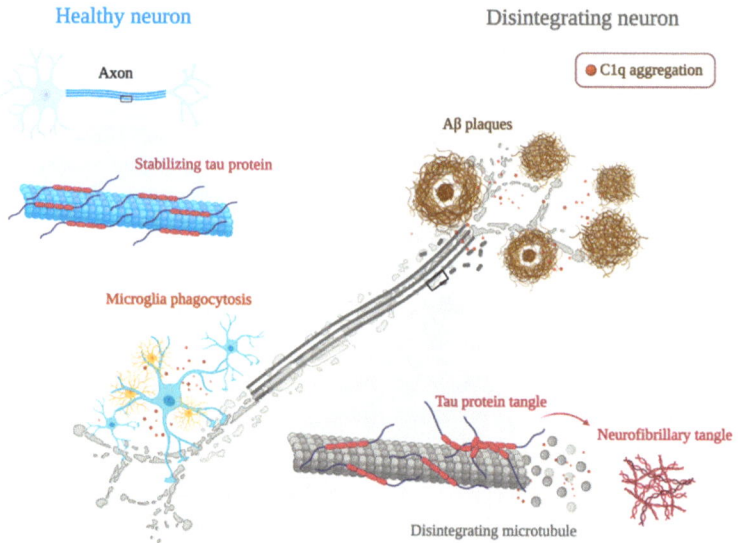

Figure 4. AD development mechanisms. Neurons with C1q aggregation show microglia engulfing healthy synapses, Aβ clumping forming plaques, hyperphosphorylated Tau proteins forming neurofibrillary tangles, and a significant decrease in their ability to bind microtubules due to Tau protein hyperphosphorylation, leading to microtubule disintegration and ultimately worsening of AD development (created with BioRender.com accessed on 12 October 2022).

5.1.1. C1q and Aβ in AD

The major component of amyloid plaques is Aβ, a peptide with 39 to 43 amino acids derived from amyloid b protein precursor (APP) [102]. Studies have shown that the imbalance between the production and clearance of Aβ and related Aβ peptides plays a fundamental role in the pathogenesis of AD [103,104]. In vitro experiments have shown that C1q interacts with Aβ through its A-chain residues 14–26 [104–107]. The complement component C1q has nearly 100% co-localization of Aβ in humans with AD and in mouse models of AD [108]. Sections of the Aβ-treated hippocampus showed a significant increase of C1q in the hippocampus [109]. When soluble Aβ oligomers were injected into the lateral ventricles of WT mice, Aβ oligomers were found to induce C1q deposition [1]. Similarly, when J20 mice were injected with a γ-secretase inhibitor that rapidly reduced Aβ production, it significantly reduced soluble Aβ levels in mice with a corresponding reduction in C1q deposition. When C1q knockdown was followed by Aβ injection, the synaptic loss induced by Aβ was significantly reduced [2]. The use of anti-C1q antibodies similarly prevented Aβ-induced synaptic loss in mice [1], suggesting that C1q is required for Aβ-induced synaptic loss in vivo. Notably, C1q knockdown does not affect Aβ deposition [110], so C1q may function downstream of Aβ. Aβ appears abnormally as early as 20 years before the onset of overt clinical symptoms [111]. Aβ deposition is the beginning of neurodegenerative lesions, but the accumulation of hyperphosphorylated Tau proteins is the main driver of the deteriorating pathological process.

5.1.2. C1q and Tau in AD

In AD and other Tau lesions, Tau aggregates in an abnormally phosphorylated form in the torso region of neurons and can localize to synapses, where it disrupts synaptic plasticity and leads to synaptic loss [112]. Positron emission tomography (PET) imaging targeting Aβ and Tau has unveiled a consequential relationship: the velocity of amyloid aggregation forecasts the advent of Tau accumulation, which in turn heralds the initiation of cognitive decline [113]. In AD, Tau protein aggregation may begin in the entorhinal cortex and then propagate to the hippocampus, as well as within the limbic cortex, reflecting the progression of AD patients from asymptomatic, mildly symptomatic, to full dementia [114]. It has been shown that hyperphosphorylated Tau protein induces more C1q aggregation at the synapse than Aβ plaques [101]. In the mouse model, increased Tau phosphorylation and accumulation were accompanied by a dose-dependent increase in C1q [115]. It has been shown that knockout of the granule protein precursor gene PGRN significantly reduces Aβ plaque production, but deletion of PGRN enhances C1q deposition at the synapse while increasing the accumulation of hyperphosphorylated Tau protein in the hippocampus [116]. Interestingly, knockdown of the transmembrane immune signaling adaptor TYROBP showed opposite results, where knockdown of TYROBP resulted in a significant reduction in C1q and improvement in memory cognition impairment, hyperphosphorylated Tau protein was not reduced by the decrease in C1q, but instead, its spread was further expanded and Tau protein phosphorylation levels were increased. Suggesting that when there are multiple competing effects occurring simultaneously, the deleterious effects of increased Tau protein phosphorylation levels and diffusion can be overcome as long as the beneficial effect of a significant decrease in C1q is large enough [117]. It may give insights into the target role of C1q in regulating the progression of AD pathology and cognitive loss.

5.2. Parkinson Disease

PD is clinically characterized by an akinetic rigid syndrome related to reduced. This syndrome is entwined with a decline in dopamine levels within the striatum, arising from the gradual demise of terminals belonging to degenerating neuromelanin-containing dopaminergic neurons in the substantia nigra pars compacta [118]. A handful of investigations have scrutinized the complement system within the context of the PD brain. The steady manifestation of C1q was discernible only within microglial cells spanning the cerebral expanse. After MPTP (1-methyl-4-phenyl-1,2,3,6-tetrahydropyridine) exposure, there was an early and temporary elevation in microglial C1q expression within the substantia nigra and striatum, as unveiled through techniques of immunohistochemistry and in situ hybridization. Notably, Rozemuller and collaborators found no immunostaining indicative of C1q within cortical Lewy bodies [119]. Concurrently, mice devoid of the C1q protein exhibited no substantial differences in terms of the loss of nigral dopaminergic neurons, striatal dopaminergic fibers, and dopamine levels induced by MPTP in comparison to their control counterparts [120,121]. This shows that C1q is not a major contributor to cognitive impairment in PD. Simultaneously, within the substantia nigra pars compacta (SNc) of PD cases, there manifested an augmented accumulation of extracellular neuromelanin within the tissue, a manifestation arising from the degeneration of dopaminergic neurons. In this milieu, neuromelanin granules and fragments from deteriorated neurons appeared to be tagged by C1q, thus becoming subject to phagocytosis by C1q-positive microglia and macrophages situated both within the tissue and around perivascular spaces. Notably, cells bearing neuromelanin and C1q also adhered to the inner surfaces of blood vessels in the SNc in the context of PD [8]. Hence, microglia demonstrate the capability to engulf and eliminate cellular detritus emanating from degenerating neurons within the SNc, effectively orchestrating this process through a pathway facilitated by C1q, a phenomenon that occurs within the context of PD. Although C1q may not play a direct pathological role in PD, it can affect the disease process through microglia phagocytosis, etc. Therefore, when we focus on the role of C1q in PD, we should not only look at its expression but also pay attention to the related pathways or effects on other cells.

5.3. Huntington's Disease

HD is an autosomal-dominant neurodegenerative disorder characterized by a relentless progression, culminating in targeted neuronal attrition and impairment, predominantly within the striatal and cortical regions [122]. Within the striatal milieu of HD, a convergence was observed wherein neurons, myelin, and astrocytes demonstrated a spatial overlap with C1q. In contrast, no C1q was found in the normal striatum. In normal control brains, the abundance of C1q mRNA ranged from 2 to 5 times lower when juxtaposed with the levels identified in the striatum affected by HD. The course of HD is marked by a neuroinflammatory progression orchestrated by the activation of microglia within the cerebral domain [123]. Astrogliosis and microgliosis were apparent in all caudate and internal capsule samples from individuals with HD, a phenomenon absent in normal brain tissue. Microglia of the M1 phenotype within the HD context produced C1q, which was subsequently triggered on neuronal membranes. This dual action of C1q not only facilitated neuronal necrosis but also contributed to proinflammatory activities [124]. Meanwhile, it has been reported that the secretion of cytokines C1q upon M1 microglial activation can induce the generation of reactive A1 astrocytes at neuronal structures, which play a major role in brain motor coordination [125,126]. These intricate processes are believed to precipitate neurodegenerative events within the brain, ultimately giving rise to the motor dysfunctions that become manifest in the later stages of this neurological affliction. Kaempferol, a natural antioxidant found in vegetables and fruits consumed as part of human nutrition, has exhibited the capacity to forestall the proteolytic activation of complement C1q protein and the subsequent emergence of reactive A1 astrocytes. This phenomenon has been observed in the context of 3-nitro propionic acid-induced injury within the striatum and hippocampus. Cognitive–behavioral deficits in experimental animals significantly improved when microglia secretion of C1q was reduced in an animal model of HD [127].

5.4. Traumatic Brain Injury

TBI emerges as the most potent environmental catalyst in the emergence of AD and other neurodegenerative disorders linked to dementia. The initial trauma sustained by the brain impairs the integrity of the BBB, consequently permitting the infiltration of peripheral circulating macrophages into the cerebral milieu. This occurrence subsequently accentuates the inflammatory response [128]. The prevailing notion suggests that a transition between the M1 and M2 microglial phenotypes transpires within the framework of TBI. However, it appears that there exists a proclivity towards favoring the M1 phenotype over the M2 phenotype in the context of TBI-associated secondary injury [129]. In pathological scenarios encompassing TBI, there is substantiated evidence suggesting that C1q plays a contributory role in steering a shift toward the M1 phenotype [78]. In tandem with the direct harm incited by M1 microglia, the C1q they release can also instigate the activation of astrocytes [130]. A prominent constituent of the inflammatory pathway, the complement system, often escapes notice, yet it too undergoes activation as an integral facet of the neuroinflammatory rejoinder in TBI [131]. The intrinsic complement system within the CNS undergoes activation, with this activation further amplified by an influx of complement components from the bloodstream, facilitated by the disruption of the BBB. In parallel, certain investigations have demonstrated a noteworthy accumulation of C1q on synapses located in the hippocampus. This accumulation aligns temporally with the loss of synapses 30 days after the injury. Significantly, both genetic interventions and the implementation of pharmacological measures to obstruct the complement pathway yielded the prevention of memory deficits in aged animals subjected to injury [132,133]. Therefore, strategically focusing on the modulation of C1q emerges as a substantial avenue for potential clinical intervention after TBI within the aging demographic (Table 2).

Table 2. Characteristics of neurodegenerative diseases.

Neurodegenerative Diseases	Animal/Cellular Model	Characteristics	C1q Effects	Ref.
AD	Tg2576 animals (APP) with C1q-deficient mice	Aβ plaques	Aβ co-localizes with C1q	[2,108,109]
	PS19 mice overexpressing the P301S mutant of human Tau/Hek cells	Tau protein misfolding and assembly	Tau protein co-localizes with C1q	[113–115]
	Tg2576 animals (APP) with C1q-deficient mice	Synapse elimination	Synapse co-localizes with C1q	[2,3,62]
PD	-	Depigmentation of the substantia nigra and locus coeruleus	C1q was restricted to microglia throughout the brain	[118]
	Autopsies from PD patients	Neuronal loss in the pars compacta of the substantia nigra		[8,120]
HD	Early HD patients	CAG trinucleotide repeat expansion in the huntingtin gene on chromosome 4	C1q produced locally by M1-type microglia is activated on the membranes of neurons	[124,134]
TBI	Sections of brains obtained at autopsy from 25 cases following closed TBI	Traumatic brain injury disrupts the BBB	C1q prompts the transformation of M2-type microglia into M1-type microglia and enhances complement system activation	[78,131]

6. Efficacy of Dietary Food Related to C1q for Memory Improvement

As one of the most important mechanisms of CNS, C1q plays an important role in the regulation of brain environment balance via the classical complement pathway, as discussed above. Recently, a body of literature has demonstrated that numerous food compositions exert neuroprotective effects via regulating C1q, providing evidence for the CNS of food related to C1q. Several common dietary food components related to the regulation of C1q for CNS health are shown in Figure 5.

Artemisia annua L., a herbaceous plant with heat-clearing properties, has garnered renown due to its antimalarial compound, artemisinin [135]. Moreover, it has garnered heightened interest owing to its demonstrated anti-inflammatory and immunoregulatory capabilities. Intriguingly, the acidic homogeneous polysaccharides derived from *Artemisia annua* have exhibited noteworthy efficacy in anticomplement activities through the classical pathway and alternative pathway. *Prunella vulgaris*, a perennial plant with a broad geographical distribution encompassing China, Japan, and Europe, has been employed for its spikes in a pivotal role within an herbal tea cherished in southern China for its ability to dissipate pathogenic heat from the bloodstream [136]. Interestingly, homogeneous acidic polysaccharides extracted from the spikes of *Prunella vulgaris* exhibit a capacity to interact with C1q, exerting an influence on the C2, C3, C5, and C9 constituents of the complement system. This property renders it potentially valuable in addressing ailments correlated with the excessive activation of the complement system. *Viola tianshanica Maxim*, a perennial herbaceous plant, finds its distribution primarily in Central Asia, notably within the Xinjiang Uygur Autonomous Region of China [137]. An investigation revealed that the ethanol extract derived from this herb showcased noteworthy anti-complement activity. Specifically, it targeted C1q, thereby impeding the classical pathway and the alternative pathway. This finding positions it as a promising contender for the role of potent anticomplement agents. Within China, *Taraxacum mongolicum Hand.-Mazz.*, a constituent of the Asteraceae family, holds eminence as a renowned medicinal plant [138]. It is often harnessed in addressing viral infections and inflammatory maladies. From this herb, a uniform water-soluble polysaccharide has been extracted. Mechanistic analyses have revealed that this compound curtails complement activation through the impediment of C1q. This trait renders it of significance in the context of managing conditions attributed to excessive activation of the complement system. Such actives currently express an inhibitory effect on C1q via the complement pathway but have not been specifically studied in the CNS and could be further investigated subsequently.

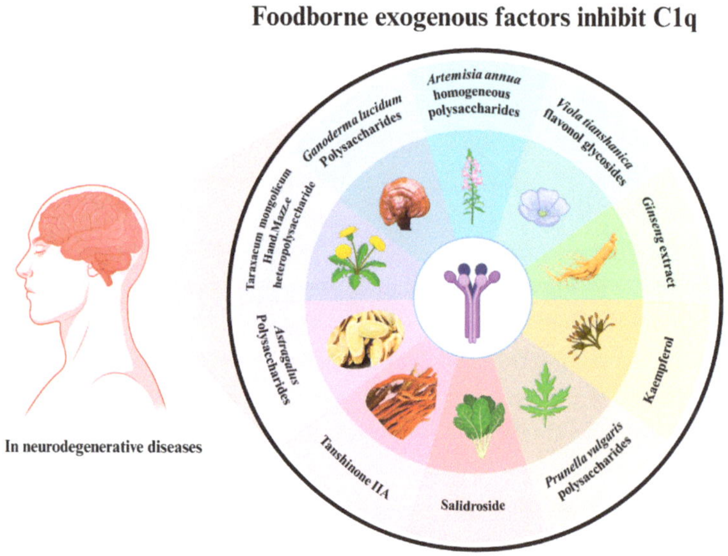

Figure 5. Inhibition of C1q aggregation by functional food factors (created with BioRender.com accessed on 28 May 2023).

Ganoderma lucidum, a medicinal fungus, finds clinical utilization across numerous Asian countries as a means to bolster health and foster longevity [139]. Studies have shown that Ganoderma lucidum has neuroprotective effects, and aqueous extracts of Ganoderma lucidum significantly attenuate Aβ-induced synaptotoxicity by protecting synaptophysin. Likewise, the examination unveiled that *Ganoderma lucidum* polysaccharides (GLP) elicit a decrease in pro-inflammatory cytokines provoked by LPS or Aβ while concurrently fostering the expression of anti-inflammatory cytokines in BV-2 and primary microglial cells. Moreover, GLP mitigates the migratory propensity of microglia linked to inflammation, curtails morphological modifications, and diminishes the likelihood of phagocytosis. Remarkably, it also substantially reduces the expression of C1q [140]. Kaempferol, an innate antioxidant found in vegetables and fruits integral to human nutrition, displays a noteworthy capacity. Specifically, when administered, it hampers the proteolytic activation of complement C3 protein and the consequent emergence of reactive A1 astrocytes triggered by NPA in the striatum and hippocampus. Furthermore, it thwarts the augmentation of NF-κB expression and the heightened secretion of cytokines IL-1α, TNFα, and C1q, all of which are associated with the formation of reactive A1 astrocytes. Beyond this, kaempferol administration also averts the exacerbated production of amyloid β peptides within the striatum and hippocampus [127]. Cellular senescence, recognized as a pivotal hallmark of aging, entails an irreversible cessation of the cell cycle and becomes expedited during the aging trajectory. Intriguingly, black ginseng, a derivative of fresh ginseng achieved through a cyclical procedure of steaming and drying carried out nine times, has emerged under the spotlight owing to its physiological advantages in counteracting reactive oxygen species, inflammation, and oncogenic processes [141]. These mechanisms are frequently implicated in the onset of aging. Black ginseng attenuates cellular senescence by downregulating complement C1q and β-catenin signaling and its downstream activator in the senescence pathway, p53-p21/p16, to downregulated age-related inflammatory genes, especially in the complement system.

Astragalus polysaccharides are one of the key active components of *Astragalus* membranaceus [87]. Pharmacological investigations have demonstrated that *Astragalus* polysaccharides exhibit a diverse range of pharmacological impacts, encompassing anti-inflammatory, antitumor, and immune regulatory properties. *Astragalus* polysaccharides regulate the polarization of microglia from M1 to M2 phenotype, reduce the secretion of inflammatory factors IL-1α, TNF-α, and C1q, and inhibit the activation of A1 neurotoxic astrocytes, thus effectively inhibiting neuroinflammation and demyelination in experimental autoimmune encephalomyelitis.

Tanshinone, a prominent lipid-soluble constituent of *Salvia miltiorrhiza*, takes shape as a substantial active ingredient, notably as TanIIA [142]. Extensive research has unveiled its pharmacological effects, particularly in the realm of neuroprotection. In the context of the rat brain, TanIIA emerges as a safeguard against Aβ-induced inflammation-induced neuronal impairment. A gamut of neuroprotective attributes can be ascribed to TanIIA, encompassing the attenuation of overactive glial cell response and the inhibition of inflammatory mediators such as IL-1β, IL-6, C1q, C3c, and C3d. Simultaneously, C1q surfaces as a countermeasure against the toxicity induced by oligomeric forms of Aβ. Its early upregulation in the aftermath of injury, distinct from the coordinated induction of other complement components, facilitates the orchestration of a gene expression program that fosters neuroprotection. This program, in turn, exhibits the potential to shield against Aβ-related pathologies during the preclinical phases of AD and other neurodegenerative processes.

Salidroside, a bioactive constituent sourced from *Rhodiola rosea*, is currently under scrutiny as a promising therapeutic avenue for addressing ischemic stroke. Particularly noteworthy is its potential effectiveness in curtailing the inflammatory response in the context of cerebral ischemia-reperfusion injury (IRI), as evidenced by studies conducted within the 24 h timeframe following the occurrence of ischemic brain events [143]. In the wake of cerebral IRI, there emerges a prompt escalation in the accumulation of immunoglobulin M, mannose-binding lectin 2, and annexin IV on cerebral endothelial cells. This is accompanied by the induction of complement components C3 and C3a within 24 h post-IRI. Subsequently, at the 48 h mark, a substantial surge is observed in the complement component C1q. Salicin affected these proteins and reversed their changes after 24 h of IRI. Salidroside operates as a neuroprotective agent by curtailing the premature activation of the lectin pathway on cerebral endothelial cells and impeding the gradual activation of the classical pathway following cerebral IRI. This protracted neuroprotection seems to be linked, at least in part, to the elevated expression of genes associated with neuroplasticity. This enhanced gene expression is facilitated by the mitigation of complement activation [144]. In a similar vein, Salidroside plays a role in diminishing inflammation and neuronal impairment after middle cerebral artery occlusion and reperfusion. This effect is, in part, attributed to the inhibition of cerebral complement C3 activation. Furthermore, Salidroside's impact on astrocytes and microglial BV2 cells following oxygen–glucose deprivation and subsequent restoration did not extend to influencing C1q, C2, or C3 levels [145]. Within human umbilical vein endothelial cells (HUVEC), Salidroside served to safeguard against the decline of CD46 and CD59 while concurrently mitigating the elevation of VCAM-1, ICAM-1, P-selectin, and E-selectin. These effects correlated with reduced LDH release and an enhanced Bcl-2/Bax ratio. Crucially, these protective outcomes of Salidroside manifested only in the context of oxygen–glucose restoration.

Significant progress in the relationship between C1q and CNS has been made in recent years, suggesting that C1q and complement pathways are regarded as potential therapeutic targets for CNS disorders. People tend to opt for dietary choices as intervention measures in addressing these ailments. Importantly, our limited grasp of the intricate mechanisms underlying C1q and complement-mediated neurodegenerative conditions has contributed to a considerable rate of unsuccessful endeavors in formulating dietary interventions for CNS disorders. The summary of current natural products or food components regulating C1q in CNS is shown in Table 3. There is a growing need for further research to explore food components as a specific and effective intervention targeting complement-related neurodegenerative diseases.

Table 3. Effect of functional food factors on C1q.

Sources	Main Active Ingredients	Mechanism of Action	Function	Ref.
Artemisia annua L.	Acidic homogeneous polysaccharides	Inhibited the classical pathway and the alternative pathway	Anti-complement activity	[135]
Prunella vulgaris	Homogeneous acidic polysaccharides	Reduced excessive activation of the complement system	Anti-complement activity	[136]
Viola tianshanica flavonol glycosides	Flavonol glycosides and other phenolic compounds	Inhibited the classical pathway and the alternative pathway	Anti-complement activity	[137]
Taraxacum mongolicum Hand.-Mazz. heteropolysaccharide	Heteropolysaccharide	Inhibited excessive activation of the complement system	Anti-complement activity	[138]
Ganoderma lcidum	Polysaccharides	Down-regulates LPS- or Aβ-induced pro-inflammatory cytokines, promotes anti-inflammatory cytokine expressions in BV-2 and primary microglia and reduces C1q expression	Neuroprotective	[140]
Black Ginseng	Panax ginseng	Downregulated age-related inflammatory genes, included in the complement system	Ameliorates cellular senescence	[141]
Astragalus	Polysaccharides	Regulates the polarization of microglia from M1 to M2 phenotype by inhibiting the miR-155, reduces the secretion of inflammatory factors, and inhibits the activation of neurotoxic astrocytes	Inhibit neuroinflammation and demyelination in experimental autoimmune encephalomyelitis	[87]
Salvia miltiorrhiza	Tanshinone IIA	Reduced the number of astrocytes and microglial cells and induced C1q decreased in the brain of Alzheimer's disease model rats	Reduced inflammation levels of AD rats	[142]
Rhodiola Rosea	Salidroside	Reducing early activation of the lectin pathway on the cerebral endothelium and inhibiting the gradual activation of the classical pathway after cerebral IR	Neuroprotective	[144]
Rhodiola Rosea	Salidroside	Inhibited classical complement activation and increased CD46 and CD59	The protection afforded in cerebral ischemia-reperfusion injury	[145]
Vegetables and fruits	Kaempferol	Blocked the NPA-induced increase of NF-κB expression and enhanced secretion of cytokines IL-1α, TNFα, and C1q	Prevents the activation of complement C3 protein and the generation of reactive A1 astrocytes	[127]

7. Discussion and Conclusions

With the increasing prevalence of neurodegenerative diseases and the frequent occurrence of their complications, people are becoming increasingly interested in obtaining safe, active ingredients from natural foods to replace the medications used for neurodegenerative disease treatment.

C1q plays an important role in the early stages of the disease by labeling and eliminating cellular debris and microbes, orchestrating immune responses, signaling "danger", and then activating the complement pathway that rapidly reacts to defend the body against external pathogens. In addition, C1q plays a key role in the mechanism by which glial cells regulate synaptic pruning by activating the complement pathway that contributes to CNS development. C1q is not only involved in synaptic growth and development but also plays distinct roles in the diverse stages of neurodegenerative diseases. Neuronal and glial cell death, as well as impaired cognitive function because of aging or genetic mutations manifested in neurodegenerative diseases, have all been shown to be inextricably linked to C1q. Thus, taking full advantage of C1q and complement-related mechanisms in physiological and pathophysiological conditions of CNS has become a new strategy for improving human health. Although significant progress in complement pathways in CNS has been made over the last decade, there are several issues that require further investigation. For example, how does C1q tagged and located on synapses and then activate microglia phagocytosis? There is limited knowledge of the ligands on synapse interact with C1q. How may we balance the crucial role of C1q in apoptotic cell debris clearance and synapse loss? Additionally, since complement inhibitors are ineffective against C1q, inhibitors and activators targeting C1q in vivo need to be discovered in further studies.

Currently, few studies have been conducted on C1q and brain health in the food industry. Studies that focus on daily food component-mediated C1q and complement-related diseases have a lot of untapped potential. Studies on the function of diverse dietary components related to C1q on CNS disorders are valuable for the clinical application prospects for disease intervention and control, especially in memory improvement and brain health in AD and others. Absolutely, various functional food factors could exert a neuroprotective role against brain injury by regulating C1q, like *Ganoderma lucidum* polysaccharides and Kaempferol. However, the specific underlying mechanisms have not been fully explained. Therefore, further studies are needed in the future to investigate the mechanism of targeting C1q to delay neurodegenerative diseases by key food functional components in the daily diet.

Author Contributions: Writing—original draft preparation, Y.X.; writing—review and editing, X.W.; visualization, D.Z.; conceptualization, J.W. and C.L.; methodology, D.W.; software, X.L.; investigation, Y.X.; resources, L.F.; supervision, X.W.; project administration, W.M.; funding acquisition, X.W. All authors have read and agreed to the published version of the manuscript.

Funding: This research was funded by the Science and Technology Research Project of Jilin Province, grant number JJKH20220347KJ and The Science and Technology Development Project of Jilin Province was funded by 20230202055NC.

Data Availability Statement: Data is contained within the article.

Conflicts of Interest: The authors declare no conflict of interest.

References

1. Hong, S.; Beja-Glasser, V.F.; Nfonoyim, B.M.; Frouin, A.; Li, S.; Ramakrishnan, S.; Merry, K.M.; Shi, Q.; Rosenthal, A.; Barres, B.A.; et al. Complement and microglia mediate early synapse loss in Alzheimer mouse models. *Science* **2016**, *352*, 712–716. [CrossRef]
2. Fonseca, M.I.; Zhou, J.; Botto, M.; Tenner, A.J. Absence of C1q leads to less neuropathology in transgenic mouse models of Alzheimer's disease. *J. Neurosci.* **2004**, *24*, 6457–6465. [CrossRef]
3. Stevens, B.; Allen, N.J.; Vazquez, L.E.; Howell, G.R.; Christopherson, K.S.; Nouri, N.; Micheva, K.D.; Mehalow, A.K.; Huberman, A.D.; Stafford, B.; et al. The classical complement cascade mediates CNS synapse elimination. *Cell* **2007**, *131*, 1164–1178. [CrossRef]
4. Pisalyaput, K.; Tenner, A.J. Complement component C1q inhibits β-amyloid- and serum amyloid P-induced neurotoxicity via caspase- and calpain-independent mechanisms. *J. Neurochem.* **2008**, *104*, 696–707. [CrossRef]
5. Poulose, S.M.; Fisher, D.R.; Larson, J.; Bielinski, D.F.; Rimando, A.M.; Carey, A.N.; Schauss, A.G.; Shukitt-Hale, B. Anthocyanin-rich Açai (*Euterpe oleracea* Mart.) Fruit Pulp Fractions Attenuate Inflammatory Stress Signaling in Mouse Brain BV-2 Microglial Cells. *J. Agric. Food Chem.* **2012**, *60*, 1084–1093. [CrossRef]
6. Tenner, A.J.; Stevens, B.; Woodruff, T.M. New tricks for an ancient system: Physiological and pathological roles of complement in the CNS. *Mol. Immunol.* **2018**, *102*, 3–13. [CrossRef]
7. Tolosa, E.; Garrido, A.; Scholz, S.W.; Poewe, W. Challenges in the diagnosis of Parkinson's disease. *Lancet Neurol.* **2021**, *20*, 385–397. [CrossRef]
8. Depboylu, C.; Schäfer, M.K.H.; Arias-Carrión, O.; Oertel, W.H.; Weihe, E.; Höglinger, G.U. Possible Involvement of Complement Factor C1q in the Clearance of Extracellular Neuromelanin from the Substantia Nigra in Parkinson Disease. *J. Neuropathol. Exp. Neurol.* **2011**, *70*, 125–132. [CrossRef]
9. Ye, J.; Yang, P.; Yang, Y.; Xia, S. Complement C1s as a diagnostic marker and therapeutic target: Progress and propective. *Front. Immunol.* **2022**, *13*, 1015128. [CrossRef]
10. Kishore, U.; Reid, K.B. Modular organization of proteins containing C1q-like globular domain. *Immunopharmacology* **1999**, *42*, 15–21. [CrossRef]

11. Kishore, U.; Ghai, R.; Greenhough, T.J.; Shrive, A.K.; Bonifati, D.M.; Gadjeva, M.G.; Waters, P.; Kojouharova, M.S.; Chakraborty, T.; Agrawal, A. Structural and functional anatomy of the globular domain of complement protein C1q. *Immunol. Lett.* **2004**, *95*, 113–128. [CrossRef]
12. Nayak, A.; Ferluga, J.; Tsolaki, A.G.; Kishore, U. The non-classical functions of the classical complement pathway recognition subcomponent C1q. *Immunol. Lett.* **2010**, *131*, 139–150. [CrossRef]
13. Gaboriaud, C.; Teillet, F.; Gregory, L.A.; Thielens, N.M.; Arlaud, G.J. Assembly of C1 and the MBL- and ficolin-MASP complexes: Structural insights. *Immunobiology* **2007**, *212*, 279–288. [CrossRef]
14. Kishore, U.; Gupta, S.K.; Perdikoulis, M.V.; Kojouharova, M.S.; Urban, B.C.; Reid, K.B. Modular organization of the carboxyl-terminal, globular head region of human C1q A, B, and C chains. *J. Immunol.* **2003**, *171*, 812–820. [CrossRef]
15. Paidassi, H.; Tacnet-Delorme, P.; Garlatti, V.; Darnault, C.; Ghebrehiwet, B.; Gaboriaud, C.; Arlaud, G.J.; Frachet, P. C1q binds phosphatidylserine and likely acts as a multiligand-bridging molecule in apoptotic cell recognition. *J. Immunol.* **2008**, *180*, 2329–2338. [CrossRef]
16. Gaboriaud, C.; Juanhuix, J.; Gruez, A.; Lacroix, M.; Darnault, C.; Pignol, D.; Verger, D.; Fontecilla-Camps, J.C.; Arlaud, G.J. The Crystal Structure of the Globular Head of Complement Protein C1q Provides a Basis for Its Versatile Recognition Properties. *J. Biol. Chem.* **2003**, *278*, 46974–46982. [CrossRef]
17. Peake, P.W.; Shen, Y.; Walther, A.; Charlesworth, J.A. Adiponectin binds C1q and activates the classical pathway of complement. *Biochem. Biophys. Res. Commun.* **2008**, *367*, 560–565. [CrossRef]
18. Kölm, R.; Schaller, M.; Roumenina, L.T.; Niemiec, I.; Kremer Hovinga, J.A.; Khanicheh, E.; Kaufmann, B.A.; Hopfer, H.; Trendelenburg, M. Von Willebrand Factor Interacts with Surface-Bound C1q and Induces Platelet Rolling. *J. Immunol.* **2016**, *197*, 3669–3679. [CrossRef]
19. Jiang, H.; Robey, F.A.; Gewurz, H. Localization of sites through which C-reactive protein binds and activates complement to residues 14–26 and 76–92 of the human C1q A chain. *J. Exp. Med.* **1992**, *175*, 1373–1379. [CrossRef]
20. McGrath, F.D.G.; Brouwer, M.C.; Arlaud, G.R.J.; Daha, M.R.; Hack, C.E.; Roos, A. Evidence That Complement Protein C1q Interacts with C-Reactive Protein through Its Globular Head Region. *J. Immunol.* **2006**, *176*, 2950–2957. [CrossRef]
21. Ying, S.C.; Gewurz, A.T.; Jiang, H.; Gewurz, H. Human serum amyloid P component oligomers bind and activate the classical complement pathway via residues 14–26 and 76–92 of the A chain collagen-like region of C1q. *J. Immunol.* **1993**, *150*, 169–176. [CrossRef]
22. Jiang, H.; Cooper, B.; Robey, F.A.; Gewurz, H. DNA binds and activates complement via residues 14-26 of the human C1q A chain. *J. Biol. Chem.* **1992**, *267*, 25597–25601. [CrossRef]
23. Roumenina, L.T.; Radanova, M.; Atanasov, B.P.; Popov, K.T.; Kaveri, S.V.; Lacroix-Desmazes, S.; Frémeaux-Bacchi, V.; Dimitrov, J.D. Heme Interacts with C1q and Inhibits the Classical Complement Pathway. *J. Biol. Chem.* **2011**, *286*, 16459–16469. [CrossRef]
24. Beurskens, F.J.; van Schaarenburg, R.A.; Trouw, L.A. C1q, antibodies and anti-C1q autoantibodies. *Mol. Immunol.* **2015**, *68*, 6–13. [CrossRef]
25. Duncan, A.R.; Winter, G. The binding site for C1q on IgG. *Nature* **1988**, *332*, 738–740. [CrossRef]
26. Roumenina, L.T.; Popov, K.T.; Bureeva, S.V.; Kojouharova, M.; Gadjeva, M.; Rabheru, S.; Thakrar, R.; Kaplun, A.; Kishore, U. Interaction of the globular domain of human C1q with Salmonella typhimurium lipopolysaccharide. *Biochim. Biophys. Acta (BBA) Proteins Proteom.* **2008**, *1784*, 1271–1276. [CrossRef]
27. Terrasse, R.; Tacnet-Delorme, P.; Moriscot, C.; Pérard, J.; Schoehn, G.; Vernet, T.; Thielens, N.M.; Di Guilmi, A.M.; Frachet, P. Human and Pneumococcal Cell Surface Glyceraldehyde-3-phosphate Dehydrogenase (GAPDH) Proteins Are Both Ligands of Human C1q Protein. *J. Biol. Chem.* **2012**, *287*, 42620–42633. [CrossRef]
28. Peerschke, E.I.; Yin, W.; Grigg, S.E.; Ghebrehiwet, B. Blood platelets activate the classical pathway of human complement. *J. Thromb. Haemost.* **2006**, *4*, 2035–2042. [CrossRef]
29. Isliker, H.; Bing, D.H.; Lahan, J.; Hynes, R.O. Fibronectin interacts with Clq, a subcomponent of the first component of complement. *Immunol. Lett.* **1982**, *4*, 39–43. [CrossRef]
30. Takahashi, K.; Rochford, C.D.P.; Neumann, H. Clearance of apoptotic neurons without inflammation by microglial triggering receptor expressed on myeloid cells-2. *J. Exp. Med.* **2005**, *201*, 647–657. [CrossRef]
31. Jiang, J.; Ding, Y.; Wu, M.; Lyu, X.; Wang, H.; Chen, Y.; Wang, H.; Teng, L. Identification of TYROBP and C1QB as Two Novel Key Genes with Prognostic Value in Gastric Cancer by Network Analysis. *Front. Oncol.* **2020**, *10*, 1765. [CrossRef] [PubMed]
32. Audrain, M.; Haure-Mirande, J.V.; Mleczko, J.; Wang, M.; Griffin, J.K.; St George-Hyslop, P.H.; Fraser, P.; Zhang, B.; Gandy, S.; Ehrlich, M.E. Reactive or transgenic increase in microglial TYROBP reveals a TREM2-independent TYROBP–APOE link in wild-type and Alzheimer's-related mice. *Alzheimer's Dement.* **2020**, *17*, 149–163. [CrossRef] [PubMed]
33. Linnartz-Gerlach, B.; Bodea, L.G.; Klaus, C.; Ginolhac, A.; Halder, R.; Sinkkonen, L.; Walter, J.; Colonna, M.; Neumann, H. TREM2 triggers microglial density and age-related neuronal loss. *Glia* **2018**, *67*, 539–550. [CrossRef] [PubMed]
34. Ghai, R.; Waters, P.; Roumenina, L.T.; Gadjeva, M.; Kojouharova, M.S.; Reid, K.B.; Sim, R.B.; Kishore, U. C1q and its growing family. *Immunobiology* **2007**, *212*, 253–266. [CrossRef] [PubMed]
35. Kojouharova, M.S.; Gadjeva, M.G.; Tsacheva, I.G.; Zlatarova, A.; Roumenina, L.T.; Tchorbadjieva, M.I.; Atanasov, B.P.; Waters, P.; Urban, B.C.; Sim, R.B.; et al. Mutational Analyses of the Recombinant Globular Regions of Human C1q A, B, and C Chains Suggest an Essential Role for Arginine and Histidine Residues in the C1q-IgG Interaction. *J. Immunol.* **2004**, *172*, 4351–4358. [CrossRef] [PubMed]

36. Ghebrehiwet, B.; Kandov, E.; Kishore, U.; Peerschke, E.I.B. Is the A-Chain the Engine That Drives the Diversity of C1q Functions? Revisiting Its Unique Structure. *Front. Immunol.* **2018**, *9*, 162. [CrossRef]
37. Siegelt, R.C.; Schumaker, V.N. Measurement of the association constants of the complexes formed between intact C1q or pepsin-treated C1q stalks and the unactivated or activated $C1r_2C1s_2$ tetramers. *Mol. Immunol.* **1983**, *20*, 53–66. [CrossRef]
38. Eggleton, P.; Tenner, A.J.; Reid, K.B.M. C1q receptors. *Clin. Exp. Immunol.* **2000**, *120*, 406–412. [CrossRef]
39. Gaboriaud, C.; Frachet, P.; Thielens, N.M.; Arlaud, G.J. The Human C1q Globular Domain: Structure and Recognition of Non-Immune Self Ligands. *Front. Immunol.* **2012**, *2*, 92. [CrossRef]
40. Ugurlar, D.; Howes, S.C.; de Kreuk, B.-J.; Koning, R.I.; de Jong, R.N.; Beurskens, F.J.; Schuurman, J.; Koster, A.J.; Sharp, T.H.; Parren, P.W.H.I.; et al. Structures of C1-IgG1 provide insights into how danger pattern recognition activates complement. *Science* **2018**, *359*, 794–797. [CrossRef]
41. Nauta, A.J.; Bottazzi, B.; Mantovani, A.; Salvatori, G.; Kishore, U.; Schwaeble, W.J.; Gingras, A.R.; Tzima, S.; Vivanco, F.; Egido, J.; et al. Biochemical and functional characterization of the interaction between pentraxin 3 and C1q. *Eur. J. Immunol.* **2003**, *33*, 465–473. [CrossRef] [PubMed]
42. Ghiran, I. Expression and Function of C1q Receptors and C1q Binding Proteins at the Cell Surface. *Immunobiology* **2002**, *205*, 407–420. [CrossRef] [PubMed]
43. Verneret, M.; Tacnet-Delorme, P.; Osman, R.; Awad, R.; Grichine, A.; Kleman, J.-P.; Frachet, P. Relative Contribution of C1q and Apoptotic Cell-Surface Calreticulin to Macrophage Phagocytosis. *J. Innate Immun.* **2014**, *6*, 426–434. [CrossRef] [PubMed]
44. Garlatti, V.; Chouquet, A.; Lunardi, T.; Vivès, R.; Païdassi, H.; Lortat-Jacob, H.; Thielens, N.M.; Arlaud, G.J.; Gaboriaud, C. Cutting Edge: C1q Binds Deoxyribose and Heparan Sulfate through Neighboring Sites of Its Recognition Domain. *J. Immunol.* **2010**, *185*, 808–812. [CrossRef] [PubMed]
45. Yin, C.; Ackermann, S.; Ma, Z.; Mohanta, S.K.; Zhang, C.; Li, Y.; Nietzsche, S.; Westermann, M.; Peng, L.; Hu, D.; et al. ApoE attenuates unresolvable inflammation by complex formation with activated C1q. *Nat. Med.* **2019**, *25*, 496–506. [CrossRef]
46. Sokolova, D.; Childs, T.; Hong, S. Insight into the role of phosphatidylserine in complement-mediated synapse loss in Alzheimer's disease. *Fac. Rev.* **2021**, *10*, 19. [CrossRef]
47. Païdassi, H.; Tacnet-Delorme, P.; Verneret, M.; Gaboriaud, C.; Houen, G.; Duus, K.; Ling, W.L.; Arlaud, G.J.; Frachet, P. Investigations on the C1q–Calreticulin–Phosphatidylserine Interactions Yield New Insights into Apoptotic Cell Recognition. *J. Mol. Biol.* **2011**, *408*, 277–290. [CrossRef]
48. van Schaarenburg, R.A.; Schejbel, L.; Truedsson, L.; Topaloglu, R.; Al-Mayouf, S.M.; Riordan, A.; Simon, A.; Kallel-Sellami, M.; Arkwright, P.D.; Åhlin, A.; et al. Marked variability in clinical presentation and outcome of patients with C1q immunodeficiency. *J. Autoimmun.* **2015**, *62*, 39–44. [CrossRef]
49. Walport, M.J.; Mackay, I.R.; Rosen, F.S. Complement. *N. Engl. J. Med.* **2001**, *344*, 1058–1066. [CrossRef]
50. Nauta, A.J.; Trouw, L.A.; Daha, M.R.; Tijsma, O.; Nieuwland, R.; Schwaeble, W.J.; Gingras, A.R.; Mantovani, A.; Hack, E.C.; Roos, A. Direct binding of C1q to apoptotic cells and cell blebs induces complement activation. *Eur. J. Immunol.* **2002**, *32*, 1726–1736. [CrossRef]
51. Botto, M.; Dell' Agnola, C.; Bygrave, A.E.; Thompson, E.M.; Cook, H.T.; Petry, F.; Loos, M.; Pandolfi, P.P.; Walport, M.J. Homozygous C1q deficiency causes glomerulonephritis associated with multiple apoptotic bodies. *Nat. Genet.* **1998**, *19*, 56–59. [CrossRef] [PubMed]
52. Ling, G.S.; Crawford, G.; Buang, N.; Bartok, I.; Tian, K.; Thielens, N.M.; Bally, I.; Harker, J.A.; Ashton-Rickardt, P.G.; Rutschmann, S.; et al. C1q restrains autoimmunity and viral infection by regulating CD8+T cell metabolism. *Science* **2018**, *360*, 558–563. [CrossRef] [PubMed]
53. Yuan, X.; Chang, C.-Y.; You, R.; Shan, M.; Gu, B.H.; Madison, M.C.; Diehl, G.; Perusich, S.; Song, L.-Z.; Cornwell, L.; et al. Cigarette smoke–induced reduction of C1q promotes emphysema. *JCI Insight* **2019**, *4*, e124317. [CrossRef] [PubMed]
54. Gomez-Arboledas, A.; Acharya, M.M.; Tenner, A.J. The Role of Complement in Synaptic Pruning and Neurodegeneration. *Immunotargets Ther.* **2021**, *10*, 373–386. [CrossRef]
55. Schartz, N.D.; Tenner, A.J. The good, the bad, and the opportunities of the complement system in neurodegenerative disease. *J. Neuroinflamm.* **2020**, *17*, 354. [CrossRef]
56. Luo, L.; O'Leary, D.D. Axon retraction and degeneration in development and disease. *Annu. Rev. Neurosci.* **2005**, *28*, 127–156. [CrossRef]
57. Schafer, D.P.; Lehrman, E.K.; Kautzman, A.G.; Koyama, R.; Mardinly, A.R.; Yamasaki, R.; Ransohoff, R.M.; Greenberg, M.E.; Barres, B.A.; Stevens, B. Microglia sculpt postnatal neural circuits in an activity and complement-dependent manner. *Neuron* **2012**, *74*, 691–705. [CrossRef]
58. Gyorffy, B.A.; Kun, J.; Torok, G.; Bulyaki, E.; Borhegyi, Z.; Gulyassy, P.; Kis, V.; Szocsics, P.; Micsonai, A.; Matko, J.; et al. Local apoptotic-like mechanisms underlie complement-mediated synaptic pruning. *Proc. Natl. Acad. Sci. USA* **2018**, *115*, 6303–6308. [CrossRef]
59. Fraser, D.A.; Laust, A.K.; Nelson, E.L.; Tenner, A.J. C1q differentially modulates phagocytosis and cytokine responses during ingestion of apoptotic cells by human monocytes, macrophages, and dendritic cells. *J. Immunol.* **2009**, *183*, 6175–6185. [CrossRef]
60. Fraser, D.A.; Pisalyaput, K.; Tenner, A.J. C1q enhances microglial clearance of apoptotic neurons and neuronal blebs, and modulates subsequent inflammatory cytokine production. *J. Neurochem.* **2010**, *112*, 733–743. [CrossRef]

61. Zhan, Y.; Paolicelli, R.C.; Sforazzini, F.; Weinhard, L.; Bolasco, G.; Pagani, F.; Vyssotski, A.L.; Bifone, A.; Gozzi, A.; Ragozzino, D.; et al. Deficient neuron-microglia signaling results in impaired functional brain connectivity and social behavior. *Nat. Neurosci.* **2014**, *17*, 400–406. [CrossRef] [PubMed]
62. Chu, Y.; Jin, X.; Parada, I.; Pesic, A.; Stevens, B.; Barres, B.; Prince, D.A. Enhanced synaptic connectivity and epilepsy in C1q knockout mice. *Proc. Natl. Acad. Sci. USA* **2010**, *107*, 7975–7980. [CrossRef] [PubMed]
63. Zabel, M.K.; Kirsch, W.M. From development to dysfunction: Microglia and the complement cascade in CNS homeostasis. *Ageing Res. Rev.* **2013**, *12*, 749–756. [CrossRef] [PubMed]
64. Reichwald, J.; Danner, S.; Wiederhold, K.-H.; Staufenbiel, M. Expression of complement system components during aging and amyloid deposition in APP transgenic mice. *J. Neuroinflamm.* **2009**, *6*, 35. [CrossRef]
65. Naito, A.T.; Sumida, T.; Nomura, S.; Liu, M.L.; Higo, T.; Nakagawa, A.; Okada, K.; Sakai, T.; Hashimoto, A.; Hara, Y.; et al. Complement C1q activates canonical Wnt signaling and promotes aging-related phenotypes. *Cell* **2012**, *149*, 1298–1313. [CrossRef] [PubMed]
66. Smyth, M.D.; Cribbs, D.H.; Tenner, A.J.; Shankle, W.R.; Dick, M.; Kesslak, J.P.; Cotman, C.W. Decreased levels of C1q in cerebrospinal fluid of living Alzheimer patients correlate with disease state. *Neurobiol. Aging* **1994**, *15*, 609–614. [CrossRef]
67. Stephan, A.H.; Madison, D.V.; Mateos, J.M.; Fraser, D.A.; Lovelett, E.A.; Coutellier, L.; Kim, L.; Tsai, H.H.; Huang, E.J.; Rowitch, D.H.; et al. A dramatic increase of C1q protein in the CNS during normal aging. *J. Neurosci.* **2013**, *33*, 13460–13474. [CrossRef]
68. Botto, M. C1q, Autoimmunity and Apoptosis. *Immunobiology* **2002**, *205*, 395–406. [CrossRef]
69. Thomas, S.; Smatti, M.K.; Ouhtit, A.; Cyprian, F.S.; Almaslamani, M.A.; Thani, A.A.; Yassine, H.M. Antibody-Dependent Enhancement (ADE) and the role of complement system in disease pathogenesis. *Mol. Immunol.* **2022**, *152*, 172–182. [CrossRef]
70. Lynch, N.J.; Willis, C.L.; Nolan, C.C.; Roscher, S.; Fowler, M.J.; Weihe, E.; Ray, D.E.; Schwaeble, W.J. Microglial activation and increased synthesis of complement component C1q precedes blood-brain barrier dysfunction in rats. *Mol. Immunol.* **2004**, *40*, 709–716. [CrossRef]
71. Leigh, L.E.; Ghebrehiwet, B.; Perera, T.P.; Bird, I.N.; Strong, P.; Kishore, U.; Reid, K.B.; Eggleton, P. C1q-mediated chemotaxis by human neutrophils: Involvement of gClqR and G-protein signalling mechanisms. *Biochem. J.* **1998**, *330 Pt 1*, 247–254. [CrossRef] [PubMed]
72. Tenner, A.J.; Fonseca, M.I. The double-edged flower: Roles of complement protein C1q in neurodegenerative diseases. *Adv. Exp. Med. Biol.* **2006**, *586*, 153–176. [CrossRef]
73. Lansita, J.A.; Mease, K.M.; Qiu, H.; Yednock, T.; Sankaranarayanan, S.; Kramer, S. Nonclinical Development of ANX005: A Humanized Anti-C1q Antibody for Treatment of Autoimmune and Neurodegenerative Diseases. *Int. J. Toxicol.* **2017**, *36*, 449–462. [CrossRef] [PubMed]
74. Bensa, J.C.; Reboul, A.; Colomb, M.G. Biosynthesis in vitro of complement subcomponents C1q, C1s and C1 inhibitor by resting and stimulated human monocytes. *Biochem. J.* **1983**, *216*, 385–392. [CrossRef] [PubMed]
75. Benoit, M.E.; Hernandez, M.X.; Dinh, M.L.; Benavente, F.; Vasquez, O.; Tenner, A.J. C1q-induced LRP1B and GPR6 proteins expressed early in Alzheimer disease mouse models, are essential for the C1q-mediated protection against amyloid-β neurotoxicity. *J. Biol. Chem.* **2013**, *288*, 654–665. [CrossRef] [PubMed]
76. Pontecorvo, M.J.; Devous, M.D.; Kennedy, I.; Navitsky, M.; Lu, M.; Galante, N.; Salloway, S.; Doraiswamy, P.M.; Southekal, S.; Arora, A.K.; et al. A multicentre longitudinal study of flortaucipir (18F) in normal ageing, mild cognitive impairment and Alzheimer's disease dementia. *Brain* **2019**, *142*, 1723–1735. [CrossRef]
77. Greenhalgh, A.D.; David, S.; Bennett, F.C. Immune cell regulation of glia during CNS injury and disease. *Nat. Rev. Neurosci.* **2020**, *21*, 139–152. [CrossRef] [PubMed]
78. Farber, K.; Cheung, G.; Mitchell, D.; Wallis, R.; Weihe, E.; Schwaeble, W.; Kettenmann, H. C1q, the recognition subcomponent of the classical pathway of complement, drives microglial activation. *J. Neurosci. Res.* **2009**, *87*, 644–652. [CrossRef]
79. Wu, Y.; Dissing-Olesen, L.; MacVicar, B.A.; Stevens, B. Microglia: Dynamic Mediators of Synapse Development and Plasticity. *Trends Immunol.* **2015**, *36*, 605–613. [CrossRef]
80. Zhou, X.; Chu, X.; Xin, D.; Li, T.; Bai, X.; Qiu, J.; Yuan, H.; Liu, D.; Wang, D.; Wang, Z. L-Cysteine-Derived H_2S Promotes Microglia M2 Polarization via Activation of the AMPK Pathway in Hypoxia-Ischemic Neonatal Mice. *Front. Mol. Neurosci.* **2019**, *12*, 58. [CrossRef]
81. Holden, S.S.; Grandi, F.C.; Aboubakr, O.; Higashikubo, B.; Cho, F.S.; Chang, A.H.; Forero, A.O.; Morningstar, A.R.; Mathur, V.; Kuhn, L.J.; et al. Complement factor C1q mediates sleep spindle loss and epileptic spikes after mild brain injury. *Science* **2021**, *373*, eabj2685. [CrossRef] [PubMed]
82. Brachova, L.; Lue, L.F.; Schultz, J.; el Rashidy, T.; Rogers, J. Association cortex, cerebellum, and serum concentrations of C1q and factor B in Alzheimer's disease. *Brain Res. Mol. Brain Res.* **1993**, *18*, 329–334. [CrossRef] [PubMed]
83. Lue, L.F.; Rydel, R.; Brigham, E.F.; Yang, L.B.; Hampel, H.; Murphy, G.M., Jr.; Brachova, L.; Yan, S.D.; Walker, D.G.; Shen, Y.; et al. Inflammatory repertoire of Alzheimer's disease and nondemented elderly microglia in vitro. *Glia* **2001**, *35*, 72–79. [CrossRef]
84. Zhang, Y.; Barres, B.A. Astrocyte heterogeneity: An underappreciated topic in neurobiology. *Curr. Opin. Neurobiol.* **2010**, *20*, 588–594. [CrossRef] [PubMed]
85. Sofroniew, M.V.; Vinters, H.V. Astrocytes: Biology and pathology. *Acta Neuropathol.* **2010**, *119*, 7–35. [CrossRef]
86. Clarke, L.E.; Liddelow, S.A.; Chakraborty, C.; Munch, A.E.; Heiman, M.; Barres, B.A. Normal aging induces A1-like astrocyte reactivity. *Proc. Natl. Acad. Sci. USA* **2018**, *115*, E1896–E1905. [CrossRef] [PubMed]

87. Liu, X.; Ma, J.; Ding, G.; Gong, Q.; Wang, Y.; Yu, H.; Cheng, X. Microglia Polarization from M1 toward M2 Phenotype Is Promoted by *Astragalus Polysaccharides* Mediated through Inhibition of miR-155 in Experimental Autoimmune Encephalomyelitis. *Oxid. Med. Cell. Longev.* **2021**, *2021*, 5753452. [CrossRef]
88. Ingram, G.; Loveless, S.; Howell, O.W.; Hakobyan, S.; Dancey, B.; Harris, C.L.; Robertson, N.P.; Neal, J.W.; Morgan, B.P. Complement activation in multiple sclerosis plaques: An immunohistochemical analysis. *Acta Neuropathol. Commun.* **2014**, *2*, 53. [CrossRef]
89. Cho, K.J.; Cheon, S.Y.; Kim, G.W. Apoptosis signal-regulating kinase 1 mediates striatal degeneration via the regulation of C1q. *Sci. Rep.* **2016**, *6*, 18840. [CrossRef]
90. Chen, L.; Yang, N.; Li, Y.; Li, Y.; Hong, J.; Wang, Q.; Liu, K.; Han, D.; Han, Y.; Mi, X.; et al. Cholecystokinin octapeptide improves hippocampal glutamatergic synaptogenesis and postoperative cognition by inhibiting induction of A1 reactive astrocytes in aged mice. *CNS Neurosci. Ther.* **2021**, *27*, 1374–1384. [CrossRef]
91. Verkhratsky, A.; Ho, M.S.; Parpura, V. Evolution of Neuroglia. *Adv. Exp. Med. Biol.* **2019**, *1175*, 15–44. [CrossRef] [PubMed]
92. Thomas, A.; Gasque, P.; Vaudry, D.; Gonzalez, B.; Fontaine, M. Expression of a complete and functional complement system by human neuronal cells in vitro. *Int. Immunol.* **2000**, *12*, 1015–1023. [CrossRef] [PubMed]
93. Terai, K.; Walker, D.G.; McGeer, E.G.; McGeer, P.L. Neurons express proteins of the classical complement pathway in Alzheimer disease. *Brain Res.* **1997**, *769*, 385–390. [CrossRef] [PubMed]
94. Rupprecht, T.A.; Angele, B.; Klein, M.; Heesemann, J.; Pfister, H.-W.; Botto, M.; Koedel, U. Complement C1q and C3 Are Critical for the Innate Immune Response to Streptococcus pneumoniae in the Central Nervous System. *J. Immunol.* **2007**, *178*, 1861–1869. [CrossRef]
95. Mahajan, S.D.; Aalinkeel, R.; Parikh, N.U.; Jacob, A.; Cwiklinski, K.; Sandhu, P.; Le, K.; Loftus, A.W.; Schwartz, S.A.; Quigg, R.J.; et al. Immunomodulatory Role of Complement Proteins in the Neuropathology Associated with Opiate Abuse and HIV-1 Co-Morbidity. *Immunol. Investig.* **2017**, *46*, 816–832. [CrossRef]
96. Benoit, M.E.; Tenner, A.J. Complement protein C1q-mediated neuroprotection is correlated with regulation of neuronal gene and microRNA expression. *J. Neurosci.* **2011**, *31*, 3459–3469. [CrossRef]
97. Scheff, S.W.; Price, D.A.; Schmitt, F.A.; Mufson, E.J. Hippocampal synaptic loss in early Alzheimer's disease and mild cognitive impairment. *Neurobiol. Aging* **2006**, *27*, 1372–1384. [CrossRef]
98. Davies, C.A.; Mann, D.M.; Sumpter, P.Q.; Yates, P.O. A quantitative morphometric analysis of the neuronal and synaptic content of the frontal and temporal cortex in patients with Alzheimer's disease. *J. Neurol. Sci.* **1987**, *78*, 151–164. [CrossRef]
99. DeKosky, S.T.; Scheff, S.W. Synapse loss in frontal cortex biopsies in Alzheimer's disease: Correlation with cognitive severity. *Ann. Neurol.* **1990**, *27*, 457–464. [CrossRef]
100. Terry, R.D.; Masliah, E.; Salmon, D.P.; Butters, N.; DeTeresa, R.; Hill, R.; Hansen, L.A.; Katzman, R. Physical basis of cognitive alterations in Alzheimer's disease: Synapse loss is the major correlate of cognitive impairment. *Ann. Neurol.* **1991**, *30*, 572–580. [CrossRef]
101. Dejanovic, B.; Huntley, M.A.; De Maziere, A.; Meilandt, W.J.; Wu, T.; Srinivasan, K.; Jiang, Z.; Gandham, V.; Friedman, B.A.; Ngu, H.; et al. Changes in the Synaptic Proteome in Tauopathy and Rescue of Tau-Induced Synapse Loss by C1q Antibodies. *Neuron* **2018**, *100*, 1322–1336.e1327. [CrossRef] [PubMed]
102. Shen, Y.; Zhang, G.; Liu, L.; Xu, S. Suppressive effects of melatonin on amyloid-β-induced glial activation in rat hippocampus. *Arch. Med. Res.* **2007**, *38*, 284–290. [CrossRef] [PubMed]
103. Selkoe, D.J.; Hardy, J. The amyloid hypothesis of Alzheimer's disease at 25 years. *EMBO Mol. Med.* **2016**, *8*, 595–608. [CrossRef]
104. Rogers, J.; Cooper, N.R.; Webster, S.; Schultz, J.; McGeer, P.L.; Styren, S.D.; Civin, W.H.; Brachova, L.; Bradt, B.; Ward, P. Complement activation by beta-amyloid in Alzheimer disease. *Proc. Natl. Acad. Sci. USA* **1992**, *89*, 10016–10020. [CrossRef] [PubMed]
105. Daly, J.t.; Kotwal, G.J. Pro-inflammatory complement activation by the Aβ peptide of Alzheimer's disease is biologically significant and can be blocked by vaccinia virus complement control protein. *Neurobiol. Aging* **1998**, *19*, 619–627. [CrossRef] [PubMed]
106. Tacnet-Delorme, P.; Chevallier, S.; Arlaud, G.J. β-amyloid fibrils activate the C1 complex of complement under physiological conditions: Evidence for a binding site for Aβ on the C1q globular regions. *J. Immunol.* **2001**, *167*, 6374–6381. [CrossRef]
107. Jiang, H.; Burdick, D.; Glabe, C.G.; Cotman, C.W.; Tenner, A.J. β-Amyloid activates complement by binding to a specific region of the collagen-like domain of the C1q A chain. *J. Immunol.* **1994**, *152*, 5050–5059. [CrossRef]
108. Lui, H.; Zhang, J.; Makinson, S.R.; Cahill, M.K.; Kelley, K.W.; Huang, H.-Y.; Shang, Y.; Oldham, M.C.; Martens, L.H.; Gao, F.; et al. Progranulin Deficiency Promotes Circuit-Specific Synaptic Pruning by Microglia via Complement Activation. *Cell* **2016**, *165*, 921–935. [CrossRef]
109. Fan, R.; Tenner, A.J. Complement C1q expression induced by Aβ in rat hippocampal organotypic slice cultures. *Exp. Neurol.* **2004**, *185*, 241–253. [CrossRef]
110. Fonseca, M.I.; Chu, S.H.; Hernandez, M.X.; Fang, M.J.; Modarresi, L.; Selvan, P.; MacGregor, G.R.; Tenner, A.J. Cell-specific deletion of C1qa identifies microglia as the dominant source of C1q in mouse brain. *J. Neuroinflamm.* **2017**, *14*, 48. [CrossRef]
111. Ghebrehiwet, B.; Hosszu, K.H.; Peerschke, E.I. C1q as an autocrine and paracrine regulator of cellular functions. *Mol. Immunol.* **2017**, *84*, 26–33. [CrossRef] [PubMed]

112. Biernat, J.; Gustke, N.; Drewes, G.; Mandelkow, E.M.; Mandelkow, E. Phosphorylation of Ser262 strongly reduces binding of tau to microtubules: Distinction between PHF-like immunoreactivity and microtubule binding. *Neuron* **1993**, *11*, 153–163. [CrossRef] [PubMed]
113. Long, J.M.; Holtzman, D.M. Alzheimer Disease: An Update on Pathobiology and Treatment Strategies. *Cell* **2019**, *179*, 312–339. [CrossRef] [PubMed]
114. Duyckaerts, C.; Bennecib, M.; Grignon, Y.; Uchihara, T.; He, Y.; Piette, F.; Hauw, J.J. Modeling the relation between neurofibrillary tangles and intellectual status. *Neurobiol. Aging* **1997**, *18*, 267–273. [CrossRef]
115. Brody, A.H.; Nies, S.H.; Guan, F.; Smith, L.M.; Mukherjee, B.; Salazar, S.A.; Lee, S.; Lam, T.K.T.; Strittmatter, S.M. Alzheimer risk gene product Pyk2 suppresses tau phosphorylation and phenotypic effects of tauopathy. *Mol. Neurodegen.* **2022**, *17*, 32. [CrossRef]
116. Takahashi, H.; Klein, Z.A.; Bhagat, S.M.; Kaufman, A.C.; Kostylev, M.A.; Ikezu, T.; Strittmatter, S.M.; Alzheimer's Disease Neuroimaging, I. Opposing effects of progranulin deficiency on amyloid and tau pathologies via microglial TYROBP network. *Acta Neuropathol.* **2017**, *133*, 785–807. [CrossRef]
117. Audrain, M.; Haure-Mirande, J.V.; Wang, M.; Kim, S.H.; Fanutza, T.; Chakrabarty, P.; Fraser, P.; St George-Hyslop, P.H.; Golde, T.E.; Blitzer, R.D.; et al. Integrative approach to sporadic Alzheimer's disease: Deficiency of TYROBP in a tauopathy mouse model reduces C1q and normalizes clinical phenotype while increasing spread and state of phosphorylation of tau. *Mol. Psychiatry* **2019**, *24*, 1383–1397. [CrossRef]
118. Hayes, M.T. Parkinson's Disease and Parkinsonism. *Am. J. Med.* **2019**, *132*, 802–807. [CrossRef]
119. Rozemuller, A.J.M.; Eikelenboom, P.; Theeuwes, J.W.; Jansen Steur, E.N.H.; de Vos, R.A.I. Activated microglial cells and complement factors are unrelated to cortical Lewy bodies. *Acta Neuropathol.* **2000**, *100*, 701–708. [CrossRef]
120. Depboylu, C.; Schorlemmer, K.; Klietz, M.; Oertel, W.H.; Weihe, E.; Höglinger, G.U.; Schäfer, M.K.H. Upregulation of microglial C1q expression has no effects on nigrostriatal dopaminergic injury in the MPTP mouse model of Parkinson disease. *J. Neuroimmunol.* **2011**, *236*, 39–46. [CrossRef]
121. Carbutt, S.; Duff, J.; Yarnall, A.; Burn, D.J.; Hudson, G. Variation in complement protein C1q is not a major contributor to cognitive impairment in Parkinson's disease. *Neurosci. Lett.* **2015**, *594*, 66–69. [CrossRef] [PubMed]
122. McColgan, P.; Tabrizi, S.J. Huntington's disease: A clinical review. *Eur. J. Neurol.* **2018**, *25*, 24–34. [CrossRef] [PubMed]
123. Crotti, A.; Glass, C.K. The choreography of neuroinflammation in Huntington's disease. *Trends Immunol.* **2015**, *36*, 364–373. [CrossRef] [PubMed]
124. Singhrao, S.K.; Neal, J.W.; Morgan, B.P.; Gasque, P. Increased Complement Biosynthesis by Microglia and Complement Activation on Neurons in Huntington's Disease. *Exp. Neurol.* **1999**, *159*, 362–376. [CrossRef]
125. Liddelow, S.A.; Guttenplan, K.A.; Clarke, L.E.; Bennett, F.C.; Bohlen, C.J.; Schirmer, L.; Bennett, M.L.; Munch, A.E.; Chung, W.S.; Peterson, T.C.; et al. Neurotoxic reactive astrocytes are induced by activated microglia. *Nature* **2017**, *541*, 481–487. [CrossRef]
126. Lopez-Sanchez, C.; Garcia-Martinez, V.; Poejo, J.; Garcia-Lopez, V.; Salazar, J.; Gutierrez-Merino, C. Early Reactive A1 Astrocytes Induction by the Neurotoxin 3-Nitropropionic Acid in Rat Brain. *Int. J. Mol. Sci.* **2020**, *21*, 3609. [CrossRef]
127. Lopez-Sanchez, C.; Poejo, J.; Garcia-Lopez, V.; Salazar, J.; Garcia-Martinez, V.; Gutierrez-Merino, C. Kaempferol prevents the activation of complement C3 protein and the generation of reactive A1 astrocytes that mediate rat brain degeneration induced by 3-nitropropionic acid. *Food Chem. Toxicol.* **2022**, *164*, 113017. [CrossRef]
128. Beschorner, R.; Nguyen, T.D.; Gözalan, F.; Pedal, I.; Mattern, R.; Schluesener, H.J.; Meyermann, R.; Schwab, J.M. CD14 expression by activated parenchymal microglia/macrophages and infiltrating monocytes following human traumatic brain injury. *Acta Neuropathol.* **2002**, *103*, 541–549. [CrossRef]
129. Kumar, A.; Loane, D.J. Neuroinflammation after traumatic brain injury: Opportunities for therapeutic intervention. *Brain Behav. Immun.* **2012**, *26*, 1191–1201. [CrossRef]
130. Pearn, M.L.; Niesman, I.R.; Egawa, J.; Sawada, A.; Almenar-Queralt, A.; Shah, S.B.; Duckworth, J.L.; Head, B.P. Pathophysiology Associated with Traumatic Brain Injury: Current Treatments and Potential Novel Therapeutics. *Cell. Mol. Neurobiol.* **2016**, *37*, 571–585. [CrossRef]
131. Bellander, B.-M.; Singhrao, S.K.; Ohlsson, M.; Mattsson, P.; Svensson, M. Complement Activation in the Human Brain after Traumatic Head Injury. *J. Neurotrauma* **2001**, *18*, 1295–1311. [CrossRef] [PubMed]
132. Krukowski, K.; Chou, A.; Feng, X.; Tiret, B.; Paladini, M.-S.; Riparip, L.-K.; Chaumeil, M.; Lemere, C.; Rosi, S. Traumatic Brain Injury in Aged Mice Induces Chronic Microglia Activation, Synapse Loss, and Complement-Dependent Memory Deficits. *Int. J. Mol. Sci.* **2018**, *19*, 3753. [CrossRef] [PubMed]
133. Ritzel, R.M.; Doran, S.J.; Glaser, E.P.; Meadows, V.E.; Faden, A.I.; Stoica, B.A.; Loane, D.J. Old age increases microglial senescence, exacerbates secondary neuroinflammation, and worsens neurological outcomes after acute traumatic brain injury in mice. *Neurobiol. Aging* **2019**, *77*, 194–206. [CrossRef]
134. Tabrizi, S.J.; Scahill, R.I.; Durr, A.; Roos, R.A.C.; Leavitt, B.R.; Jones, R.; Landwehrmeyer, G.B.; Fox, N.C.; Johnson, H.; Hicks, S.L.; et al. Biological and clinical changes in premanifest and early stage Huntington's disease in the TRACK-HD study: The 12-month longitudinal analysis. *Lancet Neurol.* **2011**, *10*, 31–42. [CrossRef] [PubMed]
135. Huo, J.; Lu, Y.; Xia, L.; Chen, D. Structural characterization and anticomplement activities of three acidic homogeneous polysaccharides from Artemisia annua. *J. Ethnopharmacol.* **2020**, *247*, 112281. [CrossRef]

136. Du, D.; Lu, Y.; Cheng, Z.; Chen, D. Structure characterization of two novel polysaccharides isolated from the spikes of *Prunella vulgaris* and their anticomplement activities. *J. Ethnopharmacol.* **2016**, *193*, 345–353. [CrossRef]
137. Qin, Y.; Wen, Q.; Cao, J.; Yin, C.; Chen, D.; Cheng, Z. Flavonol glycosides and other phenolic compounds from *Viola tianshanica* and their anti-complement activities. *Pharm. Biol.* **2016**, *54*, 1140–1147. [CrossRef]
138. Chen, M.; Wu, J.; Shi, S.; Chen, Y.; Wang, H.; Fan, H.; Wang, S. Structure analysis of a heteropolysaccharide from *Taraxacum mongolicum Hand.-Mazz.* and anticomplementary activity of its sulfated derivatives. *Carbohydr. Polym.* **2016**, *152*, 241–252. [CrossRef]
139. Lai, C.S.; Yu, M.S.; Yuen, W.H.; So, K.F.; Zee, S.Y.; Chang, R.C. Antagonizing β-amyloid peptide neurotoxicity of the anti-aging fungus *Ganoderma lucidum*. *Brain Res.* **2008**, *1190*, 215–224. [CrossRef]
140. Cai, Q.; Li, Y.; Pei, G. Polysaccharides from *Ganoderma lucidum* attenuate microglia-mediated neuroinflammation and modulate microglial phagocytosis and behavioural response. *J. Neuroinflamm.* **2017**, *14*, 63. [CrossRef]
141. Lee, S.J.; Lee, D.Y.; O'Connell, J.F.; Egan, J.M.; Kim, Y. Black Ginseng Ameliorates Cellular Senescence via p53-p21/p16 Pathway in Aged Mice. *Biology* **2022**, *11*, 1108. [CrossRef]
142. Lu, B.L.; Li, J.; Zhou, J.; Li, W.W.; Wu, H.F. Tanshinone IIA decreases the levels of inflammation induced by $A\beta_{1-42}$ in brain tissues of Alzheimer's disease model rats. *Neuroreport* **2016**, *27*, 883–893. [CrossRef] [PubMed]
143. Wei, Y.; Hong, H.; Zhang, X.; Lai, W.; Wang, Y.; Chu, K.; Brown, J.; Hong, G.; Chen, L. Salidroside Inhibits Inflammation through PI3K/Akt/HIF Signaling after Focal Cerebral Ischemia in Rats. *Inflammation* **2017**, *40*, 1297–1309. [CrossRef] [PubMed]
144. Lai, W.; Xie, X.; Zhang, X.; Wang, Y.; Chu, K.; Brown, J.; Chen, L.; Hong, G. Inhibition of Complement Drives Increase in Early Growth Response Proteins and Neuroprotection Mediated by Salidroside After Cerebral Ischemia. *Inflammation* **2018**, *41*, 449–463. [CrossRef]
145. Wang, Y.; Su, Y.; Lai, W.; Huang, X.; Chu, K.; Brown, J.; Hong, G. Salidroside Restores an Anti-inflammatory Endothelial Phenotype by Selectively Inhibiting Endothelial Complement After Oxidative Stress. *Inflammation* **2020**, *43*, 310–325. [CrossRef] [PubMed]

Disclaimer/Publisher's Note: The statements, opinions and data contained in all publications are solely those of the individual author(s) and contributor(s) and not of MDPI and/or the editor(s). MDPI and/or the editor(s) disclaim responsibility for any injury to people or property resulting from any ideas, methods, instructions or products referred to in the content.

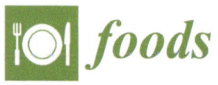

Review

Isolation and Extraction of Monomers from Insoluble Dietary Fiber

Junyao Wang [1,2], Jiarui Zhang [1,2], Sainan Wang [1,2], Wenhao Liu [1,2], Wendan Jing [1,2,*] and Hansong Yu [1,2,*]

1. College of Food Science and Engineering, Jilin Agricultural University, Changchun 130118, China; wjunyaon1@163.com (J.W.); jiarui197@163.com (J.Z.); lwh1766850992@163.com (W.L.)
2. National Soybean Industry Technology System Processing Laboratory, Changchun 130118, China
* Correspondence: jwddoc@163.com (W.J.); yuhansong@163.com (H.Y.); Tel./Fax: +86-0431-84533104 (H.Y.)

Abstract: Insoluble dietary fiber is a macromolecular polysaccharide aggregate composed of pectin, glycoproteins, lignin, cellulose, and hemicellulose. All agricultural by-products contain significant levels of insoluble dietary fiber. With the recognition of the increasing scarcity of non-renewable energy sources, the conversion of single components of dietary fiber into renewable energy sources and their use has become an ongoing concern. The isolation and extraction of single fractions from insoluble dietary fiber is one of the most important recent research directions. The continuous development of technologies for the separation and extraction of single components is aimed at expanding the use of cellulose, hemicellulose, and lignin for food, industrial, cosmetic, biomedical, and other applications. Here, to expand the use of single components to meet the new needs of future development, separation and extraction methods for single components are summarized, in addition to the prospects of new raw materials in the future.

Keywords: insoluble dietary fiber; cellulose; hemicellulose; lignin; mono-component modification

Citation: Wang, J.; Zhang, J.; Wang, S.; Liu, W.; Jing, W.; Yu, H. Isolation and Extraction of Monomers from Insoluble Dietary Fiber. *Foods* **2023**, *12*, 2473. https://doi.org/10.3390/foods12132473

Academic Editor: Luis Arturo Bello Pérez

Received: 24 May 2023
Revised: 14 June 2023
Accepted: 20 June 2023
Published: 24 June 2023

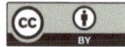

Copyright: © 2023 by the authors. Licensee MDPI, Basel, Switzerland. This article is an open access article distributed under the terms and conditions of the Creative Commons Attribution (CC BY) license (https://creativecommons.org/licenses/by/4.0/).

1. Introduction

The most basic description of dietary fiber is given in the GB/Z21922 "Basic Terminology of Food Nutrients" developed by China [1]. The definition of dietary fiber in its statutes is as follows: polymers of carbohydrates that are naturally present in plants, extracted from plants, or directly synthesized with a degree of polymerization ≥ 3; edible yet not digested or absorbed by the human small intestine; and of health significance to humans [2,3]. The "Chinese Dietary Guidelines for Residents 2016" recommends a daily intake of 25–30 g of dietary fiber, which should include grains, potatoes, vegetables, fruits, meat, eggs, dairy products, soybeans, and nuts in one's daily diet. Dietary fiber can be divided into water-soluble and non-water-soluble forms, and is mainly composed of non-starch polysaccharides from various plant substances, including cellulose, lignin, wax, chitosan, pectin, beta-glucan, inulin, and oligosaccharides [4]. Cellulose, hemicellulose, and lignin are the main components of insoluble dietary fiber, whereas pectin is a form of soluble dietary fiber found in non-fibrous substances, such as barley, legumes, carrots, citrus, flax, oats, and oat bran [5].

Dietary fiber is defined as the "seventh macronutrient" in terms of its physiological function [6]. As the standard of living and awareness increases, many people are consuming dietary fiber, which can increase stool volume, promote intestinal peristalsis, and improve bowel patterns [7]. It can also lower total and LDL cholesterol levels in the blood to prevent coronary heart disease, lower fasting and postprandial blood sugar and insulin levels, and improve insulin sensitivity [8]. Finally, it can provide energy-producing metabolites to the colon, increase the quantity and activity of beneficial bacteria, and suppress obesity [9]. IDF is important as a functional food ingredient with multiple health and nutritional benefits [10]. Dietary fiber is incorporated into bread products to increase their nutritional value and sensory quality [11], and into beverages to compensate for dietary deficiencies to a certain extent [12]. Ginseng-IDF has a typical hydrolyzed fiber structure, polysaccharide functional groups, and cellulose crystal structure, and can also be used as an ideal functional ingredient for food processing [13]. It is also used in the production of meat products to obtain high-dietary fiber, low-calorie, low-fat products; it can make the meat taste richer [14]. Developing economically viable and sustainable technologies for converting corn fiber into liquid fuels is widely seen as a promising approach to achieve improved ethanol titers and integrated utilization of byproducts in the traditional corn dry milling process [15].

Research on and the development of dietary fiber can significantly improve the economic value of agricultural products, which has profound significance for improving the health of the population and the economic efficiency of agriculture. The importance of dietary fiber in people's lives has been confirmed, and if the insoluble component of dietary fiber can be exploited, it could also be used as a substitute in the material industry, in textiles, and in nano-materials. Therefore, this review aims to provide guiding information using selected literature and experimental data, focusing on the isolation and extraction of cellulose, hemicellulose, and lignin from insoluble dietary fiber, and to discuss techniques for the modification of single components.

2. Insoluble Dietary Fiber

Insoluble dietary fiber is a type of non-starch polysaccharide that is insoluble in water and cannot be digested in the small intestine or fermented in the colon, and this includes cellulose, hemicellulose, and lignin [16]. Insoluble dietary fiber, which is the main component of the cell wall, can be extracted using physical, chemical, enzymatic, and combined enzyme–chemical methods. Further, it is completely hydrolyzed to form various monosaccharides [17], including glucose, xylose, galactose, arabinoxylan, and galacturonic acid. In terms of its chemical composition (Figure 1), the chemical structures of the various monosaccharide molecules that comprise the macromolecules are not different. Modified insoluble dietary fiber has a larger specific surface area, higher water-holding and swelling capacities, and greater functionality, based on adding or enhancing functions that were previously absent or weak. However, different binding methods produce insoluble dietary fiber-specific physicochemical properties, which in turn affect physiological functions. Functional groups (such as hydroxyl, carboxyl, amino, and acetyl) in insoluble dietary fiber confer strong hydrophilic, lipophilic, swelling, and metal ion adsorption properties [18]. In addition, these compounds have physical and chemical properties that include thermal stability, rheological properties, ion exchange capacity, and particle distribution. The water-holding and swelling forces are mainly related to the hydrophilic groups on the surface of insoluble dietary fiber and the honeycomb porous structure; its water-holding capacity is approximately 1.5–25 h based on its weight, whereas its oil-holding capacity is mainly related to the hydrophobic zone of fibers and the pore-like structure formed by cross-linking between different components [19]. Insoluble dietary fiber contains side chain groups, such as amino and carboxyl groups, which are reversibly exchanged with heavy metal ions, causing harmful ions to be adsorbed on the fiber and then eliminated in feces. These properties are closely related to the physiological functions of insoluble dietary fiber in the human body. Therefore, there is an urgent need to analyze the monocomponent structures of insoluble dietary fiber.

Cellulose, one of the important components of insoluble dietary fiber, is a polysaccharide polymer consisting of linear chains of D-glucose units linked by $\beta(1\rightarrow4)$ glycosidic bonds [20]. Cellulose has a fibrous porous structure and is a commercially important biopolymer with a good physical structure [21]. Its advantages include high crystallinity, high polymerization, a high specific surface area, and good adsorption properties, which offer a great scope for the development of renewable energy. As the most abundant natural polymer, efforts have been made to isolate and extract cellulose for use in new materials [22]; specifically, some of the cellulose is exploited in daily food, decoration, ceramic, paint, tobacco agriculture, explosive, electrical, and construction materials [23]. There is also a portion of fiber that is mainly found in fruits and vegetables, as foods that are consumed by humans. However, modified cellulose is mostly used to adsorb heavy metal ions from wastewater for recycling purposes, owing to its enhanced adsorption capacity [24]. Many companies have separated, purified, and dissolved raw cellulose materials to produce rayon, acetate, sodium carboxymethylcellulose derivatives, methylcellulose, and cellulose membranes.

Unlike cellulose, hemicellulose is a general term used to describe a variety of complex sugars [3]. The basic structural units of hemicellulose are D-arabinose, D-galactose, D-glucose, D-xylose, D-mannose, D-galacturonic acid, D-glucuronic acid, and 4-O-methylglucuronic acid, with small amounts of L-amylose and L-rhamnose [25]. They occur in various structural forms and are divided into four major groups: xylans, mannose, mixed-link-glucans, and xyloglucans [26]. Hemicellulose has a special chemical structure and unique physiological functions. It can be used for fermentation to produce ethanol [27], for microbial screening [28], and as a thermoplastic and water-resistant material [29]. Hemicellulose, one of the main components of insoluble dietary fiber, is abundant, biodegradable, renewable, and biocompatible in nature. Moreover, it is widely used in many fields, such as food packaging materials [30], paper coatings [31], chemicals [32], environmental energy, and biomedicine.

Another important component of insoluble dietary fiber, lignin, is mainly composed of three elements: carbon (C), hydrogen (H), and oxygen (O). It can also contain small amounts of nitrogen (N) and sulfur (S) depending on the source and extraction method [33]. Lignin is tightly complexed with cellulose and hemicellulose, and is a biopolymer with a three-dimensional network structure formed by three benzene propane units interconnected by ether and C-C bonds; moreover, it is rich in aromatic ring structures, aliphatic and aromatic hydroxyl groups, quinone groups, and other reactive groups [34]. Lignin is used to prevent cardiovascular diseases due to its ability to modify the activity of microorganisms in the intestinal system and to lower cholesterol and blood sugar levels. In addition, it has antioxidant activity [29] and possesses functions such as cancer cell-inhibitory activity. In addition to its physiological functions, lignin is used in the production of composite materials because it is abundant, cheap, renewable, degradable, and non-toxic. It is also used as a filler in biomass materials, such as rubber and hydrogel [35].

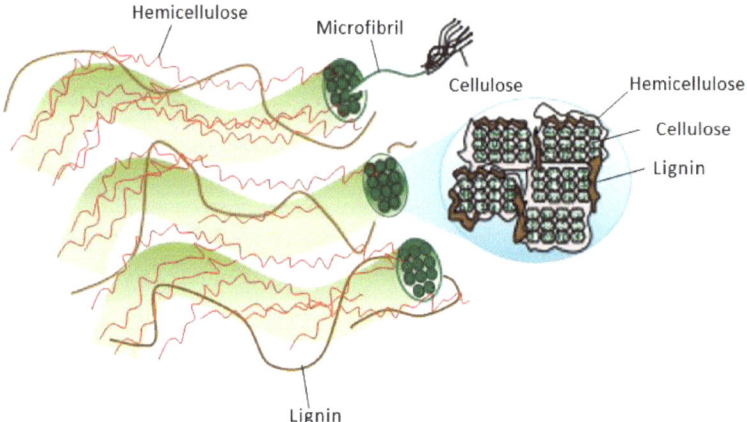

Figure 1. Plant cell wall structure and microfibril cross-section (strands of cellulose molecules embedded in a matrix of hemicellulose and lignin) [36].

3. Cellulose

3.1. Separation and Extraction Methods

Cellulose is a renewable and degradable biopolymer with high thermal stability. Depending on the separation and extraction method, cellulose has been used in food processing [37], plastic bags, cling films, the textile industry, and the bio-pharmaceutical industry [38]. Different separation and extraction methods are required in order to obtain cellulose from this biopolymer for various applications. This section provides an overview of this, based on various separation and extraction methods.

3.1.1. Acid Hydrolysis Method

The acid hydrolysis separation method involves hydrolysis of the amorphous regions of cellulose in dietary fibers, leaving the compact and dense crystalline regions intact. The rice husk is soaked overnight in 4 wt% NaOH, and the lignin and hemicellulose in the rice husk fibers are removed via acid hydrolysis (H_2SO_4). The mixture is then transferred to a round-bottomed flask and refluxed for 2 h (Figure 2). Next, the solid is filtered and washed three times with distilled water, which has been found to result in a cellulose content of approximately 31%. Acid hydrolysis is the most widely used method for preparing cellulose and cellulose-derived cellulose nanocrystals, cellulose filaments, and nanosized cellulose [39]. Through pre-treatment with bagasse, a 50% bagasse cellulose content was obtained after acid hydrolysis at 45 °C for 75 min. Owing to the long acid hydrolysis time, the crystalline structure of cellulose was completely destroyed, resulting in the formation of a needle-like structure [40]. The increase in available energy consumption in recent years has intensified the development of renewable energy sources, especially palm empty fruit bunch fibers, which are present in large quantities and have a high cellulose content [41]. Palm oil empty fruit bundles were then hydrolyzed by adding acid, at a 55% concentration, for 3 h at 45 °C to obtain cellulose with a purity of 14.98% [42]. The production of cellulose with a controlled structure, based on its isolation and extraction from bamboo and representing a dietary fiber of plant origin, has been studied as an important method to obtain good sustainability. Cellulose was successfully extracted by immersing 50 g of treated bamboo powder in a 7.5% $NaClO_2$ solution (w/v) and incubating it at 80 °C for 2 h under acidic conditions (pH = 3.8–4.0). However, the cellulose was found to exhibit different shapes depending on the acid concentration used for hydrolysis [43].

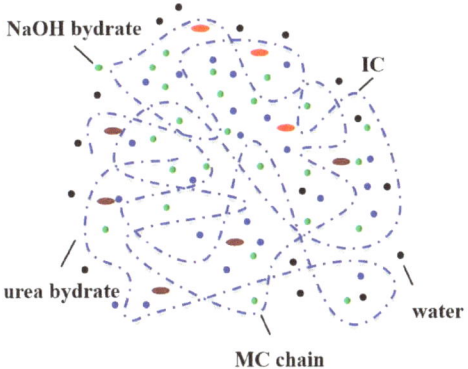

Figure 2. Interaction between NaOH/urea and cellulose [44].

3.1.2. Steam Blasting Method

Steam blasting is a physical separation method that is used for cellulose extraction. The principle behind this method is to break down the cell wall's structure. The effective heat carrier steam rapidly heats the raw material to a specified temperature; after a period of contact, the steam penetrates the raw material and immediately releases pressure, which results in the degradation of a small portion of cellulose and hemicellulose in the raw material into monosaccharides [45]. Typical steam blasting process temperatures range from 160 to 260 °C, corresponding to pressures of 0.69–4.83 MPa. Agricultural wastes, such as wheat straw and corn straw; specialized energy crops, including manzanita; and willow have been proposed as biomass resources for xylose release to produce xylitol, and the initial xylose hydrolysis products have been found to be released up to 94% under steam blast treatment with 12 Pa for 3 min with 1.2% phosphoric acid and 500 g of substrate [46]. The effects of steam blasting—with citric acid, sodium hydroxide, and water as catalysts—on the chemical properties, structural properties, and enzymatic processes of sugarcane bagasse were investigated. During the citric acid-catalyzed blast treatment, cracks appeared in the fiber cell walls and the maximum hemicellulose removal rate reached 41.5%, whereas in the NaOH-catalyzed steam blast treatment, the bagasse fibers were complete destroyed and the lignin removal rate reached 65%; the water treatment obtained a maximum cellulose yield of 97.5% [47]. By combining the steam blasting process with the traditional scraping method, the upper waterproof layer, which adversely affects the steam blasting process, was removed from the fresh blades and cut for steam blasting treatment, yielding 85.4% cellulose [48].

3.1.3. Deep Eutectic Solvent (DES) Method

The DES comprises mixtures of two or three safe and inexpensive compounds bonded to each other via hydrogen bonding to form salt solutions [49]. Considering food safety and acceptability, cellulose extraction using a DES is the best choice. Choline chloride-glycerol, choline chloride-urea, and choline chloride-oxalic acid were heated and stirred for 2 h at 80 °C, according to a certain molar ratio, to obtain a homogeneous and clarified DES solvent. Then, 2 g of ramie fiber was added to 200 g of DES, the suspension was heated in a closed flask at 100 °C in an oil bath, and the mixture was stirred and mixed at a predetermined temperature for 2–10 h. The purity of the obtained cellulose was 73–78% [50] (Figure 3). Three DES solvents were prepared, and 0.1 g of the sample was mixed with the prepared DES, heated, and stirred in an oil bath at 130 °C for 3 h. The DES prepared with ChCl-LA was the best choice for cellulose extraction. In addition to the well-known sugarcane, straw, and bamboo, in which the dietary fiber content is high, the insoluble dietary fiber component of okara is also rich, with a purity of 90% or higher [51]. The application of DES in agro-industrial treatments can be developed for industrial use. To simplify the defatting, deproteinization, and cellulose extraction steps during the cellulose pretreatment of okara, a new method for cellulose extraction, by preparing a DES solvent via a heating method, was established. Treatment of okara with the DES solution ChCl-O had a significant effect on extracted okara cellulose, improving the thermal stability and cellulose content to 92.6% [52]. To achieve an economic and ecological balance, cheaper methods for cellulose extraction must be explored. A low-eutectic solvent (DES) system of ChCl-EG was used as the solubilizing solvent. DES was used as the reaction medium and mixed with the insoluble dietary fiber of okara at 120 °C for 2 h. The yield of raw cellulose was 84–87% [53].

3.1.4. Comparison of Different Methods

Each method for separating and extracting cellulose has its own advantages and disadvantages. Table 1 presents a detailed visual comparison of the three methods for separating single components, which can provide a theoretical basis for selecting the most suitable method for future experiments.

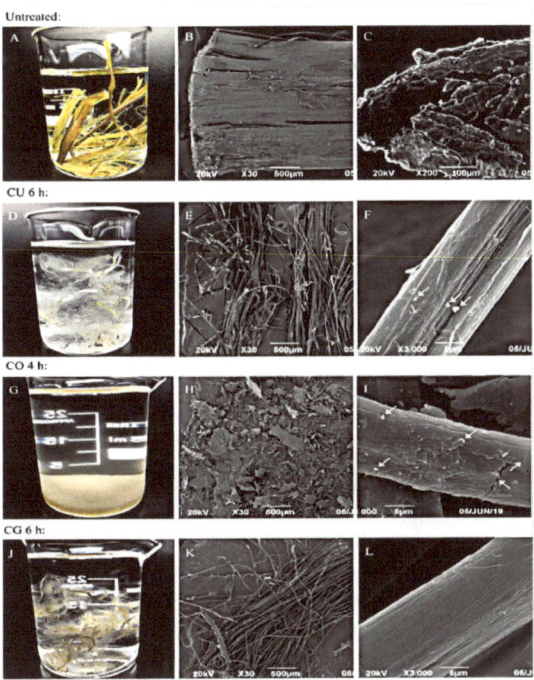

Figure 3. Deep eutectic solvent (DES) treatment of ramie raw fiber [50]. (**A–L**) Digital photographs and SEM images of raw RFs and pretreated RFs.

Table 1. Comparison of different methods to separate single components from fiber.

Extraction Methods	Advantages	Disadvantages
Acid hydrolysis method	(1) Simple process (2) Easy operation and no danger (3) Cellulose becomes nano-sized (4) Cellulose has high thermal (5) Stability and uniform particle size	(1) Large quantities of acid and impurities remain in the reactants (2) Difficult to recover and can cause environmental pollution (3) Can cause damage to the structure of cellulose
Steam blasting treatment	(1) Low energy input (2) Does not require recycling reagents (3) Little impact on the environment (4) Adding acid or bases improves the treatment efficiency	(1) Prone to Merad reaction under high temperature and pressure (2) Target products are readily degradable (3) Sample volume increases
Deep eutectic solvent method	(1) Simple preparation (2) Recyclable (3) Method (4) Non-toxic and degradable (5) Consistent with the concept of sustainability	(1) Easily soluble in water and in large amounts

3.2. Modification Technology

Plant cellulose is a natural renewable resource, and its modification is a popular research topic. This section provides a brief overview of the modification methods for cellulose, including physical, chemical, and biological approaches. The most important methods include esterification, sulfonation, etherification, ether esterification, cross-linking, and graft copolymerization. The chemical modification of cellulose refers to the use of coupling agents (e.g., citric acid, malic acid, and tartaric acid) to replace the hydroxyl groups on the surface, thus reducing the content of hydroxyl groups on the cellulose surface and weakening the cellulose and hemicellulose [54]. A series of reactions usually involves a hydroxyl group in the structure. Through modification, a series of ionic groups is introduced which enhances the hydrophilicity of cellulose. The most widely used method is the chemical modification of cellulose, and chemically modified cellulose-based nano-materials are considered one of the best nano-materials [55].

3.2.1. Physical Modification Method

The physical modification of cellulose involves changing its morphology and surface structure via physical and mechanical means, without changing its chemical composition or the chemical reaction. The most commonly used physical method is polyelectrolyte adsorption, which is the only method described in the following section [56], and it can be divided into two categories: polyelectrolytes and nonelectrolytes physically adsorbed on the cellulose surface. Uncharged polymers can bind to cellulose via van der Waals and hydrogen-bonding forces. The modified nanocellulose was firstly adsorbed with the cationic polyelectrolytes poly(DMDAAC), poly(allylamine hydrochloride), and poly(PEI), and, alternatively, the anionic polyelectrolyte poly (4-sodium allyl sulfonate); then, the modified nanocellulose was adsorbed with cationic polyelectrolytes; and finally, the complex material of nanocellulose and nano-silver was prepared by loading silver nanoparticles [57]. The results obtained from studying the antimicrobial activity of this complex material against *Staphylococcus aureus* and *Klebsiella pneumoniae* showed that both the polyelectrolytes and nanosilver were effective; however, the antimicrobial effect of nanosilver was crucial. Finally, it was used as a filler for starch-based coating-modified eucalyptus blue paper, and the application potential of the antibacterial paper products was studied. Thermally responsive nanocellulose was prepared via the adsorption of thermally responsive polyelectrolytes onto nanocellulose. Three block copolymers consisting of quaternized poly(2-dimethylamino) ethyl methacrylate (PDMAEMA) as the polyelectrolyte block and poly(ethylene glycol) methyl ether methacrylate (PDEGMA) as the thermoresponsive block were synthesized [56]. Block copolymers were synthesized through two-atom transfer radical polymerization (ATRP), in which PDMAEMA macromolecular chains were first synthesized as macromolecular initiators for the synthesis of PDEGMA polymers. Among the three block copolymers, the lengths and charges of the PDMAEMA blocks remained the same, whereas the molecular weights of the three PDEGMA blocks were different. PDMAEMA block quaternization introduced a positive charge; then, the block copolymer was adsorbed onto the negatively charged nanocellulose dispersed in water. It was also shown that a polyelectrolyte was present in nanocellulose. The modified nanocellulose exhibited thermally responsive behavior in solution upon heating and cooling, indicating that the properties of the polyelectrolyte could be transferred to cellulose. Non-electrolyte adsorption involves the physical binding of cellulose to a non-electrolyte polymer. Examples of cellulose surface-adsorption copolymers have been reviewed, some of which have a better ability to bind cellulose [58] (Figure 4).

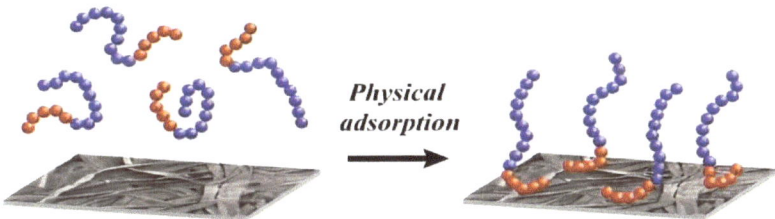

Figure 4. Physical adsorption [58].

3.2.2. Chemical Modification Method

The chemical modification of cellulose occurs mainly through a chemical reaction involving -OH of the cellulose molecular chain and compound esterification, an etherification reaction, to produce cellulose ethers and other derivatives. The surface properties of cellulose fibers can be modified by chemical reactions on the surfaces of the fibers, which can introduce small molecular groups (polar or non-polar) or polymers. The active sites where chemical reactions occur are generally the hydroxyl groups of cellulose fibers or the functional groups generated before or during cellulose fiber pretreatment. Cellulose fiber pretreatment is primarily used to reduce energy consumption, whereas cellulose fiber surface modification is used to improve the compatibility or dispersion between cellulose and other substances.

However, cellulose modification is prone to carboxylation. The 2,2,6,6-tetramethylpiperidin-1-oxyl radical (TEMPO) oxidizer is a pretreatment agent that promotes nanofiber separation by selectively introducing carboxyl (acidic) groups at the C6 position of the glucose unit [59]. This method was used as a pretreatment to enhance the mechanical decomposition of cellulose, during which cellulose secondary alcohols were first oxidized to aldehyde groups by sodium iodate and then converted to carboxyl groups with sodium chlorite during the reaction. The degree of nanofibrillation of hardwood cellulose pulp was improved via homogenization using a periodate-chlorite continuous-zone selective oxygenation method. When the carboxyl group content in the oxidized cellulose was in the range of 0.38–1.75 mmol/g, the nanofibers formed high-viscosity transparent gels with a yield of 85–100% without blocking the homogenizer. Based on the field emission scanning electron microscopy images, the typical width of the obtained nanofibers was approximately 25 ± 6 nm. Based on the wide-angle X-ray diffraction results, all nanofiber samples maintained the crystalline structure of cellulose I, with a crystallinity index of approximately 40% [60].

Cellulose can be esterified with organic acids, acyl halides, acid anhydrides, and inorganic acids to produce mono-, di-, and tri-substituted cellulose esters, but from the point of view of process and industrial applications, the most important of these is cellulose nitrate. The effects of the mixed acid composition, mass ratio, nitration temperature, and time on the properties and yield of cellulose nitrate prepared from unconventional raw materials, such as oat hulls from large-tonnage grain processing residues, were investigated. Cellulose nitrates were prepared under optimal synthesis conditions with 98% solubility in alcohol–ether mixtures [61].

3.2.3. Comparison of Different Modification Methods

The physical method of cellulose pretreatment is simple, convenient, and easy to operate, but the performance of modified products is unstable and the modifier easily falls off from the cellulose, resulting in a reduction in product performance. The chemical method is a better modification method, and it results in other properties of cellulose without changing its performance. Regarding the advantages and disadvantages of each cellulose modification method, a detailed comparison of the physical and chemical modification methods is presented in Table 2, which provides a theoretical basis for future modification methods for different samples. With improvements in the processing technology of cellulose materials, it will be possible to gradually replace traditional petroleum products to alleviate energy and environmental pressures as needed in the future.

Table 2. Comparison of different modification methods.

Extraction Methods	Advantages	Disadvantages
Physical modification method	Simple and convenient pre-processing, easy to operate	(1) Unstable product performance (2) Modifier easily comes off from the cellulose, resulting in a decrease in product performance
Chemical modification method	Imparting other properties to cellulose without changing its properties	(1) Pollution of the environment (2) Has reagent residue

4. Hemicellulose

Hemicelluloses represent promising renewable biomass as plant cell wall polysaccharides synthesized by glycosyltransferases on Golgi cell membranes and biopolymers; they are second only to cellulose in plant fibers. The hexose in hemicellulose is used in fermentation to produce fuel alcohol [62]. It also results in a reduction in sorbitol production [63]. Further, hemicellulose has been produced using xylose [64], xylitol [65], furfural [66], and feed yeast [67].

4.1. Separation and Extraction Methods

4.1.1. Alkali Treatment Method

The solid residue obtained from hydrothermal pretreatment was loaded into the reactor with 100 g of pretreated corn stover fibers and 900 mL of deionized water containing NaOH after pretreatment. After 2 h, the insoluble residue was recovered via filtration, washed to neutrality, and dried to a constant weight at 45 °C. The pH of the combined filtrates was adjusted to 5.0 using 6 mol of HCl. Three times the volume of 95% ethanol (v/v) was then added to precipitate hemicellulose for 2 h [43]. After filtration, the solid residue was freeze-dried to obtain the hemicellulose. Sweet sorghum stem hemicellulose can be extracted using similar methods. In one study, sweet sorghum stems were soaked in a 2.0% KOH aqueous solution at 90 °C for 3 h of continuous extraction with water; solids were filtered through a Bronsted funnel; and 60% ethanol was used for precipitation to obtain hemicellulose with a content of 76.3% [45]. In the ultrasonically-assisted alkaline extraction of hemicellulose from sugarcane bagasse pith, the total hemicellulose yield was up to 23.05% under the optimal conditions of an ultrasonic treatment time of 28 min, a KOH mass concentration of 3.7%, and an extraction temperature of 53 °C. The total hemicellulose yield was significantly increased by 3.24% compared with the case without ultrasonically-assisted extraction [68]. Alkaline peroxides can cause hemicellulose to be released into the sample under certain conditions, and this treatment does not change the overall structure of the hemicellulose. For the isolation and purification of hemicellulose polysaccharides from the dietary fiber of okara, which is rich in dietary fiber, the method comprised mixing the sample with 21.2 mL of 10% NaOH after pre-treatment at 35.5 °C and extraction for 5.3 h. Under these conditions, the yield of polysaccharides reached 30.21% [69]. At present, the separation and extraction of hemicellulose from insoluble dietary fiber has a low extraction rate and low quality, and cannot meet industry demands.

4.1.2. Separation and Extraction of Organic Solvents

Unlike the alkali treatment method, organic solvent separation and extraction can separate and extract hemicellulose without pretreatment or the separation of cellulose and lignin. Organic solvents can effectively prevent the removal of acetyl groups from the hemicellulose functional groups in plant cells, resulting in high purity and proximity to the original hemicellulose structure [70]. Currently, dimethyl sulfoxide is the organic solvent used for the separation and extraction of hemicellulose. The effect of the aqueous extraction of hemicellulose from wheat straw using a mixture of formic acid, acetic acid, and ethanol on its content was investigated. Formic acid–acetic acid–H_2O was the best system, producing 76.5% of the original hemicellulose from wheat straw. Moreover, organic solvent extraction is the most convenient and produces the highest hemicellulose content among all available separation and extraction methods [49]. In this study, the hemicellulose content extracted from barley straw and corn stalk cell walls using organic solvent extraction was visualized. Aqueous solutions of 90% neutral dioxane, 80% dioxane (containing 0.05 mol HCl), dimethyl sulfoxide, and 8% KOH were used to successfully extract 94.6% and 96.4% of the original hemicellulose from barley straw and corn stalks, respectively [71].

4.1.3. Basic Hydrogen Peroxide Extraction Method

Alkaline hydrogen peroxide extraction is a common method for separating plant hemicellulose. Hydrogen peroxide, under alkaline conditions, not only has a removal and bleaching effect on lignin, but also improves the solubility of large-molecular-size hemicelluloses [72]. Thus, it can be used as a mild hemicellulose solubilizer. A comparative study of two methods for the separation of hemicellulose from rice straw using alkali extraction and alkaline hydrogen peroxide showed that 67.2% hemicellulose could be obtained with alkali extraction alone, and the addition of different concentrations of hydrogen peroxide increased the hemicellulose content to 88.5%. It also had a whiter color [73]. The optimal conditions for the extraction of bagasse hemicellulose from alkaline hydrogen peroxide solution were investigated in depth, and the best reaction conditions were determined to be 6% H_2O_2 mass fraction, 4 h reaction time, 20 °C reaction temperature, and 0.5% magnesium sulfate addition, under which the hemicellulose content reached 86% and the product contained very little conjugated lignin (only 5.9%) [52].

4.1.4. Comparison of Different Isolation and Extraction Methods

Regarding the advantages and disadvantages of each hemicellulose separation and extraction method, a detailed comparison of the three methods (alkali treatment, organic solvent extraction, and alkaline hydrogen peroxide method) is presented in Table 3 to provide a theoretical basis for the future separation and extraction of hemicellulose, as well as for the development of insoluble dietary fiber hemicellulose from okara.

Table 3. Comparison of different isolation and extraction methods.

Extraction Methods	Advantages	Disadvantages
Alkali treatment method	(1) Low cost (2) Pure and non-polluting products	(1) Stronger bases generate new amino acids
Organic solvent extraction method	(1) Low cost (2) Pure and non-polluting products (3) Removal of lignin and bleaching	(1) Peroxide has strong oxidizing properties and the possibility of combustion
Alkaline hydrogen peroxide method	(1) Direct and effective (2) Closest to the original structure	(1) High energy efficiency consumption (2) Some chemical reagents will produce precipitation

4.2. Modification

Unmodified hemicellulose cannot be fully utilized because of the complexity of its structure. To explore the potential applications of hemicellulose, its modifications have been investigated both domestically and internationally. Because of the presence of numerous hydroxyl groups in both the main and side chains of hemicellulose [74], semifibers can be modified by oxidation, esterification [75], etherification [76,77], and grafting copolymerization [78].

Oxidation is the process of converting alcohol hydroxyl groups of hemicellulose into aldehyde or carboxyl groups. Oxidative modification can create carboxylic acids, the further reactive modification of which can solve the problem of the poor stability of hemicellulose-based materials. Carbonylated anionic galacturonic acid derivatives were prepared using a combined biological enzyme-oxidation reaction system [79]. When hemicellulose is combined with hydrophobic materials as a raw material, the hydrophilic property limits its interfacial integration with the resin, which in turn affects the mechanical properties of the synthesized product [80], and the esterified hemicellulose can solve the problem of excessive hydrophilicity [81]. The hydrophilic properties and polysaccharide attributes of hemicellulose make it advantageous for food preservation, microbial culture, and biopharmaceuticals. However, the excessive hydrolytic properties of hemicellulose under conditions of high humidity also limit its application, especially as a biopharmaceutical membrane material which requires good stability and surface activity; therefore, modification via etherification is necessary [82]. Copolymerization modification can also cause hemicellulose to acquire the properties of some grafting groups: i.e., grafting halogen groups to improve flame retardancy; grafting hydroxyl and aldehyde groups to improve hydrophilicity; and grafting acyl groups to increase the hydrophobicity of the material [83].

4.2.1. Etherification Modification

One of the most common methods for carboxymethylation in etherification reactions involves changing the properties of hemicellulose by introducing a carboxymethyl group into its hydroxyl group. In the case of konjac glucomannan, the hydrogen in the glucomannan molecule is replaced by a carboxymethyl group (etherification) during the reaction with chloroacetic acid in a sodium hydroxide solution, resulting in carboxymethyl glucomannan [84]. For the preparation of co-blended membranes from quaternate hemicellulose (QH) and carboxymethyl cellulose (CMC), the QH and CMC solutions were first mixed to form a homogeneous suspension and then dried under a vacuum to prepare the hybrid film. From the results of the mechanical properties and water vapor permeability (WVP), the blended film exhibited good tensile strength and transmittance and low WVP for applications in coatings and packaging [85].

4.2.2. Transesterification Modification

In addition to etherification, the hemicellulose esterification reaction results in new functions for hemicellulose, with its advantages including water resistance, hydrophilicity, thermal stability, and surface activity. Hemicellulose can be esterified using a variety of compounds, such as sulfuric acid reagents, chloride, and acid anhydride. The sulfation of hemicellulose is a process in which the hydroxyl group of hemicellulose reacts with the sulfonic acid group to dehydrate it. Xylan sulfate was obtained from alkali-soluble bagasse via sulfation with chlorosulfonic acid and N,N-dimethylformamide. Previously, a product with a degree of substitution of 1.49 and a molecular weight of up to 148,217 could be obtained in a flow system, even at room temperature, within 10 min [86].

4.2.3. Comparison of Different Modification Methods

The advantages and disadvantages of hemicellulose modification methods for both etherification and esterification reactions are listed in Table 4. With the development of technology, the extraction of hemicellulose will become increasingly easier, and there will be an increasing number of modification methods. Moreover, the modified hemicellulose can be widely used in various industries, which will bring great social and economic benefits.

Table 4. Comparison of different modification methods.

Extraction Methods		Advantages		Disadvantages
Etherification modification	(1) (2)	Strong cationic properties Strongly water-soluble	(1) (2)	Decrease in water content Increase in hydrophobicity
Esterification modification	(1) (2) (3)	Results in new properties for hemicellulose Enhanced water resistance and hydrophilicity Increased thermal stability and surface activity	(1)	Reaction is reversible

5. Lignin

5.1. Separation and Extraction Methods

Lignin separation and extraction are prerequisites which are important for the high-value utilization of lignin. Lignin has a complex molecular structure, containing crosslinked polymers of phenolic monomers, particularly p-coumaryl alcohol, coniferyl alcohol, and sinapyl alcohol [36] (Figure 5). Lignin can be used for different industrial and biomedical applications, including chemical substances, polymers, biofuels, and drug delivery, which are applications for the development of nano-materials [87]. Currently, lignin is mainly used as a binder, dispersant, chelating agent, stabilizer, emulsifier, and composite material, but associated research is still limited. Previously, the market share was low [88]. However, recently, the colloidal nature of lignin has attracted widespread attention for industrial applications, and the preparation of lignin for stabilizing emulsions [89] and the delivery of hydrophobic molecules shows promise as an alternative to toxic nanoparticles [90]. Based on this, several lignin extraction methods have been discussed, including DES, organic acid extraction, and ionic liquid (IL) treatment.

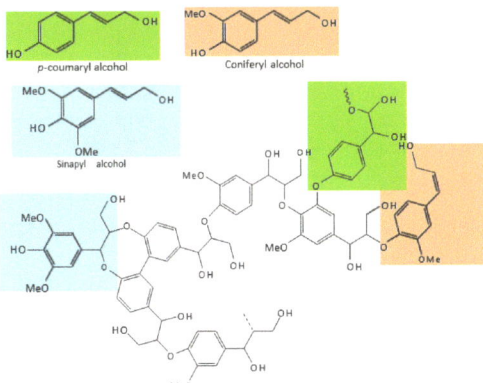

Figure 5. Chemical structures of lignin (p-coumaryl alcohol, coniferyl alcohol, and sinapyl alcohol) [36].

5.1.1. DES Method

The DES method is characterized by the formation of a homogeneous and clarified solvent mixture by heating a hydrogen bond acceptor, choline chloride, with a different hydrogen bond donor while stirring at higher temperatures [91]. When a dietary fiber component is separated and extracted, the hydrogen bond donor is replaced to achieve the desired result. DESs have become promising for lignocellulosic biomass fractionation because of their high selectivity and environmentally friendly nature [92]. ChCl and LA were mixed in a sealed glass vial at 60 °C at a 1:2 molar ratio in a vacuum oven for 2 h, with regular stirring, until a homogeneous and clear liquid was obtained. Lignin was not consistently separated during pretreatment with hot water. A lignin content of 30.97% was successfully extracted from red winter wheat straw using a synergistic DES solvent-assisted hot water synergistic treatment. However, the complex interlocking structures of cellulose, hemicellulose, and lignin and the unique properties of lignin limit its value-added utilization [93]. The preparation of DES has been achieved from choline chloride-lactic acid (ChCl-LA) to extract lignin nanoparticles from herbal biomass (wheat straw) [94] (Figure 6). Further, the DES was found to be able to extract high-purity lignin (up to 94.8%) from wheat straw.

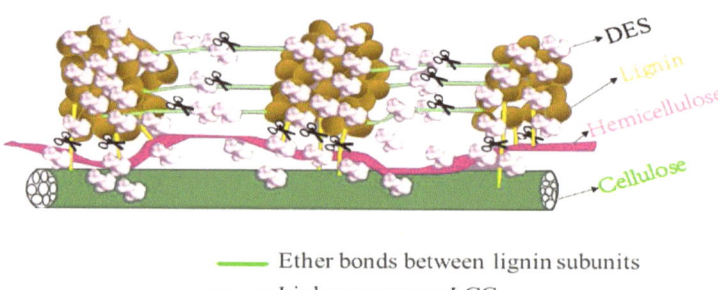

Figure 6. Link between deep eutectic solvent (DES) and single components [95].

5.1.2. Organic Acid Processing

The difficulty of isolating lignin is attributed to its complex structure, including non-hydrolyzable monomers and isomerism. Organic acid treatment is one of the most effective methods for separating lignin, and it promotes the degradation of carbohydrates during the treatment process [95]. Lignin can also be extracted from sugarcane bagasse using a phosphorylation solution. Bagasse was placed in a conical flask and heated in a water bath. The solid–liquid ratio was determined to be 1:20, and the reaction was carried out at 80 °C for 20 min using a p-TSOH solution with a concentration of 80%. Further, sugarcane bagasse achieved 88.81% lignin removal after phosphorylation [96]. Different preparation conditions are used to separate lignin from biomass depending on the production needs, as well as the production purpose. When the pretreatment effect is unsatisfactory, an organic acid treatment is used. The separation of cellulose fibers and lignin from red hemp bast using microwave-assisted organic acid treatment has also been studied [97]. Red hemp bast (12 g) was placed into four different solvents, including lactic acid, formic acid, acetic-acid, and a formic acid/acetic acid/water mixture, with a liquid–solid ratio of 20:1 and a removal rate of 94.68% after heating and stirring at 130 °C for 30 min [98].

5.1.3. IL Treatment Method

ILs are organic salts composed of organic cations or anions in a liquid state at room temperature, and can also be called room-temperature ILs [99]. These represent a new type of solvent with the advantages of almost no vapor pressure, non-flammability, non-volatility, and good chemical stability and recyclability. This is thus referred to as a "green chemical solvent", which can also be used as an alternative to low eutectic solvents. Preliminarily, it was shown that IL pretreatment could effectively disrupt the macromolecular structure of lignin and achieve its initial depolymerization. Lignins comprise various aromatic and phenolic compounds. In one study, an ionic ($H_2PO_4^-$) solution was mixed with wheat straw and rice husks, which dissolved 73% of the lignin at 100 °C for 2 h [100].

5.1.4. Comparison of Different Methods

The advantages and disadvantages of different lignin extraction methods are shown in Table 5.

Table 5. Comparison of different lignin extraction methods.

Extraction Methods	Advantages	Disadvantages
DES method	See Section 3.1.4 for details	See Section 3.1.4 for details
Organic acid extraction	(1) Obtains lignin quickly (2) High-purity lignin is obtained	(1) Organic solvents are not easily recovered (2) Pollutes the environment
Ionic liquid method	Similar to DES method	Similar to DES method

5.2. Modification Technology

Lignin contains many active functional groups, including carbonyl, methoxy, and hydroxyl groups. Several chemical modification methods for lignin have been discussed, including etherification and graft co-polymerization. Lignin can also be used as an antioxidant [101,102] and flame retardant [103]. Combined with polymer materials, this can reduce the production cost of polymer materials and the plasticity and fluidity of the products, thus increasing the performance and adding value to the products.

5.2.1. Etherification Modification

The most commonly used etherification method involves the modification of propylene oxide in an alkaline solution to prepare lignin-based epoxy resins. The resulting solution is treated with epichlorohydrin and cured via crosslinking with m-phenylenediamine [104]. Etherification reactions can produce new polyols, and are among the most promising modification methods available [105]. Insoluble lignin and other solids can be converted into water-soluble polyols through treatment with various organic solvents. This method has been used extensively for different biopolymers and bio-based materials containing hydroxyl groups, such as chitosan [106], corky [107], corn starch [108], and beet pulp [109,110]. This modification method allows for the extraction of a wide range of polyols from various biomass residues, which can be used to produce new polymeric materials, such as polyurethane foams [111]. The addition of lignin improves the mechanical and thermal properties of epoxy resins, which is attributed to the presence of aromatic groups in the lignin structure [112].

5.2.2. Graft Co-Polymerization Modification

Graft co-polymerization is the formation of a chain bond between polymer B and polymer A, which can be expressed as A-graft-B or A-g-B. Graft copolymers improve the mechanical properties of composites, reduce friction, and decrease flammability. Insoluble dietary fiber is one of the main components of okara. A single fraction of insoluble dietary fiber isolated from okara was used to produce graft polymers. This was performed by mixing okara with water in a 75% suspension, followed by homogenization. This suspension was placed in a 250 mL triangular flask equipped with a stirrer and a nitrogen line, and the suspension was treated with nitrogen for 15 min and then heated to 70 °C for 15 min under a stream of nitrogen. After adding the initiator APS (144 g) and maintaining it at 70 °C for 30 min under a stream of N_2, a solution was prepared by adding 7.2 g of AA to 16.6 mL of water. The reaction mixture was maintained under N_2 at 70 °C for 5 h. After graft polymerization was complete, the reaction mixture became a viscous product called Ok-PAA. Then, 10.3 g of the resulting viscous product was suspended in deionized water and centrifuged at 11,000 rpm for 20 min. The precipitate was collected, washed with water, centrifuged for 3 h, freeze-dried, and named OK-PAA (pre) (yield: 0.588 g). The supernatants were collected, combined, freeze-dried, and named Ok-PAA (sup) (yield: 0.815 g) [113] (Figure 7).

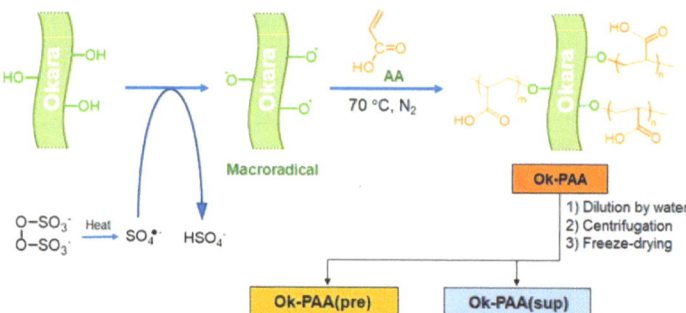

Figure 7. Synthesis and post-treatment procedures for Ok−PAA graft polymers [113].

Graft polymerization involves the addition of different initiators to the polymer to be grafted, and the final reaction product after graft polymerization is obtained by heating and stirring the mixture for a certain period. Lignin's co-polymerization with vinyl improves the reactivity of lignin and generates new graft copolymers. Previously, the polymerization reaction was initiated with ferrous chloride and hydrogen peroxide, and the grafting efficiency was maintained at approximately 18%, independent of the mass fraction of the initiator [114]. The grafting efficiency of methyl methacrylate with lignin was reduced by side reactions with phenolic hydroxyl groups when free-radical initiators were used [115]. This method provides a foundation for the preparation of lignin–graft co-polymers.

5.2.3. Comparison of Different Modification Methods

Etherification and graft co-polymerization are the most commonly used methods for modifying lignin. The advantages and disadvantages of both methods are listed in Table 6. However, this chemical modification method is difficult to use for the development of edible lignin. Therefore, further research on lignin will be of great significance for achieving green development.

Table 6. Comparison of different modification methods.

Extraction Methods	Advantages	Disadvantages
Etherification modification	Better dissolution of lignin	(1) Not friendly to the environment (2) Highly polluting
Graft co-polymerization method	Increased lignin reactivity	(1) Most initiators are toxic

6. Conclusions

In the current world of energy scarcity and severe environmental pollution, sustainable development is imperative. This paper reviews methods for the separation and extraction of cellulose, hemicellulose, and lignin from insoluble dietary fiber. Further, technology for the modification of single components in insoluble dietary fibers is discussed scientifically, allowing for a detailed understanding of this topic.

Although this review describes a variety of methods for the isolation and extraction of insoluble dietary fiber monomers, the most commonly used methods involve sugarcane and bamboo. However, these gramineous plants are not as rich in dietary fiber. For example, sugarcane contains only 0.60 g of dietary fiber per 100 g. The soybean consumption level in China is among the highest in the world, and most okara is currently discarded as feed or waste and is not fully and reasonably utilized. Many resources are wasted, which also pollutes the environment. Currently, there are few methods or theoretical bases for separating and extracting single fractions of insoluble dietary fiber from okara, making this the foundation for future development. For example, cellulose in insoluble dietary fiber from soybean residue is a renewable biomass resource that can be converted into biofuels such as biogas, bioethanol, and biodiesel through biomass energy conversion technology in the near future, which may be used as a secondary energy source. In addition, cellulose can also be converted into energy sources such as biohydrogen and biomethane through biomass fermentation technology, and can also be used to produce chemicals and materials. Therefore, the application of okara-insoluble dietary fiber to separate and extract single components has improved in various industries. For example, it can be used in food packaging bags, nano-materials, and sensors. This application also improves the utilization value of okara-insoluble dietary fiber. Okara-insoluble dietary fiber can also be used to produce rubber and bioindicators using modified technology. The use of okara-insoluble dietary fiber represents the rational use of byproducts to meet the need to conserve resources, as well as for sustainable human development.

Author Contributions: Writing—original draft preparation, J.W.; validation, J.Z.; visualization, W.L.; data curation, S.W.; funding acquisition, W.J. and H.Y. All authors have read and agreed to the published version of the manuscript.

Funding: This work was supported by the China Agriculture Research System of MOF and MARA (CARS-04), the Young & Middle-Aged Technological Innovation Outstanding Talent (team) Project (Innovation) (20210509015RQ), and Changbai Mountain Leading Team Project (ZZ202010098810020102).

Data Availability Statement: Raw data can be provided by the corresponding author upon request.

Conflicts of Interest: The authors declare no conflict of interest.

References

1. *GB Z21922-2008*; Fundermental Terminology and Definition of Nutritional Component in Foods. Standardization Administration of China: Beijng, China, 2008.
2. DeVries, J.W. Dietary Fiber: The Influence of Definition on Analysis and Regulation. *J. AOAC Int.* **2004**, *87*, 682–706. [CrossRef] [PubMed]
3. Hemicellulose Biosynthesis | SpringerLink. Available online: https://link.springer.com/article/10.1007/s00425-013-1921-1 (accessed on 4 March 2023).
4. Slavin, J.L. Carbohydrates, Dietary Fiber, and Resistant Starch in White Vegetables: Links to Health Outcomes. *Adv. Nutr.* **2013**, *4*, 351S–355S. [CrossRef] [PubMed]
5. Tosh, S.M.; Yada, S. Dietary Fibres in Pulse Seeds and Fractions: Characterization, Functional Attributes, and Applications. *Food Res. Int.* **2010**, *43*, 450–460. [CrossRef]
6. Swallah, M.S.; Fan, H.; Wang, S.; Yu, H.; Piao, C. Prebiotic Impacts of Soybean Residue (Okara) on Eubiosis/Dysbiosis Condition of the Gut and the Possible Effects on Liver and Kidney Functions. *Molecules* **2021**, *26*, 326. [CrossRef] [PubMed]
7. Krawczyk, M.; Maciejewska, D.; Ryterska, K.; Czerwińka-Rogowska, M.; Jamioł-Milc, D.; Skoniec-zna-Żydecka, K.; Milkiewicz, P.; Raszeja-Wyszomirska, J.; Stachowska, E. Gut Permeability Might Be Improved by Dietary Fiber in Individuals with Nonalcoholic Fatty Liver Disease (NAFLD) Undergoing Weight Reduction. *Nutrients* **2018**, *10*, 1793. [CrossRef] [PubMed]
8. Brownlee, I.A. The Physiological Roles of Dietary Fibre. *Food Hydrocoll.* **2011**, *25*, 238–250. [CrossRef]
9. Wang, B.; Yu, H.; He, Y.; Wen, L.; Gu, J.; Wang, X.; Miao, X.; Qiu, G.; Wang, H. Effect of Soybean Insoluble Dietary Fiber on Prevention of Obesity in High-Fat Diet Fed Mice via Regulation of the Gut Microbiota. *Food Funct.* **2021**, *12*, 7923–7937. [CrossRef]
10. Zhang, X.; Zeng, Y.; Liu, J.; Men, Y.; Sun, Y. Effects of Three Extraction Methods on the Structural and Functional Properties of Insoluble Dietary Fibers from Mycoprotein. *Food Chem. Adv.* **2023**, *2*, 100299. [CrossRef]
11. Ranaivo, H.; Thirion, F.; Béra-Maillet, C.; Guilly, S.; Simon, C.; Sothier, M.; Van Den Berghe, L.; Feugier-Favier, N.; Lambert-Porcheron, S.; Dussous, I.; et al. Increasing the Diversity of Dietary Fibers in a Daily-Consumed Bread Modifies Gut Microbiota and Metabolic Profile in Subjects at Cardiometabolic Risk. *Gut Microbes* **2022**, *14*, 2044722. [CrossRef]
12. Sadeghifar, H.; Cui, C.; Argyropoulos, D.S. Toward Thermoplastic Lignin Polymers. Part 1. Selective Masking of Phenolic Hydroxyl Groups in Kraft Lignins via Methylation and Oxypropylation Chemistries. *Ind. Eng. Chem. Res.* **2012**, *51*, 16713–16720. [CrossRef]
13. Hua, M.; Lu, J.; Qu, D.; Liu, C.; Zhang, L.; Li, S.; Chen, J.; Sun, Y. Structure, Physicochemical Properties and Adsorption Function of Insoluble Dietary Fiber from Ginseng Residue: A Potential Functional Ingredient. *Food Chem.* **2019**, *286*, 522–529. [CrossRef]
14. Kim, H.J.; Paik, H.-D. Functionality and Application of Dietary Fiber in Meat Products. *Korean J. Food Sci. Anim. Resour.* **2012**, *32*, 695–705. [CrossRef]
15. Wang, M.; Qiao, J.; Sheng, Y.; Wei, J.; Cui, H.; Li, X.; Yue, G. Bioconversion of Corn Fiber to Bioethanol: Status and Perspectives. *Waste Management* **2023**, *157*, 256–268. [CrossRef] [PubMed]

16. Mudgil, D. Chapter 3—The Interaction Between Insoluble and Soluble Fiber. In *Dietary Fiber for the Prevention of Cardiovascular Disease*; Samaan, R.A., Ed.; Academic Press: Cambridge, MA, USA, 2017; pp. 35–59, ISBN 978-0-12-805130-6.
17. Li, B.W.; Andrews, K.W.; Pehrsson, P.R. Individual Sugars, Soluble, and Insoluble Dietary Fiber Contents of 70 High Consumption Foods. *J. Food Compos. Anal.* **2002**, *15*, 715–723. [CrossRef]
18. Zafar, M.N.; Aslam, I.; Nadeem, R.; Munir, S.; Rana, U.A.; Khan, S.U.-D. Characterization of Chemically Modified Biosorbents from Rice Bran for Biosorption of Ni(II). *J. Taiwan Inst. Chem. Eng.* **2015**, *46*, 82–88. [CrossRef]
19. Dong, J.; Wang, L.; Lü, J.; Zhu, Y.; Shen, R. Structural, Antioxidant and Adsorption Properties of Dietary Fiber from Foxtail Millet (*Setaria italica*) Bran. *J. Sci. Food Agric.* **2019**, *99*, 3886–3894. [CrossRef]
20. Dai, G.; Wang, K.; Wang, G.; Wang, S. Initial Pyrolysis Mechanism of Cellulose Revealed by In-Situ DRIFT Analysis and Theoretical Calculation. *Combust. Flame* **2019**, *208*, 273–280. [CrossRef]
21. Bhaladhare, S.; Das, D. Cellulose: A Fascinating Biopolymer for Hydrogel Synthesis. *J. Mater. Chem. B* **2022**, *10*, 1923–1945. [CrossRef]
22. Chen, Y.; Wang, Y.; Wan, J.; Ma, Y. Crystal and Pore Structure of Wheat Straw Cellulose Fiber during Recycling. *Cellulose* **2010**, *17*, 329–338. [CrossRef]
23. Jahan, M.S.; Saeed, A.; He, Z.; Ni, Y. Jute as Raw Material for the Preparation of Microcrystalline Cellulose. *Cellulose* **2011**, *18*, 451–459. [CrossRef]
24. Chen, Z.; Aziz, T.; Sun, H.; Ullah, A.; Ali, A.; Cheng, L.; Ullah, R.; Khan, F. Advances and Applications of Cellulose Bio-Composites in Biodegradable Materials. *J. Environ. Polym. Degra-Dation* **2023**, *30*, 1–12.
25. Qaseem, M.F.; Shaheen, H.; Wu, A.-M. Cell Wall Hemicellulose for Sustainable Industrial Utilization. *Renew. Sustain. Energy Rev.* **2021**, *144*, 110996. [CrossRef]
26. Khodayari, A.; Thielemans, W.; Hirn, U.; Van Vuure, A.W.; Seveno, D. Cellulose-Hemicellulose Interactions—A Nanoscale View. *Carbohydr. Polym.* **2021**, *270*, 118364. [CrossRef]
27. de Souza Queiroz, S.; Jofre, F.M.; dos Santos, H.A.; Hernández-Pérez, A.F.; Felipe, M.d.G.d.A. Xylitol and Ethanol Co-Production from Sugarcane Bagasse and Straw Hemicellulosic Hydrolysate Supplemented with Molasses. *Biomass Conv. Bioref.* **2023**, *13*, 3143–3152. [CrossRef]
28. Zhang, C.; Cai, B.; Sun, Y.; Kang, J.; Pei, F.; Ge, J. Microbial Communities That Drive the Degradation of Flax Pectin and Hemicellulose during Dew Retting with Bacillus Licheniformis HDYM-04 and Bacillus Subtilis ZC-01 Addition. *Bioresour. Technol.* **2023**, *371*, 128516. [CrossRef]
29. Ahmad, N.; Tayyeb, D.; Ali, I.; Alruwaili, N.K.; Ahmad, W.; ur Rehman, A.; Khan, A.H.; Iqbal, M.S. Development and Characterization of Hemicellulose-Based Films for Antibacterial Wound-Dressing Application. *Polymers* **2020**, *12*, 548. [CrossRef]
30. Liu, G.; Shi, K.; Sun, H. Research Progress in Hemicellulose-Based Nanocomposite Film as Food Packaging. *Polymers* **2023**, *15*, 979. [CrossRef] [PubMed]
31. Farhat, W.; Venditti, R.; Quick, A.; Taha, M.; Mignard, N.; Becquart, F.; Ayoub, A. Hemicellulose Extraction and Characterization for Applications in Paper Coatings and Adhesives. *Ind. Crops Prod.* **2017**, *107*, 370–377. [CrossRef]
32. Huang, L.-Z.; Ma, M.-G.; Ji, X.-X.; Choi, S.-E.; Si, C. Recent Developments and Applications of Hemicellulose From Wheat Straw: A Review. *Front. Bioeng. Biotechnol.* **2021**, *9*. [CrossRef]
33. Agarwal, A.; Rana, M.; Park, J.-H. Advancement in Technologies for the Depolymerization of Lignin. *Fuel Process. Technol.* **2018**, *181*, 115–132. [CrossRef]
34. Asina, F.; Brzonova, I.; Kozliak, E.; Kubátová, A.; Ji, Y. Microbial Treatment of Industrial Lignin: Successes, Problems and Challenges. *Renew. Sustain. Energy Rev.* **2017**, *77*, 1179–1205. [CrossRef]
35. Yadollahi, M.; Namazi, H.; Aghazadeh, M. Antibacterial Carboxymethyl Cellulose/Ag Nanocomposite Hydrogels Cross-Linked with Layered Double Hydroxides. *Int. J. Biol. Macromol.* **2015**, *79*, 269–277. [CrossRef] [PubMed]
36. Lee, H.V.; Hamid, S.B.A.; Zain, S.K. Conversion of Lignocellulosic Biomass to Nanocellulose: Structure and Chemical Process. *Sci. World J.* **2014**, *2014*, 1–20. [CrossRef] [PubMed]
37. Nath, P.C.; Debnath, S.; Sharma, M.; Sridhar, K.; Nayak, P.K.; Inbaraj, B.S. Recent Advances in Cellulose-Based Hydrogels: Food Applications. *Foods* **2023**, *12*, 350. [CrossRef] [PubMed]
38. Khan, R.; Jolly, R.; Fatima, T.; Shakir, M. Extraction Processes for Deriving Cellulose: A Comprehensive Review on Green Approaches. *Polym. Adv. Technol.* **2022**, *33*, 2069–2090. [CrossRef]
39. Johar, N.; Ahmad, I.; Dufresne, A. Extraction, Preparation and Characterization of Cellulose Fibres and Nanocrystals from Rice Husk. *Ind. Crops Prod.* **2012**, *37*, 93–99. [CrossRef]
40. de Morais Teixeira, E.; Bondancia, T.J.; Teodoro, K.B.R.; Corrêa, A.C.; Marconcini, J.M.; Mattoso, L.H.C. Sugarcane Bagasse Whiskers: Extraction and Characterizations. *Ind. Crops Prod.* **2011**, *33*, 63–66. [CrossRef]
41. Thi, S.; Lee, K.M. Comparison of Deep Eutectic Solvents (DES) on Pretreatment of Oil Palm Empty Fruit Bunch (OPEFB): Cellulose Digestibility, Structural and Morphology Changes. *Bioresour. Technol.* **2019**, *282*, 525–529. [CrossRef]
42. Setyaningsih, D.; Uju, Muna, N.; Isroi; Suryawan, N.B.; Nurfauzi, A.A. Cellulose Nanofiber Isolation from Palm Oil Empty Fruit Bunches (EFB) through Strong Acid Hydrolysis. *IOP Conf. Ser. Earth Environ. Sci.* **2018**, *141*, 012027. [CrossRef]
43. Zhang, P.P.; Tong, D.S.; Lin, C.X.; Yang, H.M.; Zhong, Z.K.; Yu, W.H.; Wang, H.; Zhou, C.H. Effects of Acid Treatments on Bamboo Cellulose Nanocrystals: EFFECTS OF ACID TREATMENTS ON BAMBOO CELLULOSE NANOCRYSTALS. *Asia-Pac. J. Chem. Eng.* **2014**, *9*, 686–695. [CrossRef]

44. Zainal, S.H.; Mohd, N.H.; Suhaili, N.; Anuar, F.H.; Lazim, A.M.; Othaman, R. Preparation of Cellulose-Based Hydrogel: A Review. *J. Mater. Res. Technol.* **2021**, *10*, 935–952. [CrossRef]
45. Shu, B.; Ren, Q.; Hong, L.; Xiao, Z.; Lu, X.; Wang, W.; Yu, J.; Fu, N.; Gu, Y.; Zheng, J. Effect of Steam Explosion Technology Main Parameters on Moso Bamboo and Poplar Fiber. *J. Renew. Mater.* **2021**, *9*, 585–597. [CrossRef]
46. Wang, W.; Wu, H.; Shakeel, U.; Wang, C.; Yan, T.; Xu, X.; Xu, J. Synergistic Effect of Acidity Balance and Hydrothermal Pretreatment Severity on Alkali Extraction of Hemicelluloses from Corn Stalk. *Biomass Conv. Bioref.* **2022**, *12*, 459–468. [CrossRef]
47. Sun, S.-L.; Wen, J.-L.; Ma, M.-G.; Sun, R.-C. Successive Alkali Extraction and Structural Characterization of Hemicelluloses from Sweet Sorghum Stem. *Carbohydr. Polym.* **2013**, *92*, 2224–2231. [CrossRef] [PubMed]
48. Lyu, B.; Wang, Y.; Zhang, X.; Chen, Y.; Fu, H.; Liu, T.; Hao, J.; Li, Y.; Yu, H.; Jiang, L. Changes of High-Purity Insoluble Fiber from Soybean Dregs (Okara) after Being Fermented by Colonic Flora and Its Adsorption Capacity. *Foods* **2021**, *10*, 2485. [CrossRef] [PubMed]
49. Tomé, L.I.N.; Baião, V.; da Silva, W.; Brett, C.M.A. Deep Eutectic Solvents for the Production and Application of New Materials. *Appl. Mater. Today* **2018**, *10*, 30–50. [CrossRef]
50. Yu, W.; Wang, C.; Yi, Y.; Wang, H.; Zeng, L.; Li, M.; Yang, Y.; Tan, Z. Comparison of Deep Eutectic Solvents on Pretreatment of Raw Ramie Fibers for Cellulose Nanofibril Production. *ACS Omega* **2020**, *5*, 5580–5588. [CrossRef] [PubMed]
51. Wang, S.; Sun, W.; Swallah, M.S.; Amin, K.; Lyu, B.; Fan, H.; Zhang, Z.; Yu, H. Preparation and Characterization of Soybean Insoluble Dietary Fiber and Its Prebiotic Effect on Dyslipidemia and Hepatic Steatosis in High Fat-Fed C57BL/6J Mice. *Food Funct.* **2021**, *12*, 8760–8773. [CrossRef]
52. Li, P.; Wang, Y.; Hou, Q.; Liu, H.; Lei, H.; Jian, B.; Li, X. Preparation of Cellulose Nanofibrils from Okara by High Pressure Homogenization Method Using Deep Eutectic Solvents. *Cellulose* **2020**, *27*, 2511–2520. [CrossRef]
53. Yan, M.; Tian, C.; Wu, T.; Huang, X.; Zhong, Y.; Yang, P.; Zhang, L.; Ma, J.; Lu, H.; Zhou, X. In-sights into Structure and Properties of Cellulose Nanofibrils (CNFs) Prepared by Screw Extrusion and Deep Eutectic Solvent Permeation. *Int. J. Biol. Macromol.* **2021**, *191*, 422–431. [CrossRef]
54. Yi, T.; Zhao, H.; Mo, Q.; Pan, D.; Liu, Y.; Huang, L.; Xu, H.; Hu, B.; Song, H. From Cellulose to Cellulose Nanofibrils—A Comprehensive Review of the Preparation and Modification of Cellulose Nanofibrils. *Materials* **2020**, *13*, 5062. [CrossRef] [PubMed]
55. Dias, Y.J.; Kolbasov, A.; Sinha-Ray, S.; Pourdeyhimi, B.; Yarin, A.L. Theoretical and Experimental Study of Dissolution Mechanism of Cellulose. *J. Mol. Liq.* **2020**, *312*, 113450. [CrossRef]
56. Larsson, E.; Sanchez, C.C.; Porsch, C.; Karabulut, E.; Wågberg, L.; Carlmark, A. Thermo-Responsive Nanofibrillated Cellulose by Polyelectrolyte Adsorption. *Eur. Polym. J.* **2013**, *49*, 2689–2696. [CrossRef]
57. Martins, N.C.T.; Freire, C.S.R.; Pinto, R.J.B.; Fernandes, S.C.M.; Pascoal Neto, C.; Silvestre, A.J.D.; Causio, J.; Baldi, G.; Sadocco, P.; Trindade, T. Electrostatic Assembly of Ag Nanoparticles onto Nanofibrillated Cellulose for Antibacterial Paper Products. *Cellulose* **2012**, *19*, 1425–1436. [CrossRef]
58. Hatton, F.L.; Malmström, E.; Carlmark, A. Tailor-Made Copolymers for the Adsorption to Cellulosic Surfaces. *Eur. Polym. J.* **2015**, *65*, 325–339. [CrossRef]
59. Besbes, I.; Vilar, M.R.; Boufi, S. Nanofibrillated Cellulose from Alfa, Eucalyptus and Pine Fibres: Preparation, Characteristics and Reinforcing Potential. *Carbohydr. Polym.* **2011**, *86*, 1198–1206. [CrossRef]
60. Liimatainen, H.; Visanko, M.; Sirviö, J.A.; Hormi, O.E.O.; Niinimaki, J. Enhancement of the Nano-fibrillation of Wood Cellulose through Sequential Periodate–Chlorite Oxidation. *Biomacromolecules* **2012**, *13*, 1592–1597. [CrossRef]
61. Korchagina, A.A.; Budaeva, V.V.; Kukhlenko, A.A. Esterification of Oat-Hull Cellulose. *Russ. Chem. Bull.* **2019**, *68*, 1282–1288. [CrossRef]
62. Detroy, R.W.; Cunningham, R.L.; Bothast, R.J.; Bagby, M.O.; Herman, A. Bioconversion of Wheat Straw Cellulose/Hemicellulose to Ethanol BySaccharomyces Uvarum AndPachysolen Tannophilus. *Biotechnol. Bioeng.* **1982**, *24*, 1105–1113. [CrossRef]
63. Qiu, M.; Zheng, J.; Yao, Y.; Liu, L.; Zhou, X.; Jiao, H.; Aarons, J.; Zhang, K.; Guan, Q.; Li, W. Directly Converting Cellulose into High Yield Sorbitol by Tuning the Electron Structure of Ru2P Anchored in Agricultural Straw Biochar. *J. Clean. Prod.* **2022**, *362*, 132364. [CrossRef]
64. Perez, R.F.; Fraga, M.A. Hemicellulose-Derived Chemicals: One-Step Production of Furfuryl Alcohol from Xylose. *Green Chem.* **2014**, *16*, 3942–3950. [CrossRef]
65. Ribeiro, L.S.; Delgado, J.J.; de Melo Órfão, J.J.; Pereira, M.F.R. A One-Pot Method for the Enhanced Production of Xylitol Directly from Hemicellulose (Corncob Xylan). *RSC Adv.* **2016**, *6*, 95320–95327. [CrossRef]
66. Mamman, A.S.; Lee, J.-M.; Kim, Y.-C.; Hwang, I.T.; Park, N.-J.; Hwang, Y.K.; Chang, J.-S.; Hwang, J.-S. Furfural: Hemicellulose/Xylosederived Biochemical. *Biofuels. Bioprod. Bioref.* **2008**, *2*, 438–454. [CrossRef]
67. Perez, C.L.; Milessi, T.S.; Sandri, J.P.; Foulquié-Moreno, M.R.; Giordano, R.C.; Thevelein, J.M.; de Lima Camargo Giordano, R.; Zangirolami, T.C. Unraveling Continuous 2G Ethanol Production from Xylose Using Hemicellulose Hydrolysate and Immobilized Superior Recombinant Yeast in Fixed-Bed Bioreactor. *Biochem. Eng. J.* **2021**, *169*, 107963. [CrossRef]
68. Xie, Y.; Guo, X.; Ma, Z.; Gong, J.; Wang, H.; Lv, Y. Efficient Extraction and Structural Characterization of Hemicellulose from Sugarcane Bagasse Pith. *Polymers* **2020**, *12*, 608. [CrossRef]
69. Extraction and Purification of Hemicellulose Polysaccharide from Soybean Dietary Fiber—«Modern Food Science and Technology». 2019. Available online: https://en.cnki.com.cn/Article_en/CJFDTotal-GZSP200901012.htm (accessed on 12 March 2023).

70. Sun, X.F.; Sun, R.C.; Sun, J.X. Acetylation of Sugarcane Bagasse Using NBS as a Catalyst under Mild Reaction Conditions for the Production of Oil Sorption-Active Materials. *Bioresour. Technol.* **2004**, *95*, 343–350. [CrossRef]
71. Jin, A.X.; Ren, J.L.; Peng, F.; Xu, F.; Zhou, G.Y.; Sun, R.C.; Kennedy, J.F. Comparative Characteri-zation of Degraded and Non-Degradative Hemicelluloses from Barley Straw and Maize Stems: Composition, Structure, and Thermal Properties. *Carbohydr. Polym.* **2009**, *78*, 609–619. [CrossRef]
72. Phan, D.T.; Tan, C.-S. Innovative Pretreatment of Sugarcane Bagasse Using Supercritical CO_2 Followed by Alkaline Hydrogen Peroxide. *Bioresour. Technol.* **2014**, *167*, 192–197. [CrossRef]
73. Sun, R.C.; Tomkinson, J.; Ma, P.L.; Liang, S.F. Comparative Study of Hemicelluloses from Rice Straw by Alkali and Hydrogen Peroxide Treatments. *Carbohydr. Polym.* **2000**, *42*, 111–122. [CrossRef]
74. Zhang, P.; Dong, S.-J.; Ma, H.-H.; Zhang, B.-X.; Wang, Y.-F.; Hu, X.-M. Fractionation of Corn Stov-er into Cellulose, Hemicellulose and Lignin Using a Series of Ionic Liquids. *Ind. Crops Prod.* **2015**, *76*, 688–696. [CrossRef]
75. Peng, X.; Ren, J.; Sun, R. Homogeneous Esterification of Xylan-Rich Hemicelluloses with Maleic Anhydride in Ionic Liquid. *Biomacromolecules* **2010**, *11*, 3519–3524. [CrossRef]
76. Alekhina, M.; Mikkonen, K.S.; Alén, R.; Tenkanen, M.; Sixta, H. Carboxymethylation of Alkali Extracted Xylan for Preparation of Bio-Based Packaging Films. *Carbohydr. Polym.* **2014**, *100*, 89–96. [CrossRef]
77. Ren, J.-L.; Sun, R.-C.; Peng, F. Carboxymethylation of Hemicelluloses Isolated from Sugarcane Bagasse. *Polym. Degrad. Stab.* **2008**, *93*, 786–793. [CrossRef]
78. Dong, L.; Hu, H.; Shuo, Y.; Cheng, F. Grafted Copolymerization Modification of Hemicellulose Directly in the Alkaline Peroxide Mechanical Pulping (APMP) Effluent and Its Surface Sizing Effects on Corrugated Paper. *Ind. Eng. Chem. Res.* **2014**, *53*, 6221–6229. [CrossRef]
79. Parikka, K.; Leppänen, A.-S.; Xu, C.; Pitkänen, L.; Eronen, P.; Österberg, M.; Brumer, H.; Willför, S.; Tenkanen, M. Functional and Anionic Cellulose-Interacting Polymers by Selective Chemo-Enzymatic Carboxylation of Galactose-Containing Polysaccharides. *Biomacromolecules* **2012**, *13*, 2418–2428. [CrossRef] [PubMed]
80. Hoffman, M.; Jia, Z.; Peña, M.J.; Cash, M.; Harper, A.; Blackburn, A.R.; Darvill, A.; York, W.S. Structural Analysis of Xyloglucans in the Primary Cell Walls of Plants in the Subclass Asteridae. *Carbohydr. Res.* **2005**, *340*, 1826–1840. [CrossRef]
81. Liu, L.; Paulitz, J.; Pauly, M. The Presence of Fucogalactoxyloglucan and Its Synthesis in Rice Indicates Conserved Functional Importance in Plants. *Plant Physiol.* **2015**, *168*, 549–560. [CrossRef] [PubMed]
82. Vähä-Nissi, M.; Talja, R.; Hartman, J.; Setälä, H.; Poppius-Levlin, K.; Hyvärinen, S.; Sievänen, J.; Harlin, A. Wood-Based Hemicelluloses for Packaging Materials. In Proceedings of the TAPPI European PLACE Conference, Seattle, WA, USA, 6–9 May 2012; pp. 364–386.
83. Mierczynska-Vasilev, A.; Smith, P.A. Surface Modification Influencing Adsorption of Red Wine Constituents: The Role of Functional Groups. *Appl. Surf. Sci.* **2016**, *386*, 14–23. [CrossRef]
84. Xiao, M.; Dai, S.; Wang, L.; Ni, X.; Yan, W.; Fang, Y.; Corke, H.; Jiang, F. Carboxymethyl Modification of Konjac Glucomannan Affects Water Binding Properties. *Carbohydr. Polym.* **2015**, *130*, 1–8. [CrossRef]
85. Qi, X.-M.; Liu, S.-Y.; Chu, F.-B.; Pang, S.; Liang, Y.-R.; Guan, Y.; Peng, F.; Sun, R.-C. Preparation and Characterization of Blended Films from Quaternized Hemicelluloses and Carboxymethyl Cellulose. *Materials* **2016**, *9*, 4. [CrossRef] [PubMed]
86. Ebringerová, A.; Novotná, Z.; Kačuráková, M.; Machová, E. Chemical Modification of Beechwood Xylan with P-Carboxybenzyl Bromide. *J. Appl. Polym. Sci.* **1996**, *62*, 1043–1047. [CrossRef]
87. Figueiredo, P.; Lintinen, K.; Hirvonen, J.T.; Kostiainen, M.A.; Santos, H.A. Properties and Chemical Modifications of Lignin: Towards Lignin-Based Nanomaterials for Biomedical Applications. *Prog. Mater. Sci.* **2018**, *93*, 233–269. [CrossRef]
88. Stewart, D. Lignin as a Base Material for Materials Applications: Chemistry, Application and Economics. *Ind. Crops Prod.* **2008**, *27*, 202–207. [CrossRef]
89. Frangville, C.; Rutkevičius, M.; Richter, A.P.; Velev, O.D.; Stoyanov, S.D.; Paunov, V.N. Fabrication of Environmentally Biodegradable Lignin Nanoparticles. *ChemPhysChem* **2012**, *13*, 4235–4243. [CrossRef]
90. Yang, Y.; Wei, Z.; Wang, C.; Tong, Z. Lignin-Based Pickering HIPEs for Macroporous Foams and Their Enhanced Adsorption of Copper(Ii) Ions. *Chem. Commun.* **2013**, *49*, 7144. [CrossRef] [PubMed]
91. Lynam, J.G.; Kumar, N.; Wong, M.J. Deep Eutectic Solvents' Ability to Solubilize Lignin, Cellulose, and Hemicellulose; Thermal Stability; and Density. *Bioresour. Technol.* **2017**, *238*, 684–689. [CrossRef]
92. Lou, R.; Zhang, X. Evaluation of Pretreatment Effect on Lignin Extraction from Wheat Straw by Deep Eutectic Solvent. *Bioresour. Technol.* **2022**, *344*, 126174. [CrossRef] [PubMed]
93. Huang, D.; Li, R.; Xu, P.; Li, T.; Deng, R.; Chen, S.; Zhang, Q. The Cornerstone of Realizing Lignin Value-Addition: Exploiting the Native Structure and Properties of Lignin by Extraction Methods. *Chem. Eng. J.* **2020**, *402*, 126237. [CrossRef]
94. Lou, R.; Ma, R.; Lin, K.; Ahamed, A.; Zhang, X. Facile Extraction of Wheat Straw by Deep Eutectic Solvent (DES) to Produce Lignin Nanoparticles. *ACS Sustain. Chem. Eng.* **2019**, *7*, 10248–10256. [CrossRef]
95. Zheng, W.; Lan, T.; Li, H.; Yue, G.; Zhou, H. Exploring Why Sodium Lignosulfonate Influenced Enzymatic Hydrolysis Efficiency of Cellulose from the Perspective of Substrate–Enzyme Adsorption. *Biotechnol. Biofuels* **2020**, *13*, 19. [CrossRef]
96. Feng, C.; Zhu, J.; Cao, L.; Yan, L.; Qin, C.; Liang, C.; Yao, S. Acidolysis Mechanism of Lignin from Bagasse during P-Toluenesulfonic Acid Treatment. *Ind. Crops Prod.* **2022**, *176*, 114374. [CrossRef]

97. Lv, W.; Xia, Z.; Song, Y.; Wang, P.; Liu, S.; Zhang, Y.; Ben, H.; Han, G.; Jiang, W. Using Microwave Assisted Organic Acid Treatment to Separate Cellulose Fiber and Lignin from Kenaf Bast. *Ind. Crops Prod.* **2021**, *171*, 113934. [CrossRef]
98. Vanderghem, C.; Richel, A.; Jacquet, N.; Blecker, C.; Paquot, M. Impact of Formic/Acetic Acid and Ammonia Pre-Treatments on Chemical Structure and Physico-Chemical Properties of Miscanthus x Giganteus Lignins. *Polym. Degrad. Stab.* **2011**, *96*, 1761–1770. [CrossRef]
99. Espinoza-Acosta, J.L.; Torres-Chávez, P.I.; Carvajal-Millán, E.; Ramírez-Wong, B.; Bello-Pérez, L.A.; Montaño-Leyva, B. Ionic Liquids and Organic Solvents for Recovering Lignin from Lignocellulosic Biomass. *BioResources* **2014**, *9*, 3660–3687. [CrossRef]
100. Mehmood Asim, A.; Uroos, M.; Muhammad, N. Extraction of Lignin and Quantitative Sugar Release from Biomass Using Efficient and Cost-Effective Pyridinium Protic Ionic Liquids. *RSC Adv.* **2020**, *10*, 44003–44014. [CrossRef]
101. Vinardell, M.P.; Ugartondo, V.; Mitjans, M. Potential Applications of Antioxidant Lignins from Different Sources. *Ind. Crops Prod.* **2008**, *27*, 220–223. [CrossRef]
102. Domenek, S.; Louaifi, A.; Guinault, A.; Baumberger, S. Potential of Lignins as Antioxidant Additive in Active Biodegradable Packaging Materials. *J. Polym. Environ.* **2013**, *21*, 692–701. [CrossRef]
103. De Chirico, A.; Armanini, M.; Chini, P.; Cioccolo, G.; Provasoli, F.; Audisio, G. Flame Retardants for Polypropylene Based on Lignin. *Polym. Degrad. Stab.* **2003**, *79*, 139–145. [CrossRef]
104. Hofmann, K.; Glasser, W.G. Engineering Plastics from Lignin. 21. Synthesis and Properties of Epoxidized Lignin-Poly(Propylene Oxide) Copolymers. *J. Wood Chem. Technol.* **1993**, *13*, 73–95. [CrossRef]
105. da Silva, E.A.B.; Zabkova, M.; Araújo, J.D.; Cateto, C.A.; Barreiro, M.F.; Belgacem, M.N.; Ro-drigues, A.E. An Integrated Process to Produce Vanillin and Lignin-Based Polyurethanes from Kraft Lignin. *Chem. Eng. Res. Des.* **2009**, *87*, 1276–1292. [CrossRef]
106. Fernandes, S.; Freire, C.S.R.; Neto, C.P.; Gandini, A. The Bulk Oxypropylation of Chitin and Chitosan and the Characterization of the Ensuing Polyols. *Green Chem.* **2008**, *10*, 93–97. [CrossRef]
107. Evtiouguina, M.; Margarida Barros, A.; Cruz-Pinto, J.J.; Pascoal Neto, C.; Belgacem, N.; Pavier, C.; Gandini, A. The Oxypropylation of Cork Residues: Preliminary Results. *Bioresour. Technol.* **2000**, *73*, 187–189. [CrossRef]
108. de Menezes, A.J.; Pasquini, D.; da Silva Curvelo, A.A. Self-Reinforced Composites Obtained by the Partial Oxypropylation of Cellulose Fibers. 2. Effect of Catalyst on the Mechanical and Dynamic Mechanical Properties. *Cellulose* **2009**, *16*, 239–246. [CrossRef]
109. Pavier, C.; Gandini, A. Oxypropylation of Sugar Beet Pulp. 2. Separation of the Grafted Pulp from the Propylene Oxide Homopolymer. *Carbohydr. Polym.* **2000**, *42*, 13–17. [CrossRef]
110. Pavier, C.; Gandini, A. Urethanes and Polyurethanes from Oxypropylated Sugar Beet Pulp: I. Kinetic Study in Solution. *Eur. Polym. J.* **2000**, *36*, 1653–1658. [CrossRef]
111. Aniceto, J.P.S.; Portugal, I.; Silva, C.M. Biomass-Based Polyols through Oxypropylation Reaction. *ChemSusChem* **2012**, *5*, 1358–1368. [CrossRef]
112. Matsushita, Y. Conversion of Technical Lignins to Functional Materials with Retained Polymeric Properties. *J. Wood Sci.* **2015**, *61*, 230–250. [CrossRef]
113. Zhu, J.; Song, X.; Tan, W.K.; Wen, Y.; Gao, Z.; Ong, C.N.; Loh, C.S.; Swarup, S.; Li, J. Chemical Modification of Biomass Okara Using Poly(Acrylic Acid) through Free Radical Graft Polymerization. *J. Agric. Food Chem.* **2020**, *68*, 13241–13246. [CrossRef]
114. Chen, R.; Kokta, B.V.; Valade, J.L. Graft Copolymerization of Lignosulfonate and Styrene. *J. Appl. Polym. Sci.* **1979**, *24*, 1609–1618. [CrossRef]
115. Dournel, P.; Randrianalimanana, E.; Deffieux, A.; Fontanille, M. Synthesis and Polymerization of Lignin Macromonomers—I. Anchoring of Polymerizable Groups on Lignin Model Compounds. *Eur. Polym. J.* **1988**, *24*, 843–847. [CrossRef]

Disclaimer/Publisher's Note: The statements, opinions and data contained in all publications are solely those of the individual author(s) and contributor(s) and not of MDPI and/or the editor(s). MDPI and/or the editor(s) disclaim responsibility for any injury to people or property resulting from any ideas, methods, instructions or products referred to in the content.

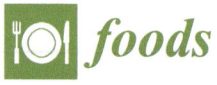

Article

Rheology, Texture and Swallowing Characteristics of a Texture-Modified Dysphagia Food Prepared Using Common Supplementary Materials

Xin Wang, Liyuan Rong, Mingyue Shen, Qiang Yu, Yi Chen, Jinwang Li and Jianhua Xie *

State Key Laboratory of Food Science and Resources, Nanchang University, Nanchang 330047, China; wx163ylfz@163.com (X.W.); rongliyuan01@163.com (L.R.); shenmingyue1107@ncu.edu.cn (M.S.); yuqiang8612@163.com (Q.Y.); chenyi-417@163.com (Y.C.); lijw202418@163.com (J.L.)
* Correspondence: jhxie@ncu.edu.cn; Tel.: +86-791-8830-4347

Abstract: A dysphagia diet is a special eating plan. The development and design of dysphagia foods should consider both swallowing safety and food nutritional qualities. In this study, the effects of four food supplements, namely vitamins, minerals, salt and sugar, on swallowing characteristics, rheological and textural properties were investigated, and a sensory evaluation of dysphagia foods made with rice starch, perilla seed oil and whey isolate protein was carried out. The results showed that all the samples belonged to foods at level 4 (pureed) in The International Dysphagia Diet Standardization Initiative (IDDSI) framework, and exhibited shear thinning behavior, which is favorable for dysphagia patients. Rheological tests showed that the viscosity of a food bolus was increased with salt and sugar (SS), while it decreased with vitamins and minerals (VM) at shear rates of 50 s^{-1}. Both SS and VM strengthened the elastic gel system, and SS enhanced the storage modulus and loss modulus. VM increased the hardness, gumminess, chewiness and color richness, but left small residues on the spoon. SS provided better water-holding, chewiness and resilience by influencing the way molecules were connected, promoting swallowing safety. SS brought a better taste to the food bolus. Dysphagia foods with both VM and 0.5% SS had the best sensory evaluation score. This study may provide a theoretical foundation for the creation and design of new dysphagia nutritional food products.

Keywords: dysphagia; IDDSI; swallowing; rheological property; sensory evaluation

1. Introduction

Dysphagia is considered to be a swallowing disorder in that food fails to pass smoothly down the esophagus from the oral cavity to the stomach, which can limit food intake and nutrient absorption [1]. In the case of newborns and the elderly who are prone to swallowing disorders, in particular, it greatly impacts their normal lives and growth [2]. An unformed food bolus or the misclosure of the pharyngeal epiglottis during oral processing caused by poor chewing and swallowing abilities increase the risk of malnutrition, choking and pneumonia in dysphagia patients [3,4]. The prevalence of dysphagia is about 13% in people over 65 years old and about 51% in institutionalized elderly [5]. Along with increased population aging, dysphagia is affecting more and more elderly in terms of their quality of life, and mental and physical health. Actually, this swallowing disorder frequently bothers patients with postoperative muscle loss, neurological impairment and Alzheimer's disease, resulting in additional time and expense required for patient treatment [6,7]. Therefore, it is necessary to work on dysphagia foods.

Thicker products such as pastes and purees are often considered more suitable for dysphagia patients because of the delayed flow of liquid and more time for safe swallowing [8]. Softer, more uniform, easier to chew and more elastic foods seem to take fewer oral efforts to swallow [9,10]. Thus, to meet these needs of special populations, the modification of food texture by adding hydrocolloids such as starches and proteins has received attention. For instance, beef patties obtained a softer texture with tapioca starch added [11], and carrot puree showed a better viscosity with xanthan gum added [12], which was more suitable for dysphagia patients. The International Dysphagia Diet Standardization Initiative (IDDSI), was established worldwide to provide better dietary recommendations for individuals with dysphagia [13]. A series of easy-to-run tests (flow test, fork drip test, spoon tilt test, etc.) are used by the IDDSI framework to evaluate the dysphagia-relevant characteristics based on food texture and flow thickness, classifying all foods from fully liquid to fully solid on a scale of 0~7, a total of 8 levels [14]. Dysphagia foods prepared with mung bean starch and flaxseed protein as gel with calcium salts added were classified as level 5 (minced and moist) and level 6 (soft and bite-sized) foods in the IDDSI framework [15]. In addition, the desirability and quantity of dysphagia foods can be increased by optimizing taste and shape, for instance by adding small doses of salt to mask the fishy flavor of fish sauce with increased chewiness and elasticity [16], and 3D printing to enhance the attractiveness and interest of thickened foods made from black fungus [17].

The texture-modified products may be poorer in nutrients and more likely to result in malnutrition and muscle weakness than ordinary foods [18,19]. A total of 18.6% of elderly with dysphagia are undernourished [20]. Energy and protein intakes were both lower in dysphagia patients receiving the texture-modified diet than those treated with a normal hospital diet [21]. For dysphagia patients, the food is usually thickened by adding hydrocolloids such as starch, xanthan gum, and guar gum as thickening agents to suit their compromised swallowing ability, thus reducing the nutrient density of original food [22]. In addition, dysphagia diets are generally deficient in fruits, vegetables and whole grains, which leads to a demand for nutritional diversity of foods for dysphagia patients [22]. Nutritional intake deficiencies occur from the energy intake of basic nutrients such as carbohydrates and proteins and the absorption of micronutrients such as vitamins and minerals [23]. Compared to vegetable oils, perilla seed oil is known to contain up to 67% α-linolenic acid, which can well meet the unsaturated fatty acid requirements of the elderly today, as well as lowering blood lipids, improving memory, liver protection and other effects that are among the reasons behind its popularity [24]. On the other hand, in Britain's aging population, vitamin B_{12} deficiency accounts for 12% and folic acid deficiency for 15% of elderly [25], and 67.8% of the over 65s have varying degrees of vitamin and mineral inadequacy [23]. Furthermore, a vicious loop is created when malnutrition exacerbates dysphagia through neuromuscular dysfunction [26]. Due to a single nutritional pattern, using dysphagia food prepared by combining carrot puree with xanthan gum and κ-carrageenan gum may make it challenging to satisfy the nutritional requirements of patients [12]. Therefore, the design of dysphagia food products should also consider the wide range of food matrices and nutritional properties [7].

More and more attention is being paid to the dysphagia population and suitable dysphagia foods. Currently, the development of most dysphagia products is focused on improving the texture properties of natural foods, which could lead to inadequate nutritional composition and single-product patterns. In this paper, the most fundamental ingredients (rice starch, whey isolate protein and perilla seed oil) were used to construct a dysphagia food bolus model based on nutritional requirements that gives more design possibilities with regard to swallowing foods. The effects of common supplements (vitamins, minerals, salt and sugar) on the swallowing characteristics and texture properties were investigated. Moreover, the correlations between rheology, texture and sensory evaluation were explored to provide a theoretical basis for developing more practical and nutritional dysphagia foods.

2. Materials and Methods

2.1. Materials and Chemicals

Rice starch (RIS) (≥99%) was obtained from Wuxi JinNong Biology Science and Technology Co. (Wuxi, China). Whey isolate protein (WPI) (protein, 89%; moisture,

4.7%; ash, 2.7%; fat, 1.3%; and lactose, 0.1%) was bought from Hilmar Corporation (Hilmar, LA, CA, USA). Perilla Seed Oil (PSO) (≥99%) was purchased from KangShanYuan Fats & Oils Co. (Nanchang, China). Salt and sugar were obtained from Tianhong supermarket (Nanchang, China). Mixed vitamins and mixed minerals were obtained from RuiPu Biotechnology Co. (Tianjin, China). The materials above were all food grade. All of the trials were conducted with Millipore ultrapure water.

2.2. Sample Preparation

2.2.1. The Design of a Simple Dysphagia Food System

RIS, WPI and PSO were used as carbohydrate, high quality protein and fatty acid suppliers, respectively and their energy coefficients were 17 kJ/g, 17 kJ/g and 37 kJ/g, respectively. The ratio of flour to water was 1:5, in each 100 g of material powder, containing PSO (X g), RIS (Yg) and WPI (Z g). According to the General Rules for Formula Food for Special Medical Purposes (GB 29922-2013) [27] and the Chinese Dietary Reference Intakes (2013) [28] published by the Chinese National Health and Family Planning Commission, dysphagia food boluses were designed to satisfy the following requirements:

(i) No less than 295 kJ energy per 100 g of ready-to-eat products:

$$37X + 17Y + 17Z \geq 295 \times (1 + 5); \tag{1}$$

(ii) At least 0.7 g protein per 100 kJ energy:

$$Z \geq [(37X + 17Y + 17Z)/100] \times 0.7; \tag{2}$$

(iii) A total of 50–65% energy from carbohydrates and 20–30% energy from fats:

$$50\% \leq 17Y/(37X + 17Y + 17Z) \leq 65\%, \tag{3}$$

$$20\% \leq 37X/(37X + 17Y + 17Z) \leq 30\%. \tag{4}$$

According to Equations (1) and (4), the PSO content is 9.73~16.45%. To simplify the formulation and calculation, PSO content was set to 10% and 15% for follow-up design.

According to Equations (2) and (3), the contents of RIS and WPI were set as follows:

A: When the PSO content is 15%, the RIS content is 58.82~76.47%, and the WPI content is 14.00~26.18%. To simplify the formulation and calculation, the RIS and WPI contents were set to 60% and 25%, 65% and 20%, and 70% and 15%, respectively.

B: When the PSO content is 10%, the RIS content is 55.88~72.65%, the WPI content is 13.30~34.12%. To simplify formulation and calculation, the RIS and WPI contents were set to 60% and 30%, 65% and 20%, and 70% and 15% respectively.

The dysphagia food bolus components are shown in Table 1.

Table 1. The design of the dysphagia food bolus.

Dysphagia Food	PSO	RIS	WPI
A	15%	60%	25%
B		65%	20%
C		70%	15%
D	10%	60%	30%
E		65%	25%
F		70%	20%

2.2.2. The Design of the Dysphagia Food Bolus with Supplementary Materials

According to the National Food Safety Standard Determination of General Rules for Formula Food for Special Medical Purposes (GB 29922-2013) [27], the vitamin, mineral, salt and sugar contents were added by relying on Tables 2 and 3. Because the weight of the supplementary materials is very small, the additional contents are on top of the RIS, PSO and WPI total weight.

Table 2. The nutrient requirements of dysphagia food (the additional contents are on the top of the RIS, PSO and WPI total weight).

Supplementary Materials		GB 29922-2013 for People over 10 Years of Age Special Medical Food Requirements for Nutrients/100 kJ	Nutrient Contents in Mixed Vitamins and Mixed Minerals/g	Additional Contents in Food Bolus
Mixed minerals	Mg (mg)	≥4.4	130	1%
	Fe (mg)	0.20–0.55	9.5	
	Zn (mg)	0.1–0.5	6	
	Ca (mg)	≥13	260	
	P (mg)	≥9.6	189	
Mixed vitamins	VA (μg)	9.3–53.8	3376	0.20%
	VB_1 (mg)	≥0.02	3.906	
	VB_2 (mg)	≥0.02	3.9	
	VB_6 (mg)	≥0.02	3.91	
	VB_{12} (μg)	≥0.03	9.8	
	VC (mg)	≥1.3	525	
	VD (μg)	0.19–0.75	4.075	
	VE (mg)	≥0.19	36	
	Nicotinic acid (mg)	≥0.05	62.5	
	Folic acid (μg)	≥5.3	1300	
	Pantothenic acid (mg)	≥0.07	12.512	
Salt		≤5.0 g/d		0.5%, 1%
Sugar		≤10.0 g/d		0.5%, 1%

Table 3. The design of dysphagia food with supplementary materials (the additional contents are on the top of RIS, PSO and WPI total weight).

Dysphagia Food	RIS:WPI:PSO	Mixed Minerals	Mixed Vitamins	Salt	Sugar
F	70%:20%:10%	-	-	-	-
F-VM		1%	0.2%	-	-
F-0.5%SS		-	-	0.5%	0.5%
F-1%SS		-	-	1%	1%
F-VM + 0.5%SS		1%	0.2%	0.5%	0.5%
F-VM + 1%SS		1%	0.2%	1%	1%

The corresponding proportions of substances were weighed and dissolved in water with stirring to obtain suspensions, which were then heated in a magnetic stirring water bath from room temperature to 95 °C for another 10 min to produce mud-like dysphagia food bolus.

2.3. Water-Holding Capacity (WHC)

The WHC of the food sample was estimated by the centrifugation method [29]. Samples weighing 5 g were centrifuged at 10,000× g for 10 min at room temperature and the supernatants were removed.

$$WHC\ (\%) = (m_2 - m_0)/(m_1 - m_0) \times 100\%, \tag{5}$$

where m_0 is the weight of the empty tube, m_1 is the total weight of the sample and tube before centrifugation, and m_2 is the total weight of the precipitate and tube after centrifugation.

2.4. IDDSI Test Methods

Definitive IDDSI levels of the food bolus were determined by the fork drip test and spoon tilt test [30]. Fork drip test: the samples were held up and examined to see if they would trickle through the tines or prongs of a fork. Spoon tilt test: the states of samples were observed when the spoon was placed steadily and tilted sideways, along with the appearance of the spoon after they slid off.

2.5. Rheological Characterization

In order to better emulate the effects of oral shear on the rheology and viscoelasticity of the food bolus, the samples were equilibrated in a water bath at 37 °C (human body temperature) for 2 h. Then, the sample was set up between parallel plates (40 mm diameter and 1.0 mm gap) equipped with clamps and finally measured by a DHR-2 rheometer (TA Instruments, New Castle, DE, USA) [28].

2.5.1. Steady-State Viscous Flow Tests

Flow sweep was used in shear rates (γ) of 0.1–100 s^{-1} with 1% strain to study the variation of viscous flow behavior, and the flow curves were fitted with a power-law model ($\eta = K\gamma^n$), where consistency K (Pa·s^n), the flow behavior index (n) and the apparent viscosity (η) at 0.1, 1, 10, 50 and 100 s^{-1} of samples were recorded [31].

2.5.2. Small Amplitude Oscillatory Shear Tests

The viscoelastic changes of the dysphagia food bolus were evaluated by the storage modulus (G') and loss modulus (G''), which were examined using an oscillatory frequency model in the frequency range of 0.1 Hz–16 Hz with 1% strain [6,31–33].

2.6. Back Extrusion Test for Swallowing the Food Bolus

The texture properties of the samples were performed using a texture analyzer (TA-XT plus, Stable Micro System Co., London, UK) for the back extrusion test after equilibrating at 37 °C for 2 h [34]. Parameter settings: cylindrical probe was P/36R, the pre-test, test and post-test speeds were 1 mm/s, compression deformation was 15%, and trigger force was 5 g.

2.7. Structural Characteristics Tests

2.7.1. Scanning Electron Microscopy (SEM)

A freeze-dried food bolus was fixed and sprayed on the sample stage with gold via a JFC-1600 ion sputtering device (JEOL Ltd., Tokyo, Japan). The gold-sprayed sample was observed using SEM (JSM6701F, Tokyo, Japan) with 5 kV accelerating voltage, and digital images were captured using XT Microscope-Control software (version FESEM 1.0, JEOL Ltd., Tokyo, Japan) [35].

2.7.2. X-ray Diffraction (XRD) Analysis

Freeze-dried samples were tested at 40 kV and 40 mA with Cu Kα radiation using an X-ray diffractometer (D8 Advance, Bruker, Karlsruhe, Germany). The determined range was from 5° to 40° with a scanning rate of 1 °/min [36].

2.7.3. Confocal Laser Scanning Microscopy (CLSM)

The food bolus (500 mg) was dissolved in 10 mL ultrapure water to prepare the suspension. Nile red solution (0.01% in methanol, *w/v*) and Nile blue A solution (0.01% in methanol, *w/v*) were first mixed in a ratio of 2:1 as the dyeing agent. Then, a 1 mL suspension was mixed with 40 µL dyeing agent for 10 min. The CLSM images were observed by confocal laser scanning microscopy (Leica TCS SP8, Leica Microsystems GmbH, Wetzlar, Germany) with excitation wavelengths of 488 nm and 633 nm, respectively [16].

2.8. Color Measurements

The boluses were laid flat on the bottoms of dishes after being balanced at 37 °C for 2 h, and color parameters (lightness, L*; redness/greenness, a*; yellowness/blueness, b*; chroma, C_{ab}^*; hue, h_{ab}^*; and color variations, ΔE*) were recorded and calculated using a portable colorimeter (HP-2136, Puxi, Shanghai, China) [37].

$$C_{ab}^* = [(a^*)^2 + (b^*)^2]^{1/2} \tag{6}$$

$$h_{ab}^* = \arctan(b^*/a^*) \tag{7}$$

$$\Delta E^* = [(\Delta L^*)^2 + (\Delta a^*)^2 + (\Delta b^*)^2]^{1/2} \tag{8}$$

2.9. Sensory Evaluation

The sensory evaluation conformed with the ethical and testing requirements in the national standard (GB/T 10220-2012) published by the Standardization Administration of China [38]. A team of 6 students aged 20–25 years, majoring in food science and having undergone courses in sensory analysis, took part in the study as panelists. Before sensory testing, the evaluation participants were trained in dysphagia, dysphagia foods and scoring criteria for each indicator to ensure that the evaluation results were informative [10,34,37]. Samples were kept at 37 °C for evaluation, and water was provided for oral rinsing after each sample was tested to avoid bias [16]. The evaluation criteria for sensory evaluation were referred from the studies by Ribes et al. [37] and Xie et al. [16], and color, organization, taste, flavor, adhesion and swallowing were selected (Table 4). The scores of every level were referred from the study by Xie et al. [16]. In order to emphasize the swallowing characteristics of the food bolus, the scores of each criterion were modified, especially the percentage of the swallowing score in the total score, which was increased.

Table 4. Score criteria for the sensory evaluation of dysphagia samples.

Criteria	Standard for Evaluation	Score
Color	Not uniform	0–6
	Generally uniform	7–11
	Very uniform	12–16
Organization	Loose structure, poor elasticity and chewiness.	0–6
	Tight structure, normal elasticity and chewiness	7–11
	Tight structure, good elasticity and chewiness	12–16
Taste	Poor taste and hard texture	0–6
	Average taste and soft texture	7–11
	Good taste and soft texture	12–16
Flavor	Strange smell and unacceptable	0–6
	Light smell and acceptable	7–11
	Good smell and very acceptable	12–16
Adhesion	More oral residue after swallowing	0–6
	Less oral residue after swallowing	7–11
	No residue in oral after swallowing	12–16
Swallowing	Hard to swallow	0–7
	Normal to swallow	8–13
	Easy to swallow	14–20

2.10. Statistical Analysis

Data are expressed as mean ± SD for at least triplicate determinations, while IBM SPSS Statistics (version 26.0, Chicago, IL, USA) and OriginPro (version 9.0, Stat-Ease Company, Northampton, MA, USA) software were used for statistical analysis, and one-way ANOVA

3. Results

3.1. Construction of the Dysphagia Food System

3.1.1. WHC and IDDSI Level of the Dysphagia Food System

The mixed suspensions of RIS, WPI and PSO were heated to form different textural dysphagia food boluses by cross-linking interactions between each other and the water molecules [39]. Under the heating process, starch molecules absorb water and expand, the crystalline structures are broken, and on cooling, starch molecules are rearranged to form a stable gel system [29]. Proteins and oils can be present in the gel network formed by the rearrangement of starch molecules to form starch–protein complexes, starch–oil complexes or starch–protein–oil complexes [40]. Evaluation of the physicochemical properties of potato-starch-based foods and their interactions with milk protein and soybean oil was carried out. When the RIS content was definite, comparing samples A and D, samples B and E, and samples C and F, it was found that WPI could give better WHC to the swallowed food bolus than PSO, which may be due to the fact that proteins with more hydrophilic groups are more likely to cross-link with starch to form more hydrogen bonds, and possess better hydrophilicity than hydrophobic oils [40] The food bolus showed the best water holding capacity when RIS was 70%, PSO was 10% and WPI was 20% (Figure 1A). The better WHC endowed the dysphagia food bolus with a softer texture and more lubrication with less resistance in accessing the esophagus and stomach [16].

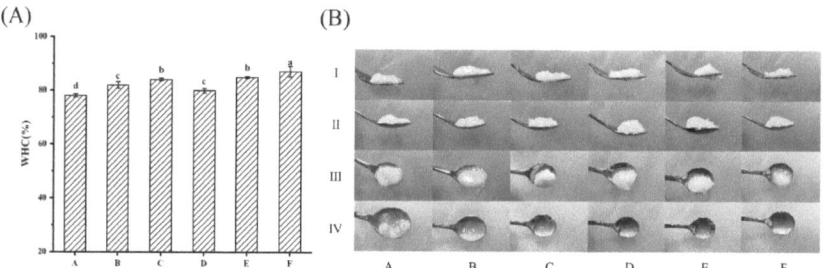

Figure 1. The water holding capacity (**A**) of gels used to construct the dysphagia food system. The different letters are significantly different ($p < 0.05$). IDDSI tests (**B**) of gels used to construct the dysphagia food system. A–F are prepared dysphagia food bulus rely on Table 1. The fork driptest (I raw) and spoon tilttest (II, III and IV raws corresponding before, during and aftertilting the spoon).

From the fork drip test (Figure 1(B-I)), all samples accumulated over the fork top and formed a fishtail shape underneath but did not drip off. In the spoon tilt test (Figure 1 (B-II~IV)), the samples were able to stack well on the spoon and slowly slide off when tilted, indicating that all six samples may be classified as level 4 (pureed) of the IDDSI framework [14]. Samples D, E and F slipped from the spoon with only a very small residue and a clear film appeared on the spoon surface, while samples A and B had much larger residues, which suggested that boluses A (PSO:RIS:WPI = 15%:60%:25%) and B (PSO:RIS:WPI = 15%:65%:20%) could be highly susceptible to residual food debris in the pharynx, with a strong risk of accidental aspiration during swallowing [1].

3.1.2. Rheological Properties

As shown in Figure 2, the apparent viscosity of all samples decreased with increasing shear rate, exhibiting a shear thinning behavior, which was suitable for dysphagia patients to slow down the swallowing process [41]. Sample F (PSO:RIS:WPI = 10%:70%:20%) exhibited the highest apparent viscosity (η) and also a lower flow behavior index ($n = 0.193 \pm 0.005$), indicating more pseudoplastic behavior and better safety of swallowing [42].

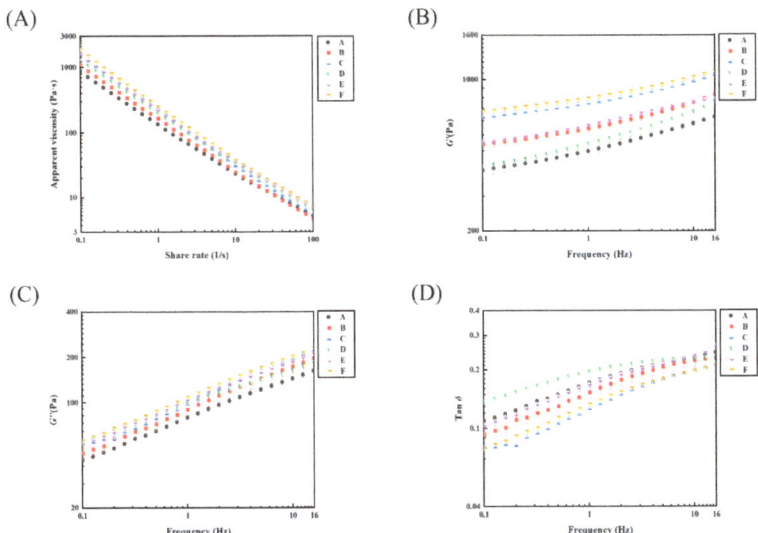

Figure 2. Apparent viscosity (**A**), storage modulus (G') (**B**), loss modulus (G'') (**C**) and loss factor (Tanδ) (**D**) curves of the dysphagia food system.

The loss factor Tanδ is the ratio of loss modulus (G'') to storage modulus (G'), which indicates the viscoelastic characteristics [42]. When the food Tanδ is higher than 1, it is harder to control for people with poor chewing and swallowing abilities, because the food tends to be more liquid and its flow rate is higher and difficult to control, so that it could easily enter the airway to cause choking and coughing [41]. For dysphagia patients, a soft gel with a Tanδ less than 1 is very suitable, not only because the flow rate is easy to control, but the food is more easily deformed and passed smoothly through the esophagus [41]. G' is greater than G'' for all samples, which is the distinctive feature of dysphagia foods [43]. Similar viscoelastic patterns are shown in Figure 2B–D, but F exhibited the highest modulus values than the others, especially G'. This shows the high elasticity property of food bolus F. The Tanδ value also indicates the energy loss of the food during chewing and compression [43] Among all samples, F had the smallest Tanδ, indicating that F could require less energy to be consumed during chewing and compression, which is easier for dysphagia patients. In order to make the swallowing of the food bolus safer, the F bolus with 70% RIS, 10% PSO and 20% WPI was chosen to continue the investigation of the effects of the supplementary materials on the texture and swallowing characteristics.

3.1.3. The CLSM of the Food Bolus

In order to verify the feasibility of the food bolus construction, CLSM was used to observe the food bolus structure, especially the distribution of oils and proteins, as the content of both was lower than that of starch. Proteins and oils were stained with Nile blue A and Nile red, respectively. Protein was marked in green (Figure 3a), and oil was marked in red (Figure 3b). From the results, the protein and oil could be uniformly dispersed in the gel system. In the combined image of them (Figure 3c), the common distribution of green and red indicates that the mixing distribution of protein and oil in food bolus F was relatively consistent, which also shows that the three materials could be well mixed in the starch-based system from the side [16]. The result indicates that the food bolus construction is successful.

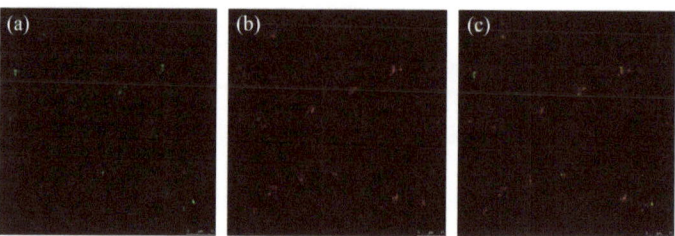

Figure 3. The CLSM images of food bolus F. From left to right are WPI staining with Nile blue A (**a**), WPI staining with Nile red (**b**), and the combination of the two (**c**), respectively.

3.2. Effects of Supplementary Materials on the WHC of the Food Bolus

The effects of different supplementary materials on the WHC of the dysphagia food bolus are shown in Figure 4A. Compared to F, VM did not significantly affect the WHC of the food system ($p < 0.05$), but the 1% SS caused a clear increase from 87.69 ± 0.49% to 90.13 ± 0.53%. In the formative dysphagia gel system, salt ions might contribute to an enhanced hydrophobic interaction that blocked the migration of free water to trap more water in gel space [44]. It has been reported that sucrose could also enhance the WHC of the system by forming some small cavities in gels [45]. However, compared to F-SS, the WHC of F-VM-SS was reduced by the addition of VM, which could be attributed to the fact that the released Ca^{2+} and Mg^{2+} resulted from the presence of Cl^- replacing Na^+. Furthermore, the Ca^{2+} increased the linkage between proteins and weakened the cross-linking among different molecules, leading to the aggregation of proteins and the formation of a rough gel structure, with a decrease in WHC [35].

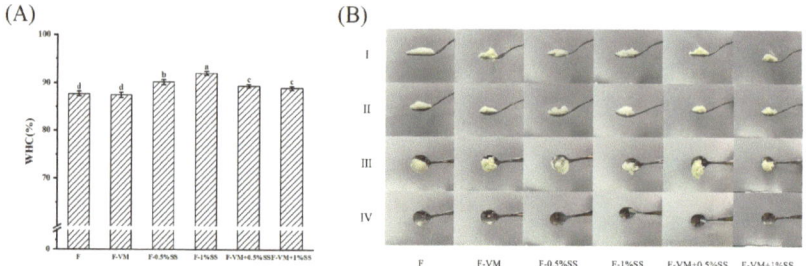

Figure 4. The WHC (**A**) of the food boluses with supplementary. The different letters are significantly different ($p < 0.05$). IDDSI tests (**B**) of the food boluses with supplementary materials. The fork driptest (I raw) and spoon tilttest (II, III and IV raws corresponding before, during and aftertilting the spoon).

3.3. Classification of the Dysphagia Food Bolus with Supplementary Materials

The results of the fork drip test and spoon tilt test for all samples based on the IDDSI framework are shown in Figure 4B. From the fork drip result, all samples could be well stacked on the top of the fork and there was no dripping from the slit. The samples could accumulate well above the spoon and slide slowly when tilted, indicating that the gels all belonged to level 4 (pureed foods) in the IDDSI framework [14]. However, after slipping down, there were still small residues of F-VM and F-VM + 1%SS sticking to the spoon surface, which is unsafe for dysphagia patients. After swallowing, less material still remained in the pharynx and did not enter the esophagus, leading to a more dispersed bolus, which could have a high probability of slipping into the trachea and causing serious aspiration [1]. Compared to the F bolus with a clear film on the spoon, F-0.5%SS, F-1%SS and F-VM + 0.5%SS were found to have better swallowing characteristics in that spoons were clearer and smoother after slipping off, making them more suitable for those suffering from dysphagia.

3.4. Rheological Analysis of the Effects of Supplementary Materials on the Food Bolus

3.4.1. Flow Rheological Properties of the Food Bolus with Supplementary Materials

Figure 5A shows the viscous flow behavior of samples with added excipient. At the shear rate of 50 s^{-1}, which was simulated for normal human oral chewing, the apparent viscosities (η) of the food bolus were enhanced with SS, while decreased with VM (Table 5). However, the elderly or dysphagia groups have impaired chewing and swallowing abilities, which prevents the oral shear rate from increasing to 50 s^{-1} [46]. Herranz et al. rheologically characterized three commercial thickening products for dysphagia patients. They highlighted the importance of measuring the viscosity at low shear rates as a transient increase in apparent viscosity of the bolus is accompanied by the decrease in shear rate associated with the swallowing process [6]. The lower shear rates of 0.1, 1 and 10 s^{-1} were chosen to compare the η values of food samples. The addition of VM increased the η of the food system compared to F, while at 50 s^{-1}, it decreased. This suggests that F-VM may be more suitable for dysphagia patients than F at lower shear rates, and also that F-VM could have stronger shear thinning. This may provide the possibility for people with varying degrees of swallowing problems to choose foods with the appropriate apparent viscosity and shear characteristics to suit them better [6] The food bolus with SS already added showed a similar tendency, where VM reduced the n at 50, 10, 1 and 0.1 s^{-1} shear rates. The strong water absorption of SS led to more water molecules present in systems with enhanced η, while the divalent mineral ions were involved in hindering intermolecular linkages resulting in a decreased η [16,35]. The flow behavior index (n) was obtained by fitting a power-law model to flow curves from six groups, and significant differences were observed ($p < 0.05$). The curves were in good agreement with R^2 higher than 0.95 [47]. As shown in Table 5, all supplementary materials decreased the n values and increased the shear thinning behaviors of the gel system. The η of thickened products would be reduced to a very small value with the increasing shear rate at a lower n value, which did not facilitate swallowing [48]. Nevertheless, the samples in this study were maintained in the range of pudding-type food consistency (K) in the NDD standard even at higher shear rates, which could enable a safe swallowing process [49].

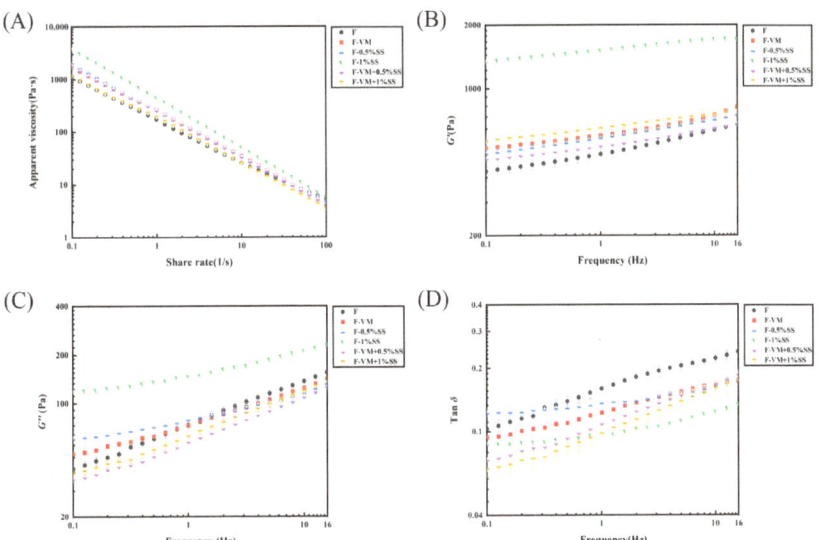

Figure 5. Apparent viscosity (**A**), storage modulus (G') (**B**), loss modulus (G'') (**C**) and loss factor (Tanδ) (**D**) curves of the food boluses with supplementary materials.

Table 5. Steady flow and dynamic rheological parameters of dysphagia food with supplementary materials.

Sample	F	F-VM	F-0.5%SS	F-1%SS	F-VM + 0.5%SS	F-VM + 1%SS
			Flow Sweep			
$\eta_{0.1}$ (Pa·s)	1124 ± 50 [c]	1740 ± 45 [b]	1857 ± 85 [b]	3863 ± 151 [a]	1850 ± 53 [b]	1155 ± 16 [c]
η_1 (Pa·s)	167.2 ± 10.3 [d]	263.6 ± 6.2 [b]	257.2 ± 5.2 [b]	462.7 ± 14.1 [a]	258.2 ± 3.3 [b]	192.0 ± 0.8 [c]
η_{10} (Pa·s)	26.70 ± 2.02 [c]	35.17 ± 0.77 [b]	33.87 ± 1.15 [b]	52.20 ± 1.47 [a]	33.74 ± 0.50 [b]	25.75 ± 0.14 [c]
η_{50} (Pa·s)	8.437 ± 0.434 [b]	7.842 ± 0.238 [b]	8.220 ± 0.450 [b]	11.39 ± 0.28 [a]	7.894 ± 0.155 [b]	6.443 ± 0.025 [c]
K (Pa·s^n)	168.9 ± 10.2 [c]	247.7 ± 3.5 [b]	258.8 ± 9.9 [b]	459.2 ± 13.7 [a]	249.3 ± 4.8 [b]	179.1 ± 2.5 [c]
n (-)	0.225 ± 0.008 [a]	0.130 ± 0.009 [c]	0.122 ± 0.005 [c]	0.055 ± 0.002 [d]	0.125 ± 0.004 [c]	0.159 ± 0.005 [b]
R^2 (Power law)	0.988	0.981	0.992	0.970	0.962	0.982
			Frequency Sweep			
G'_{1Hz} (Pa)	487.3 ± 26.7 [d]	598.1 ± 12.6 [bc]	582.9 ± 4.5 [bc]	1521 ± 44 [a]	533.1 ± 10.0 [cd]	643.7 ± 52.4 [b]
G''_{1Hz} (Pa)	74.13 ± 4.13 [b]	73.31 ± 2.08 [b]	79.72 ± 6.72 [b]	148.0 ± 2.3 [a]	58.20 ± 3.33 [c]	62.40 ± 3.06 [c]
Tan δ_{1Hz} (-)	0.159 ± 0.010 [a]	0.123 ± 0.002 [bc]	0.137 ± 0.010 [b]	0.097 ± 0.003 [d]	0.109 ± 0.004 [cd]	0.098 ± 0.009 [d]
G'_0	498.7 ± 22.2 [d]	613.2 ± 11.6 [b]	587.3 ± 10.5 [bc]	1517 ± 41 [a]	541.4 ± 9.3 [cd]	648.3 ± 50.8 [b]
n'	0.094 ± 0.005 [a]	0.075 ± 0.001 [c]	0.082 ± 0.004 [b]	0.055 ± 0.002 [e]	0.072 ± 0.003 [c]	0.065 ± 0.002 [d]
R^2 (Power law)	0.990	0.976	0.992	0.985	0.991	0.995
G''_0	74.80 ± 3.83 [b]	75.31 ± 2.16 [b]	81.00 ± 5.94 [b]	152.0 ± 3.5 [a]	58.94 ± 2.88 [c]	63.83 ± 3.31 [c]
n''	0.251 ± 0.002 [b]	0.212 ± 0.002 [c]	0.148 ± 0.010 [d]	0.134 ± 0.002 [e]	0.264 ± 0.007 [a]	0.267 ± 0.001 [a]
R^2 (Power law)	0.988	0.994	0.982	0.980	0.996	0.976

Mean values ± standard deviation. For each rheological property, mean values without the same letter in the same row are significantly different ($p < 0.05$). $\eta_{0.1}$, η_1, η_{10}, η_{50} and η_{100}, apparent viscosities at shear rates 0.1, 1, 10, 50 and 100 s^{-1}; K and n, consistency and flow behavior index from the power-law model; R^2, determination coefficient of power-law model; G'_{1Hz}, storage modulus at 1 Hz; G''_{1Hz}, loss modulus at 1 Hz; Tanδ_{1Hz}, loss factor at 1 Hz; G'_0 and G''_0, correspond to G' and G'' values with frequency (f) at 1 Hz; n' and n'', regression coefficients relating G' and G'' with frequency (f) in Hz.

3.4.2. Viscoelastic Properties of Food Boluses with Supplementary Materials

The curves of the dynamic flow properties of all samples are shown in Figure 5B–D. SS significantly increased the G' and G'' of the samples in a dose-dependent manner ($p < 0.05$). However, VM was observed to reduce the modulus increases, which was consistent with the variation in steady-state flow characteristics. In the gel system of dysphagia foods, mineral ions might interact with starch and protein molecules through hydrogen bonds or van der Waals forces to modify their own mechanical properties. Similar conclusions were obtained when Ca^{2+} was used to act on jicama starches and proteins, reducing the viscosity and gel strength [35,50,51]. In addition, the G' and G'' of all samples were increased with an increase in angular frequency, and were fitted with power-law functions ($G' = G_0' f n'$ and $G'' = G_0'' f n''$) to account for modulus dependence on frequency [6], where n' and n'' denote the dependence of G' and G'' on frequency (f), respectively. As shown in Table 5, SS induced a decrease in the n' value of gels, resulting in a lower dependence of G' on f, suggesting that SS could support stronger molecular interactions to promote more powerful gels [52]. The n' values were similar to the nectar and pudding-like products for dysphagia [53]. The VM and SS had positive effects on the elastic properties of the prepared gel system, with G'_{1Hz} increased (Table 5). Compared to the bolus with SS alone, although F-VM-SS significantly reduced the G' and G'' ($p < 0.05$), there was no significant difference in Tanδ, indicating that the equilibrium of the elastic–viscous system in the samples was not changed remarkably.

3.5. Effects of Supplementary Materials on the Mechanical Properties of the Food Bolus

The acceptability of dysphagia food is highly correlated with food texture. For dysphagia patients, better springiness, greater cohesiveness, higher softness and easier chewiness are preferred [54]. SS increased the springiness, chewiness and resilience of the food bolus (Table 6), which is beneficial for dysphagia patients, allowing food to pass smoothly through the pharynx into the esophagus. A high level of Na^+ in salt could promote molecular connection and strong water absorption could promote the formation of gels with a more solid network structure [36,55], thus improving food texture. However, the positive effect of SS was weakened when all materials were present together. In a study of calcium-ion-induced

Mesona chinensis polysaccharide–whey protein isolate gels, it was found that calcium ions increased protein–protein linkage, decreased protein–polysaccharide cross-linking, and weakened gel strength [35]. More divalent ions in VM were released to drown out Na^+, which served as the bridge to strengthen cross-linking between the same molecules and weaken that between different molecules [53]. Compared with the SS-only food bolus, chewiness and resilience were reduced, but springiness was not significantly different, suggesting that F-VM+SS was still acceptable to dysphagia patients. The cohesiveness of the six groups was no different. Although SS and VM significantly increased the hardness and gumminess of the food bolus, they decreased when all supplementary materials were present at the same time. This suggests that the risk of accidental aspiration was likely to be minimal when both SS and VM were present, while the texture of the food bolus was likely to be the softest [4]. In addition, F-VM-1%SS showed a more pronounced decrease in texture than powders containing 0.5% SS (e.g., chewiness decreased from 271.5 ± 31.4 to 182.5 ± 7.0 at 0.5% added, and from 354.7 ± 28.5 to 211.3 ± 44.1 at 1% added). There was no significant difference in mechanical properties between the F-VM + 0.5%SS and F-VM + 1%SS boluses in the study, but a better textural property was still observed than without any supplementary materials.

Table 6. Effect of supplementary materials on the textural features of food boluses.

Sample	Hardness (g)	Springiness	Cohesiveness	Gumminess	Chewiness	Resilience
F	200.9 ± 18.0 [c]	0.884 ± 0.010 [ab]	0.672 ± 0.053 [ab]	134.8 ± 13.1 [d]	119.0 ± 10.5 [d]	0.136 ± 0.008 [c]
F-VM	395.7 ± 19.2 [b]	0.940 ± 0.010 [a]	0.647 ± 0.059 [abc]	275.0 ± 18.3 [b]	241.3 ± 31.6 [bc]	0.261 ± 0.069 [ab]
F-0.5%SS	534.4 ± 10.8 [a]	0.911 ± 0.027 [a]	0.556 ± 0.038 [c]	308.8 ± 21.0 [b]	271.5 ± 31.4 [b]	0.204 ± 0.040 [abc]
F-1%SS	563.5 ± 71.5 [a]	0.929 ± 0.032 [a]	0.683 ± 0.040 [a]	382.0 ± 29.0 [a]	354.7 ± 28.5 [a]	0.281 ± 0.033 [a]
F-VM + 0.5%SS	377.0 ± 21.3 [b]	0.850 ± 0.037 [b]	0.571 ± 0.028 [bc]	217.7 ± 2.4 [c]	182.5 ± 7.0 [c]	0.165 ± 0.035 [bc]
F-VM + 1%SS	392.4 ± 76.1 [b]	0.884 ± 0.026 [ab]	0.608 ± 0.033 [abc]	206.1 ± 5.3 [c]	211.3 ± 44.1 [bc]	0.254 ± 0.070 [ab]

Mean values ± standard deviation. Mean values without the same letter in the same column are significantly different ($p < 0.05$).

3.6. Effects of Supplementary Materials on the Microstructure the Food Bolus

SEM could provide better visualization of the interior structural changes in the samples [56]. The samples without any supplementary materials showed a laminar structure with one piece pressed on top of the other (Figure 6A). The addition of VM contributed to larger holes and erratic cross-linking (Figure 6A). After SS was mixed, a few regular gel networks could be clearly observed, giving the bolus a harder texture and better gel quality. In a study of the influence of Nacl on gel properties of *Mesona chinensis* polysaccharide–maize starches, it was found that Na^+ contributed to forming honeycomb network structure gels and enhanced the interaction between starch and polysaccharide molecules through electrostatic interactions to form stronger gels [52]. Moreover, a rupture of gel structure was observed when adding VM to the system containing SS, which explains why the food softened when all supplementary materials were added. The presence of more divalent ions may induce aggregation between homo-molecules, while breaking bonds and connections between different molecules such as proteins and starches [53].

XRD is an effective method for evaluating the crystal structure of dysphagia food boluses [57]. The XRD patterns of dysphagia food were all similar, with a broader diffraction peak at 2θ of 20° owing to amorphous structures (Figure 6B). A very broad dispersion peak was shown between 2θ of 10°–30° in the XRD spectrum under the modified waxy maize starch with saturated fatty acid chlorides, which was attributed to the broken starch crystal structure finally being converted to an amorphous one [56]. The addition of supplementary materials did not affect the general view of the diffraction pattern of the gel systems.

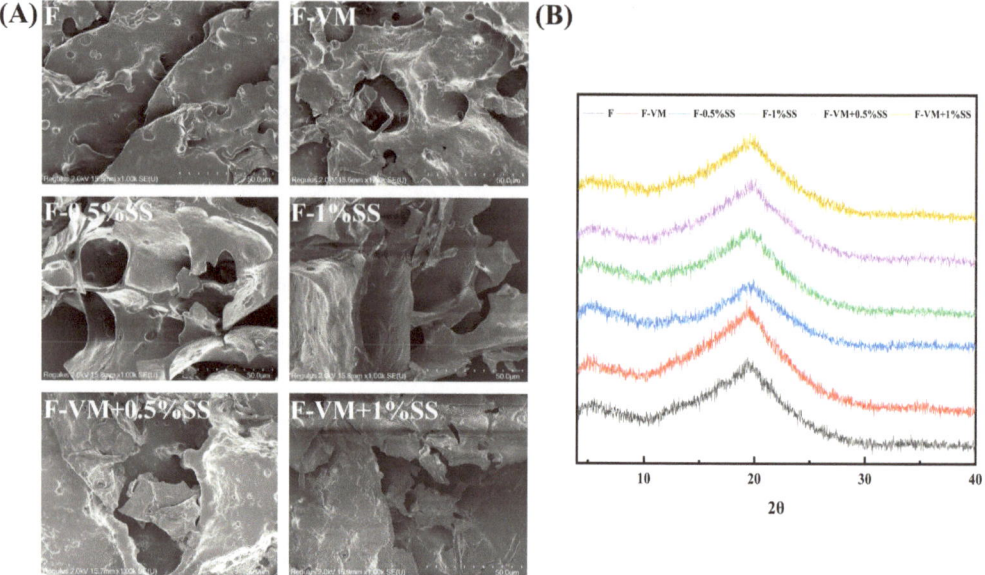

Figure 6. Scanning electron micrographs (**A**) and X-ray diffraction curves (**B**) of food boluses with supplementary materials.

3.7. Effects of Supplementary Materials on the Color Properties of the Food Bolus

In relation to color analysis (Figure 7A–C and Table 7), the b* and C_{ab}^* values of the F-VM, F-VM + 0.5%SS and F-VM + 1%SS pellets were significantly higher than those of F ($p < 0.05$), and the ΔE^* values were larger, most likely because various vitamins contained in VM added more yellow to the food bolus. In VM, VB_2, also known as riboflavin, is bright yellow and exists stably under heating in neutral conditions, VC and VA powders are generally slightly yellow, VE is yellow-green, folic acid takes the form of yellowish crystals or flakes, and pantothenic acid is a yellowish sticky material [23]. In addition, nicotinic acid and VB_2 are more stable under heating conditions, which could better maintain their nutritional properties [23]. The gel system with a network structure formed by the complexation of starch, protein, oil and water has a good protection effect on unstable VC, VE, folic acid and pantothenic acid. Proteins and oils could form a V-shaped wrapping structure through hydrogen bonding after starch molecules absorb water and expand, which could better wrap or load vitamins without being broken and protect the nutritional activity [58]. Soybean isolate protein and pectin particles formed a gel system with a definite network structure as a delivery system which could increase the encapsulation rate of VE up to 72.1 ± 5.9% and exhibit good in vitro antioxidant activity [58]. Adding VM together increased the L* of the system compared to adding SS alone to the food bolus. The L* value reflects the brightness of food. It may be attributed to the fact that the addition of VM gave the food F-SS a softer structure and a smaller particle size to scatter more light [59]. Fish sauce with repeated grinding possessed a smaller particle size and an increased specific surface area, which increased the brightness value of fish sauce by scattering more light [16]. Compared with F, in F-0.5%SS and F-1%SS it was found that SS could marginally reduce L*, b*, C_{ab}^* and h_{ab}^* values and their ΔE^* values were also smaller at 5.325 ± 0.324 and 8.364 ± 0.140. However, SS did not affect color changing and the yellow color increase brought by VM to the food, observed in F-VM + 0.5%SS and F-VM + 1%SS.

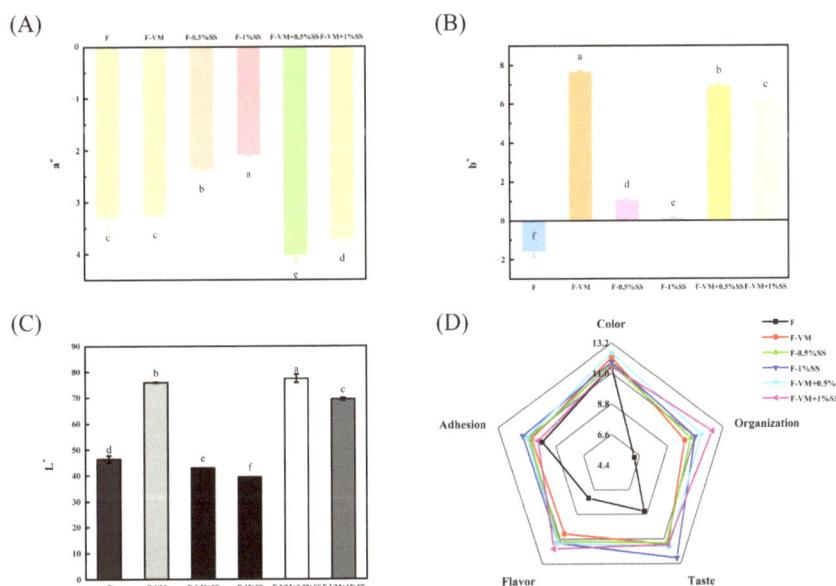

Figure 7. Redness/greenness, a* (**A**), yellowness/blueness, b* (**B**), lightness, L* (**C**) and average scores of sensory evaluations (**D**) of dysphagia food with supplementary materials. The different letters are significantly different ($p < 0.05$).

Table 7. Effect of supplementary materials on the color and sensory parameters of the dysphagia food boluses.

Sample	Chroma			Sensory Test	
	C_{ab}^*	h_{ab}^*	ΔE^*	Swallowing	Total Score
F	4.300 ± 0.654 [c]	0.422 ± 0.055 [a]	-	11.17 ± 2.27 [c]	54.50 ± 3.04 [c]
F-0VM	8.335 ± 0.068 [a]	−1.169 ± 0.010 [e]	29.84 ± 0.32 [b]	11.33 ± 1.11 [c]	66.33 ± 4.64 [b]
F-0.5%SS	2.465 ± 0.052 [d]	−0.371 ± 0.080 [c]	5.325 ± 0.324 [e]	13.00 ± 1.41 [ab]	68.67 ± 3.77 [ab]
F-1%SS	2.079 ± 0.033 [e]	−0.057 ± 0.031 [b]	8.364 ± 0.140 [d]	15.00 ± 1.63 [a]	73.17 ± 2.48 [a]
F-VM + 0.5%SS	7.999 ± 0.115 [a]	−1.048 ± 0.015 [d]	31.18 ± 1.58 [a]	14.17 ± 1.67 [a]	72.17 ± 4.74 [a]
F-VM + 1%SS	7.174 ± 0.065 [b]	−1.043 ± 0.020 [d]	23.11 ± 1.05 [c]	13.00 ± 1.15 [ab]	70.33 ± 3.59 [ab]

Mean values ± standard deviation. Mean values without the same letter in the same column are significantly different ($p < 0.05$). C_{ab}^*, chroma; h_{ab}^*, hue; ΔE^*, color variations.

3.8. Sensory Evaluation

The addition of supplementary materials could significantly increase the organization, taste and flavor of the primary food system, with no difference in color and adhesion. Among all samples, F-VM + 0.5%SS had the most consistent color, while F-VM + 1%SS provided an optimal flavor and the best organization; F-1%SS also tasted the best and had the least residue after swallowing (Figure 7D). Furthermore, F-VM + 0.5%SS obtained a higher sensory total score than F-VM + 1%SS (72.17 ± 4.74 vs. 70.33 ± 3.59) (Table 7). For swallowing ease, F-1%SS and F-VM + 0.5%SS were rated as easy to swallow and the other samples were swallowed normally. However, the swallowing scores of food groups with SS were both significantly higher than those of F and F-VM ($p < 0.05$), which is consistent with the IDDSI test results.

3.9. Relationship between Rheology, Texture and Sense

Focusing on the correlation between indexes can be beneficial for the development of dysphagia foods. As shown in Figure 8, the WHC of samples had a mostly strong positive correlation with both textural properties and rheological values (r ⩾ 0.72). This suggests that the WHC could affect the organization and gel properties of samples. The F-1%SS bolus with the best WHC obtained the highest gumminess, chewiness and rheological scores, as well as good taste in the sensory evaluation. This was most likely due to the increased molecular cross-linking, and gel cavities formed to seal in water and strengthen the gel network structure. Similarly, in a study of the effects of psyllium on corn starch properties, the gel rheology and pasting properties were modified because psyllium brought an increase in water-holding capacity [60]. The chewiness, resilience, gel strength and G' of steamed cold noodles were enhanced when the WHC of egg whites on wheat starch gel food was increased from 87% to 94%, relying on the interaction between protein and starch molecules to form a more powerful network [61]. In addition, the texture properties were generally correlated positively with the K (0.82 ⩾ r ⩾ 0.25), G' (0.78 ⩾ r ⩾ 0.42) and G'' (0.74 ⩾ r ⩾ 0.41), but negatively with n (−0.39 ⩾ r ⩾ −0.85). Among the sensory attributes, organization, taste and adhesion were all strongly correlated with hardness (0.69 ⩾ r ⩾ 0.59), chewiness (0.48 ⩾ r ⩾ 0.58) and gumminess (0.60 ⩾ r ⩾ 0.54) in texture indicators, although springiness (0.14 ⩾ r ⩾ 0.02) and cohesiveness (−0.09 ⩾ r ⩾ −0.25) were weakly correlated. It is suggested that supplementary materials affect the viscoelasticity and spatial structure of systems by influencing the contact and interaction between different components in the network, thus affecting the swallowing experiences of food gels. In the preparation of chia seed mucilage-modified soups, the maximum area value and the maximum force value in the texture test were shown to have a strong positive correlation with the oral consistency in swallowing properties [62]. At a lower shear rate of $10\ \mathrm{s}^{-1}$, there was a strong relationship between taste (r = 0.62), adhesion (r = 0.67) and apparent viscosity (η), indicating that high-viscosity food boluses are less likely to remain in the oral cavity after chewing, with less swallowing-induced malabsorption and discomfort. The Tanδ value, the information about the balance of the viscoelastic modulus, was negatively linked to sensory properties (−0.43 ⩾ r ⩾ −0.79) and swallowing ease evaluation (r = −0.76), suggesting that samples with higher G' and lower G'' might be more favored by dysphagia populations. It has been reported that foods with great resistance to deformation (high G^* values) and great elasticity (low Tanδ values) could be safe to swallow [6]. Thus, rheological and textural data can be used to provide some indication of the swallowing characteristics of foods. In this study, water-holding capacity, apparent viscosity, springiness, chewiness, consistency and loss modulus were important indicators for regulating food swallowing abilities.

In the principal component analysis (PCA) results (Figure 9), PC1 and PC2 explained 81.5% of the total variance, with PC1 accounting for 62.9% and PC2 for 18.6%, respectively. The inter-index relationship analysis in the loading plot (Figure 9A) yielded results consistent with Figure 8, where G'_{1Hz}, G''_{1Hz}, η_{10}, K, gumminess, resilience, water holding capacity, hardness and chewiness were strongly positively related with taste, organization and swallowing behavior, while strongly negatively related with η and Tanδ. The lower flow behavior index n indicates that the sample's apparent viscosity reduces more quickly with increasing shear rates, which in turn means that the sample has a correspondingly high viscosity at lower shear rates. Since dysphagia patients typically have a lower oral shear rate, chewing higher-viscosity foods helps them eat and replenish nutrients [8]. In the score plot (Figure 9B), the dot of F was visually distant from the other samples, suggesting that the addition of supplementary materials had greater effects on food system properties. VM and SS made a large difference in food groups on PC1. However, VM slowed down the promotion of salt ions on food gels, which was in line with the rheological property results. F-VM + 0.5%SS and F-VM + 1%SS do not differ either on PC1 or on PC2. However, by comparing with F-0.5%SS and F-1%SS, VM exerted a greater effect when SS content was higher, especially on PC2. Therefore, the comprehensive picture showed that the F-VM + 0.5%SS food bolus was more suitable for dysphagia patients, due to its good texture, high total sensory score and appropriate swallowing ease.

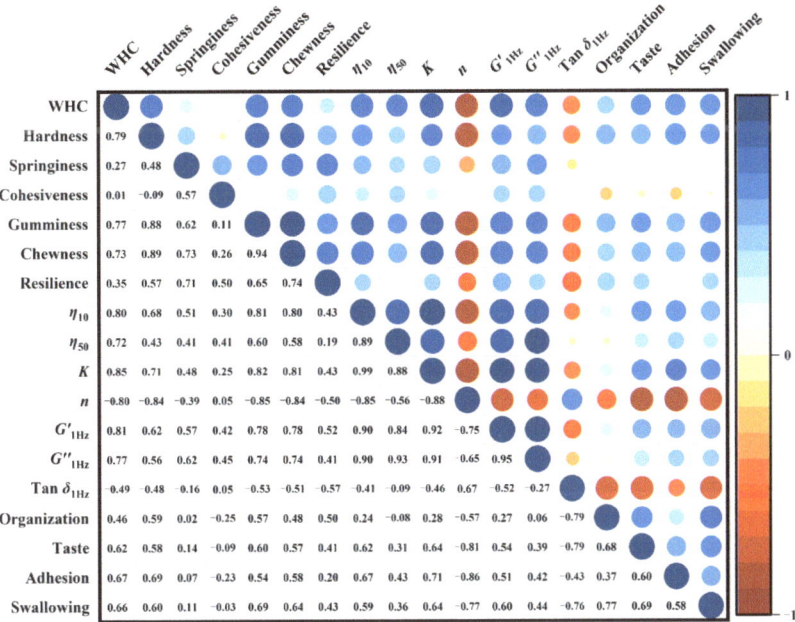

Figure 8. The correlation analysis between rheology, texture and sense of dysphagia food boluses. Blue represents a positive correlation and red represents a negative correlation.

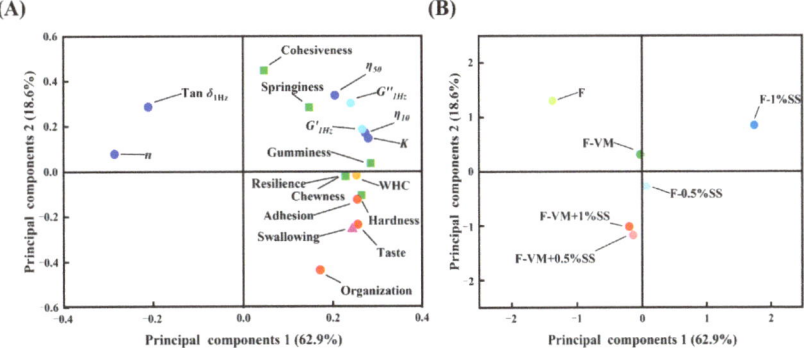

Figure 9. Principal component analysis (loading plot (**A**) and scores plot (**B**)) of dysphagia food with supplementary materials.

4. Conclusions

This work demonstrated that four supplementary materials (VM and SS) affected the texture, flow properties and swallowing characteristics of a food bolus, and all samples belonged to the pureed level 4 in the IDDSI framework. SS changed the spatial structure and viscoelasticity of the gel system by enhancing the intermolecular interaction forces, resulting in a more networked gel pattern, which increased the water-holding capacity, viscosity, storage modulus, chewiness and swallowing ability of dysphagia foods. VM could endow the food bolus with richer color characteristics but increased the residues on the spoon, with the attendant risk of accidental aspiration. F-VM + 0.5%SS obtained a better evaluation than F-VM + 1%SS in terms of sensory properties and swallowing ease. In addition, the texture and fluidity of a bolus also showed a strong correlation with swallowing characteristics. The information provided in this work should help to prepare nutritional dysphagia foods, but the mechanism of supplementary materials acting together to influence food swallowing still needs to be explored more deeply.

Author Contributions: Conceptualization, X.W. and J.X.; methodology, X.W. and J.X.; supervision and validation, J.X., Q.Y., Y.C. and M.S.; formal analysis, X.W.; resources, J.X. and M.S.; data curation, X.W.; writing—original draft, X.W.; writing—review and editing, L.R., J.L. and J.X. All authors have read and agreed to the published version of the manuscript.

Funding: This study was financially supported by the Program of the National Natural Science Foundation of China (31972034).

Institutional Review Board Statement: The sensory evaluation conformed with ethical and testing requirements in the national standard (GB/T 10220-2012) published by the Standardization Administration of China.

Data Availability Statement: The data used to support the findings of this study can be made available by the corresponding author upon request.

Conflicts of Interest: The authors declare that they have no conflict of interest.

References

1. Marconati, M.; Engmann, J.; Burbidge, A.S.; Mathieu, V.; Souchon, I.; Ramaioli, M. A review of the approaches to predict the ease of swallowing and post swallow residues. *Trends Food Sci. Technol.* **2019**, *86*, 281–297. [CrossRef]
2. Andersen, U.T.; Beck, A.M.; Kjaersgaard, A.; Hansen, T.; Poulsen, I. Systematic review and evidence based recommendations on texture modified foods and thickened fluids for adults (≥18 years) with oropharyngeal dysphagia. *e-SPEN J.* **2013**, *8*, e127–e134. [CrossRef]
3. Kou, W.; Pandolfino, J.E.; Kahrilas, P.J.; Patankar, N.A. Simulation studies of the role of esophageal mucosa in bolus transport. *Biomech. Model. Mechanobiol.* **2017**, *16*, 1001–1009. [CrossRef] [PubMed]
4. Pant, A.; Lee, A.Y.; Karyappa, R.; Lee, C.P.; An, J.; Hashimoto, M.; Tan, U.-X.; Wong, G.; Chua, C.K.; Zhang, Y. 3D food printing of fresh vegetables using food hydrocolloids for dysphagic patients. *Food Hydrocoll.* **2021**, *114*, 106546. [CrossRef]
5. Cosentino, G.; Todisco, M.; Giudice, C.; Tassorelli, C.; Alfonsi, E. Anodal transcranial direct current stimulation and intermittent theta-burst stimulation improve deglutition and swallowing reproducibility in elderly patients with dysphagia. *Neurogastroenterol. Motil.* **2020**, *32*, e13791. [CrossRef] [PubMed]
6. Herranz, B.; Criado, C.; Pozo-Bayon, M.A.; Alvarez, M.D. Effect of addition of human saliva on steady and viscoelastic rheological properties of some commercial dysphagia-oriented products. *Food Hydrocoll.* **2021**, *111*, 106403. [CrossRef]
7. Ueshima, J.; Momosaki, R.; Shimizu, A.; Motokawa, K.; Sonoi, M.; Shirai, Y.; Uno, C.; Kokura, Y.; Shimizu, M.; Nishiyama, A.; et al. Nutritional assessment in adult patients with dysphagia: A scoping review. *Nutrients* **2021**, *13*, 778. [CrossRef]
8. Cichero, J.A.Y. Adjustment of food textural properties for elderly patients. *J. Texture Stud.* **2016**, *47*, 277–283. [CrossRef]
9. Dietsch, A.M.; Pelletier, C.A.; Solomon, N.P. Saliva production and enjoyment of real-food flavors in people with and without dysphagia and/or xerostomia. *Dysphagia* **2018**, *33*, 803–808. [CrossRef]
10. Tokifuji, A.; Matsushima, Y.; Hachisuka, K.; Yoshioka, K. Texture, sensory and swallowing characteristics of high-pressure-heat-treated pork meat gel as a dysphagia diet. *Meat Sci.* **2013**, *93*, 843–848. [CrossRef]
11. Pematilleke, N.; Kaur, M.; Adhikari, B.; Torley, P.J. Investigation of the effects of addition of carboxy methyl cellulose (CMC) and tapioca starch (TS) on the beef patties targeted to the needs of people with dysphagia: A mixture design approach. *Meat Sci.* **2022**, *191*, 108868. [CrossRef] [PubMed]
12. Strother, H.; Moss, R.; McSweeney, M.B. Comparison of 3D printed and molded carrots produced with gelatin, guar gum and xanthan gum. *J. Texture Stud.* **2020**, *51*, 852–860. [CrossRef] [PubMed]
13. Cichero, J.A.Y.; Lam, P.T.; Chen, J.; Dantas, R.O.; Duivestein, J.; Hanson, B.; Kayashita, J.; Pillay, M.; Riquelme, L.F.; Steele, C.M.; et al. Release of updated International Dysphagia Diet Standardisation Initiative Framework (IDDSI 2.0). *J. Texture Stud.* **2020**, *51*, 195–196. [CrossRef] [PubMed]
14. Cichero, J.A.Y.; Lam, P.; Steele, C.M.; Hanson, B.; Chen, J.; Dantas, R.O.; Duivestein, J.; Kayashita, J.; Lecko, C.; Murray, J.; et al. Development of international terminology and definitions for texture-modified foods and thickened fluids used in dysphagia management: The IDDSI Framework. *Dysphagia* **2017**, *32*, 293–314. [CrossRef]
15. Min, C.; Yang, Q.; Pu, H.; Cao, Y.; Ma, W.; Kuang, J.; Huang, J.; Xiong, Y.L. Textural characterization of calcium salts-induced mung bean starch-flaxseed protein composite gels as dysphagia food. *Food Res. Int.* **2023**, *164*, 112355. [CrossRef]
16. Xie, Y.S.; Zhao, W.Y.; Yu, W.Y.; Lin, X.Y.; Tao, S.F.; Prakash, S.; Dong, X.P. Validating the textural characteristics of soft fish-based paste through International Dysphagia Diet Standardisation Initiative recommended tests. *J. Texture Stud.* **2021**, *52*, 240–250. [CrossRef]
17. Xing, X.; Chitrakar, B.; Hati, S.; Xie, S.; Li, H.; Li, C.; Liu, Z.; Mo, H. Development of black fungus-based 3D printed foods as dysphagia diet: Effect of gums incorporation. *Food Hydrocoll.* **2022**, *123*, 107173. [CrossRef]

18. Shimizu, A.; Maeda, K.; Tanaka, K.; Ogawa, M.; Kayashita, J. Texture-modified diets are associated with decreased muscle mass in older adults admitted to a rehabilitation ward. *Geriatr. Gerontol. Int.* **2018**, *18*, 698–704. [CrossRef]
19. Shimizu, A.; Momosaki, R.; Kayashita, J.; Fujishima, I. Impact of multiple texture-modified diets on oral intake and nutritional status in older patients with pneumonia: A retrospective cohort study. *Dysphagia* **2020**, *35*, 574–582. [CrossRef]
20. Serra-Prat, M.; Palomera, M.; Gomez, C.; Sar-Shalom, D.; Saiz, A.; Montoya, J.G.; Navajas, M.; Palomera, E.; Clave, P. Oropharyngeal dysphagia as a risk factor for malnutrition and lower respiratory tract infection in independently living older persons: A population-based prospective study. *Age Ageing* **2012**, *41*, 376–381. [CrossRef]
21. Wright, L.; Cotter, D.; Hickson, M.; Frost, G. Comparison of energy and protein intakes of older people consuming a texture modified diet with a normal hospital diet. *J. Hum. Nutr. Diet.* **2005**, *18*, 213–219. [CrossRef] [PubMed]
22. Dhillon, B.; Sodhi, N.S.; Singh, D.; Kaur, A. Analyses of functional diets formulated for dysphagia patients under international dysphagia diet standardization initiative (IDDSI) level 3 to level 7. *J. Food Meas. Charact.* **2022**, *16*, 3537–3546. [CrossRef]
23. Rodd, B.G.; Tas, A.A.; Taylor, K.D.A. Dysphagia, texture modification, the elderly and micronutrient deficiency: A review. *Crit. Rev. Food Sci. Nutr.* **2022**, *62*, 7354–7369. [CrossRef] [PubMed]
24. Hao, L.; Lv, C.; Cui, X.; Yi, F.; Su, C. Study on biological activity of perilla seed oil extracted by supercritical carbon dioxide. *LWT-Food Sci. Technol.* **2021**, *146*, 111457. [CrossRef]
25. Laird, E.J.; O'Halloran, A.M.; Carey, D.; O'Connor, D.; Kenny, R.A.; Molloy, A.M. Voluntary fortification is ineffective to maintain the vitamin B-12 and folate status of older Irish adults: Evidence from the Irish Longitudinal Study on Ageing (TILDA). *Br. J. Nutr.* **2018**, *120*, 111–120. [CrossRef] [PubMed]
26. Wirth, R.; Smoliner, C.; Jager, M.; Warnecke, T.; Leischker, A.H.; Dziewas, R.; Committee, D.S. Guideline clinical nutrition in patients with stroke. *Exp. Trans. Stroke Med.* **2013**, *5*, 14. [CrossRef] [PubMed]
27. The National Health and Family Planning Commission of China. Chinese General Guidelines for Special Medical Use Formulas GB29922-2013. In *The National Food Safety Standard Determination*; Standards Press of China: Beijing, China, 2013.
28. Cheng, Y.Y. Introduction to Chinese Dietary Reference Intakes (2013 resived). *Nutr. Sci.* **2014**, *36*, 313–317.
29. Jiang, L.; Ren, Y.M.; Shen, M.Y.; Zhang, J.H.; Yu, Q.; Chen, Y.; Zhang, H.D.; Xie, J.H. Effect of acid/alkali shifting on function, gelation properties, and microstructure of *Mesona chinensis* polysaccharide-whey protein isolate gels. *Food Hydrocoll.* **2021**, *117*, 106699. [CrossRef]
30. Pematilleke, N.; Kaur, M.; Wai, C.T.R.; Adhikari, B.; Torley, P.J. Effect of the addition of hydrocolloids on beef texture: Targeted to the needs of people with dysphagia. *Food Hydrocoll.* **2021**, *113*, 106413. [CrossRef]
31. Ren, Y.M.; Rong, L.Y.; Shen, M.Y.; Liu, W.M.; Xiao, W.H.; Luo, Y.; Xie, J.H. Interaction between rice starch and *Mesona chinensis* Benth polysaccharide gels: Pasting and gelling properties. *Carbohydr. Polym.* **2020**, *240*, 116316. [CrossRef]
32. Ren, Y.M.; Wu, Z.H.; Shen, M.Y.; Rong, L.Y.; Liu, W.M.; Xiao, W.H.; Xie, J.H. Improve properties of sweet potato starch film using dual effects: Combination *Mesona chinensis* Benth polysaccharide and sodium carbonate. *LWT-Food Sci. Technol.* **2021**, *140*, 110679. [CrossRef]
33. Cui, T.; Wu, Y.; Ni, C.; Sun, Y.; Cheng, J. Rheology and texture analysis of gelatin/dialdehyde starch hydrogel carriers for curcumin controlled release. *Carbohydr. Polym.* **2022**, *283*, 119154. [CrossRef] [PubMed]
34. Ribes, S.; Estarriaga, R.; Grau, R.; Talens, P. Physical, sensory, and simulated mastication properties of texture-modified Spanish sauce using different texturing agents. *Food Funct.* **2021**, *12*, 8181–8195. [CrossRef]
35. Zhang, J.H.; Jiang, L.; Yang, J.; Chen, X.X.; Shen, M.Y.; Yu, Q.; Chen, Y.; Xie, J.H. Effect of calcium chloride on heat-induced *Mesona chinensis* polysaccharide-whey protein isolation gels: Gel properties and interactions. *LWT-Food Sci. Technol.* **2022**, *155*, 112907. [CrossRef]
36. Huang, S.X.; Chi, C.D.; Li, X.X.; Zhang, Y.P.; Chen, L. Understanding the structure, digestibility, texture and flavor attributes of rice noodles complexation with xanthan and dodecyl gallate. *Food Hydrocoll.* **2022**, *127*, 107538. [CrossRef]
37. Ribes, S.; Gallego, M.; Barat, J.M.; Grau, R.; Talens, P. Impact of chia seed mucilage on technological, sensory, and in vitro digestibility properties of a texture-modified puree. *J. Funct. Food.* **2022**, *89*, 104943. [CrossRef]
38. The National Standardization Administration of China. Sensory evaluation GB/T 10220-2012. In *National Standards of the People's Republic of China*; Standards Press of China: Beijing, China, 2012.
39. Min, C.; Ma, W.H.; Kuang, J.W.; Huang, J.R.; Xiong, Y.L.L. Textural properties, microstructure and digestibility of mungbean starch-flaxseed protein composite gels. *Food Hydrocoll.* **2022**, *126*, 107482. [CrossRef]
40. Guan, Y.; Zhao, G.; Thaiudom, S. Evaluation of the physico-chemical properties of potato starch-based foods and their interactions with milk protein and soybean oil. *Food Chem. X* **2022**, *16*, 110495. [CrossRef]
41. Ong, J.J.X.; Steele, C.M.; Duizer, L.M. Challenges to assumptions regarding oral shear rate during oral processing and swallowing based on sensory testing with thickened liquids. *Food Hydrocoll.* **2018**, *84*, 173–180. [CrossRef] [PubMed]
42. Kong, D.; Zhang, M.; Mujumdar, A.S.; Li, J. Feasibility of hydrocolloid addition for 3D printing of Qingtuan with red bean filling as a dysphagia food. *Food Res. Int.* **2023**, *165*, 112469. [CrossRef]
43. Dafiah, P.M.; Swapna, N. Variations in the amplitude and duration of hyolaryngeal elevation during swallow: Effect of sour and carbonated liquid bolus. *Physiol. Behav.* **2020**, *224*, 113028. [CrossRef] [PubMed]
44. Li, J.H.; Li, X.; Wang, C.Y.; Zhang, M.Q.; Xu, Y.L.; Zhou, B.; Su, Y.J.; Yang, Y.J. Characteristics of gelling and water holding properties of hen egg white/yolk gel with NaCl addition. *Food Hydrocoll.* **2018**, *77*, 887–893. [CrossRef]

45. Khemakhem, M.; Attia, H.; Ayadi, M.A. The effect of pH, sucrose, salt and hydrocolloid gums on the gelling properties and water holding capacity of egg white gel. *Food Hydrocoll.* **2019**, *87*, 11–19. [CrossRef]
46. Cutler, A.N.; Morris, E.R.; Taylor, L.J. Oral perception of viscosity in fluid foods and model systems. *J. Texture Stud.* **1983**, *14*, 377–395. [CrossRef]
47. Liu, W.; Zhang, Y.; Xu, Z.; Pan, W.; Shen, M.; Han, J.; Sun, X.; Zhang, Y.; Xie, J.; Zhang, X.; et al. Cross-linked corn bran arabinoxylan improves the pasting, rheological, gelling properties of corn starch and reduces its in vitro digestibility. *Food Hydrocoll.* **2022**, *126*, 107440. [CrossRef]
48. Gallegos, C.; Quinchia, L.; Ascanio, G.; Salinas-Vázquez, M.; Brito-de la Fuente, E. Rheology and dysphagia: An overview. *Annu. Trans. Nord. Rheol. Soc.* **2012**, *20*, 3–10.
49. National Dysphagia Diet Task Force and American Dietetic Association. *National Dysphagia Diet: Standardization for Optimal Care*; American Dietetic Association: Chicago, IL, USA, 2002.
50. Contreras-Jimenez, B.; Vazquez-Contreras, G.; Cornejo-Villegas, M.D.; del Real-Lopez, A.; Rodriguez-Garcia, M.E. Structural, morphological, chemical, vibrational, pasting, rheological, and thermal characterization of isolated jicama (*Pachyrhizus* spp.) starch and jicama starch added with $Ca(OH)_{2}$. *Food Chem.* **2019**, *283*, 83–91. [CrossRef]
51. Hadde, E.K.; Nicholson, T.M.; Cichero, J.A.Y.; Deblauwe, C. Rheological characterisation of thickened milk components (protein, lactose and minerals). *J. Food Eng.* **2015**, *166*, 263–267. [CrossRef]
52. Luo, Y.; Shen, M.Y.; Han, X.Y.; Wen, H.L.; Xie, J.H. Gelation characteristics of *Mesona chinensis* polysaccharide-maize starches gels: Influences of KCl and NaCl. *J. Cereal Sci.* **2020**, *96*, 103108. [CrossRef]
53. Cornejo-Villegas, M.D.; Rincon-Londono, N.; Del Real-Lopez, A.; Rodriguez-Garcia, M.E. The effect of Ca^{2+} ions on the pasting, morphological, structural, vibrational, and mechanical properties of corn starch-water system. *J. Cereal Sci.* **2018**, *79*, 174–182. [CrossRef]
54. Hayakawa, F.; Kazami, Y.; Ishihara, S.; Nakao, S.; Nakauma, M.; Funami, T.; Nishinari, K.; Kohyama, K. Characterization of eating difficulty by sensory evaluation of hydrocolloid gels. *Food Hydrocoll.* **2014**, *38*, 95–103. [CrossRef]
55. Li, J.H.; Zhang, M.Q.; Chang, C.H.; Gu, L.P.; Peng, N.; Su, Y.J.; Yang, Y.J. Molecular forces and gelling properties of heat-set whole chicken egg protein gel as affected by NaCl or pH. *Food Chem.* **2018**, *261*, 36–41. [CrossRef] [PubMed]
56. Mirzaaghaei, M.; Nasirpour, A.; Keramat, J.; Goli, S.A.H.; Dinari, M.; Desobry, S.; Durand, A. Chemical modification of waxy maize starch by esterification with saturated fatty acid chlorides: Synthesis, physicochemical and emulsifying properties. *Food Chem.* **2022**, *393*, 133293. [CrossRef]
57. Luan, H. Exploration of the Characterization Method of Starch Crystal Structure by XRD. Master's Thesis, Tianjin University of Science and Technology, Tianjin, China, 2020.
58. Geng, M.; Feng, X.; Wu, X.; Tan, X.; Liu, Z.; Li, L.; Huang, Y.; Teng, F.; Li, Y. Encapsulating vitamins C and E using food-grade soy protein isolate and pectin particles as carrier: Insights on the vitamin additive antioxidant effects. *Food Chem.* **2023**, *418*, 135955. [CrossRef]
59. Afoakwa, E.O.; Paterson, A.; Fowler, M.; Vieira, J. Particle size distribution and compositional effects on textural properties and appearance of dark chocolates. *J. Food Eng.* **2008**, *87*, 181–190. [CrossRef]
60. Belorio, M.; Marcondes, G.; Gomez, M. Influence of psyllium versus xanthan gum in starch properties. *Food Hydrocoll.* **2020**, *105*, 105843. [CrossRef]
61. Bai, J.; Dong, M.X.; Li, J.Y.; Tian, L.J.; Xiong, D.D.; Jia, J.; Yang, L.; Liu, X.B.; Duan, X. Effects of egg white on physicochemical and functional characteristics of steamed cold noodles (a wheat starch gel food). *LWT-Food Sci. Technol.* **2022**, *169*, 114057. [CrossRef]
62. Ribes, S.; Grau, R.; Talens, P. Use of chia seed mucilage as a texturing agent: Effect on instrumental and sensory properties of texture-modified soups. *Food Hydrocoll.* **2022**, *123*, 107171. [CrossRef]

Disclaimer/Publisher's Note: The statements, opinions and data contained in all publications are solely those of the individual author(s) and contributor(s) and not of MDPI and/or the editor(s). MDPI and/or the editor(s) disclaim responsibility for any injury to people or property resulting from any ideas, methods, instructions or products referred to in the content.

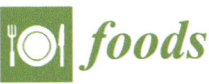

Article

Insoluble Dietary Fiber from Soybean Residue (Okara) Exerts Anti-Obesity Effects by Promoting Hepatic Mitochondrial Fatty Acid Oxidation

Jiarui Zhang [1,2], Sainan Wang [1,2], Junyao Wang [1,2], Wenhao Liu [1,2], Hao Gong [1,2], Zhao Zhang [3], Bo Lyu [2,*] and Hansong Yu [1,*]

1. College of Food Science and Engineering, Jilin Agricultural University, Changchun 130118, China
2. Division of Soybean Processing, Soybean Research & Development Center, Chinese Agricultural Research System, Changchun 130118, China
3. Sinoglory Health Food Co., Ltd., Liaocheng 252000, China
* Correspondence: lvbo@jlau.edu.cn (B.L.); yuhansong@jlau.edu.cn (H.Y.); Tel.: +86-189-4656-5410 (B.L.); +86-0431-8453-3104 (H.Y.)

Abstract: Numerous investigations have shown that insoluble dietary fiber (IDF) has a potentially positive effect on obesity due to a high-fat diet (HFD). Our previous findings based on proteomic data revealed that high-purity IDF from soybean residue (okara) (HPSIDF) prevented obesity by regulating hepatic fatty acid synthesis and degradation pathways, while its intervention mechanism is uncharted. Consequently, the goal of this work is to find out the potential regulatory mechanisms of HPSIDF on hepatic fatty acid oxidation by determining changes in fatty acid oxidation-related enzymes in mitochondria and peroxisomes, the production of oxidation intermediates and final products, the composition and content of fatty acids, and the expression levels of fatty acid oxidation-related proteins in mice fed with HFD. We found that supplementation with HPSIDF significantly ameliorated body weight gain, fat accumulation, dyslipidemia, and hepatic steatosis caused by HFD. Importantly, HPSIDF intervention promotes medium- and long-chain fatty acid oxidation in hepatic mitochondria by improving the contents of acyl-coenzyme A oxidase 1 (ACOX1), malonyl coenzyme A (Malonyl CoA), acetyl coenzyme A synthase (ACS), acetyl coenzyme A carboxylase (ACC), and carnitine palmitoyl transferase-1 (CPT-1). Moreover, HPSIDF effectively regulated the expression levels of proteins involved with hepatic fatty acid β-oxidation. Our study indicated that HPSIDF treatment prevents obesity by promoting hepatic mitochondrial fatty acid oxidation.

Keywords: insoluble dietary fiber; okara; obesity; fatty acid oxidation; regulatory mechanism

1. Introduction

Obesity is becoming a major public health issue around the world, with its prevalence rising year after year. Obesity can cause severe consequences, such as type 2 diabetes, metabolic syndrome, cardiovascular disease, and neurodegenerative diseases [1–3]. HFD is thought to increase the risk of obesity by increasing lipid synthesis, decreasing fatty acid oxidation, and impairing triglyceride (TG) export. At present, the primary methods for treating obesity are dieting, drug treatment, and surgical treatment, all of which have varying degrees of side effects. In consequence, there is a desperate demand for secure and effective ways to prevent and manage obesity.

The most active tissue for fatty acid oxidation is the liver. The oxidation of fatty acids is classified as β-oxidation and particular oxidation modes such as α-oxidation and ω-oxidation, with β-oxidation being the primary oxidation pathway [4–6]. β-oxidation occurs in the mitochondria and peroxisomes. AMP-activated protein kinase (AMPK) is a key signaling element that regulates hepatic fatty acid oxidation. When AMPK is activated, it inhibits fat accumulation and promotes fatty acid oxidation by regulating the enzymatic activities of sterol regulatory element-binding protein-1c (SREBP-1c) and peroxisome

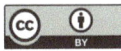

proliferator-activated receptor-α (PPARα) [7–10]. Silent mating type information regulation 2 homolog-1 (SIRT1) increases the transcriptional activity of PPARα mainly through proliferator-activated receptor gamma coactivator-1α (PGC-1α) deacetylation, which in turn promotes the β-oxidation of fatty acids in the liver. In addition, some proteins situated downstream of the AMPK pathway, such as CPT-1, are intimately related to β-oxidation. CPT-1 is localized on the outer mitochondrial surface and reduces the intracellular fatty acid concentration by catalyzing the beta-oxidation of fatty acids [11–13]. Therefore, obesity can be prevented and controlled by promoting fatty acid oxidation.

Soybean residue (okara) is the insoluble portion remaining after filtering the water-soluble portion during soymilk or soybean curd (tofu) production. Although large amounts of okara are yielded by the food industry, most of it is wasted because the high moisture content. As we all know, okara contains a variety of nutrients, especially dietary fiber (DF), which is regarded as the seventh nutrient. DF is essential for maintaining human health and is classified into soluble dietary fiber and IDF according to its water solubility. Numerous forward-looking studies have demonstrated the critical role of IDF in obesity prevention. Frank et al. discovered that insoluble cereal fiber supplementation significantly lowered weight gain and improved insulin sensitivity compared to long-term supplementation with soluble cereal fiber [14]. Another study showed that IDF from *Pleurotus eryngii* has a preventive effect on obesity through its modulation of the gut microbiota [15]. Our previous study demonstrated that high-purity IDF from okara (HPSIDF) plays a beneficial role in preventing obesity by regulating hepatic fatty acid synthesis and degradation pathways in HFD-fed mice. However, the mechanism of intervention is unclear [16].

Therefore, according to the results of previous research, this work was conducted to further explore the regulatory mechanisms of HPSIDF on fatty acid oxidation by analyzing the changes in the content of mitochondrial and peroxisomal oxidation-related enzymes, the production of oxidative intermediates and final products, fatty acid content and composition, and the expression levels of hepatic fatty acid oxidation-associated proteins in HFD induced mice.

2. Materials and Methods

2.1. Materials and Reagents

Crude soybean residue with 60% IDF content was purchased from Shandong Sinoglory Health Food Co., Ltd. (Liaocheng, China). The CDF was used to prepare the HPSIDF by the enzymatic method. The specific conditions are as follows: α-amylase at 95 °C for 35 min, neutral protease at 60 °C for 30 min, and amyloglucosidase at 60 °C for 30 min [17]. Kits for total cholesterol (TC), TG, low-density lipoprotein cholesterol (LDL-C), and high-density lipoprotein cholesterol (HDL-C) were derived from the Nanjing Jiancheng Bioengineering Institute (Nanjing, China). ELISA kits for free fatty acids (FFA), 3-hydroxybutyric acid (3-OHB), acetoacetate (ACAC), CPT1, ACOX1, ACS, Malonyl CoA, ACC, hydrogen peroxide (H_2O_2), acetyl-coenzyme A (A-CoA), citrate synthase (CS), and succinyl-coenzyme A (SCoA) were derived from Shanghai Enzyme-linked Biotechnology Co., Ltd. (Shanghai, China). HPLC-grade methyl tert-butyl ether (MTBE), methanol (MeOH), and *n*-hexane were derived from Merck (Darmstadt, Germany). Sodium chloride and phosphate were acquired from Sigma-Aldrich (St. Louis, MO, USA). A methanol solution of 15% boron trifluoride was bought from RHAWN (Shanghai, China). The antibodies to PPARα, fatty acid synthase (FAS), and long-chain acyl-coenzyme A dehydrogenase (ACADL) were derived from Wuhan Sanying Biotechnology Co., Ltd. (Wuhan, China). SREBP-1c, AMPK, CPT1, SIRT1, phosphorylated adenylate-activated protein kinase (pAMPK), PGC-1α, ACOX1, long-chain acyl-coenzyme A synthetase (ACSL), and β-actin were provided by Abcam (Cambridge, UK).

2.2. Animal Experimental Design

The research was carried out in accordance with the Laboratory Animals Guidelines of Jilin Agricultural University and authorized by the Jilin Agricultural University Laboratory

Animal Welfare and Ethics Committee (no. 2019 04 10 005). Six-week-old male C57BL/6J mice ($n = 40$; 18–22 g) were obtained from the Experimental Animal Center of Jilin Agricultural University. Mice were kept in a temperature-controlled (20–25 °C) environment with a 12-h cycle of light/darkness.

Following the first week of acclimatized feeding, mice were separated into four groups for 18 weeks: the normal diet (ND) group, the HFD group, the HFD supplemented with HP-SIDF group (HPSIDF, 1000 mg/kg [16]), and the HFD supplemented with L-carnitine group (PC, 40 mg/kg). Notably, L-carnitine has been shown to promote fatty acid metabolism in vivo, which is consistent with the pathway explored in this study, so we chose it as a positive control [18,19]. The body weight and food intake of mice in each group were recorded weekly and daily, respectively. At the end of the trial, mice were anesthetized, and blood was collected through the orbital venous plexus. Then all the animals were euthanized by carbon dioxide. The blood samples were followed by centrifugation at 3000 rpm for 15 min at 4 °C to obtain serum. The liver and fat tissues were obtained by dissection after the execution of mice, weighed, and immediately stored at −80 °C for further analysis.

2.3. Biochemical Analysis

The levels of TC, TG, LDL-C, and HDL-C in serum were determined using commercial assay kits. TC and TG levels in the liver were determined using the same kit as the serum assay. Moreover, the levels of FFA, 3-OHB, and ACAC in serum were determined using the ELISA kits.

2.4. Analysis of Enzyme Contents Related to Fatty Acid Oxidation

An amount of liver was mixed with saline at 1:9 and homogenized on ice. Then it was centrifugated at 3000 rpm for 15 min at 4 °C to obtain the supernatant. The levels of CPT-1, ACOX1, Malonyl Coenzyme A, ACC, ACS, A-CoA, CS, SCoA, and H_2O_2 were analyzed by ELISA kits.

2.5. Histological Investigation

Liver and epididymal fat were fixed in 4% paraformaldehyde, engrained in paraffin for making sections (5 μm thickness), and stained using hematoxylin and eosin (H&E).

2.6. Analysis of Hepatic Fatty Acid Composition and Content

The liver samples from each group of mice were thawed, and the samples (0.05 g) were mixed with 150 μL of MeOH, 200 μL of MTBE, and 50 μL of 36% phosphoric acid/water (precooled at −20 °C). The mixture was vortexed for 3 min at 2500 rpm and centrifuged at 12,000 rpm for 5 min at 4 °C. Then, 200 μL of supernatant was collected into a new centrifuge tube, blow dry, and 300 μL of a methanol solution of 15% boron trifluoride was added. The mixture was vortexed for 3 min at 2500 rpm and keep in the oven at 60 °C for 30 min. Then 500 μL of n-hexane and 200 μL of saturated sodium chloride solution were added accurately at room temperature. After the mixture was vortexed for 3 min and centrifuged at 12,000 rpm and 4 °C for 5 min, 100 μL of n-hexane layer solution was transferred for further GC-MS analysis.

A GC-EI-MS system was used to analyze the sample derivates. (GC, Agilent 8890 https://Agilent.com.cn/ (accessed on 13 March 2019); MS, 5977B System, https://Agilent.com.cn/ (accessed on 13 March 2019). The following were the analytical conditions: GC column, DB-5MS capillary column (30 m × 0.25 mm × 0.25 μm, Agilent); Carrier gas, highly pure argon gas (purity > 99.999%); The heating procedure was started at 40 °C (2 min), then increased at 30 °C/min to 200 °C (1 min), 10 °C/min to 240 °C (1 min), and 5 °C/min to 285 °C (3 min); traffic: 1.0 mL/min; inlet temperature: 230 °C; injection volume: 1.0 μL. EI-MS: Agilent 8890-5977B GC-MS System, Temperature: 230 °C; ionization voltage: 70eV; power transmission temperature: 240 °C; four-stage rod temp.: 150 °C; solvent postpone: 4 min; scanning method: SIM.

Qualitative and quantitative analysis. Standard solutions of different concentrations of 0.01, 0.02, 0.05, 0.1, 0.2, 0.5, 1, 2, 5, 10, 20, and 50 μg/mL were prepared, and the peak intensity data corresponding to the different concentrations of the standards were obtained to plot the standard curves. The integrated peak areas of the detected liver samples were brought to the standard curve to calculate the concentrations, which were then further calculated to give absolute content data for the different substances in the actual samples.

The fatty acid content of the sample (μg/g) = $c*V3/1000*V1/V2/m$

Meaning of the letters in the formula:

c: Concentration values obtained by substituting the integrated peak area of the sample into the standard curve (μg/mL);

V1: Volume of sample extraction solution (μL);

V2: Volume of collected supernatant (μL);

V3: Volume of resolution (μL);

m: The sample weight (g).

2.7. Western Blot Analysis

The liver was homogenized in RIPA lysis solution, centrifuged at a speed of 12,000 rpm at 4 °C for 20 min, and the supernatant was collected. The BCA kit was used to determine the content of protein, followed by routine protein blotting analysis. Briefly, protein lysates were isolated by SDS-PAGE and moved to polyvinylidene fluoride (PVDF) films. The blotting film was closed with 5% defatted skim for 1.5 h and then hatched with the corresponding elementary antibodies FAS, SREBP-1c, ACOX1, PPARα, AMPK, pAMPK, SIRT1, PGC-1α, ACADL, ACSL, and CPT1 for the whole night at 4 °C, then incubated with the relevant secondary antibodies for 1.5 h. The bands were analyzed on an iBright CL1000 imaging system using an enhanced chemiluminescence reagent (Invitrogen, Singapore). β-actin was used as a reference to standardize protein expression.

2.8. Statistical Analysis

SPSS 19.0 (SPSS, Chicago, IL, USA) was used for statistical analysis. A one-way analysis of variance (ANOVA) and Duncan's multiple range tests were used to assess the statistical significance, with $p < 0.05$ regarded as statistically significant.

3. Results

3.1. Effects of HPSIDF on Body Weight, Food Intake and Fat Accumulation in HFD-Fed Mice

As shown in Table 1, there was no remarkable difference in the initial body weight of the mice in each group. After 18 weeks of feeding, the body weight gain of mice was remarkably increased in the HFD group as opposed to the ND group ($p < 0.05$). In comparison to the HFD group, there was a decrease in body weight gain in the HPSIDF and PC groups, especially the HPSIDF group ($p < 0.05$). There was a significant 15% increase in body weight in the HFD group compared to the ND group at the end of the experiment. Compared to the HFD group, weight loss was 15% and 8% in the HPSIDF group and PC group, respectively. In terms of food intake, only the HFD group had a significantly higher food intake in contrast to the other groups ($p < 0.05$), with no significant variation between the other three groups. In addition, we found that chronic HFD caused abnormal accumulation of perirenal, subcutaneous, and epididymal fat compared to ND ($p < 0.0001$) (Figure 1A–C). However, HPSIDF treatment significantly reduced the weight of perirenal, subcutaneous, and epididymal fat induced by HFD ($p < 0.0001$), which was better than the PC group. As shown in Figure 1D, we also found significant adipocyte hypertrophy in HFD-fed mice. Interestingly, HPSIDF treatment considerably alleviated HFD-induced adipocyte hypertrophy compared to the PC group.

Table 1. The effect of HPSIDF on body weight and food intake in HFD−fed mice.

Items	ND	HFD	HPSIDF	PC
Initial body weight (g)	20.02 ± 0.93	20.80 ± 1.19	21.10 ± 1.04	21.45 ± 0.63
Final body weight (g)	27.49 ± 2.09 [b]	31.78 ± 2.77 [a]	26.90 ± 2.79 [b]	28.96 ± 2.24 [b]
Body weight gain (g)	7.47 ± 1.40 [b]	10.98 ± 2.94 [a]	5.99 ± 2.40 [c]	7.50 ± 2.57 [b]
Food intake (g)	2.13 ± 0.10 [b]	2.47 ± 0.04 [a]	2.08 ± 0.07 [b]	2.15 ± 0.13 [b]

ND—normal diet-fed group; HFD—high-fat diet-fed group; HPSIDF—high-fat diet plus HPSIDF (1000 mg/kg) fed group; PC—high-fat diet plus L-carnitine (40 mg/kg) fed group. The same column with different letters (a, b, c) are markedly different ($p < 0.05$). Results are shown as average ± SD ($n = 10$).

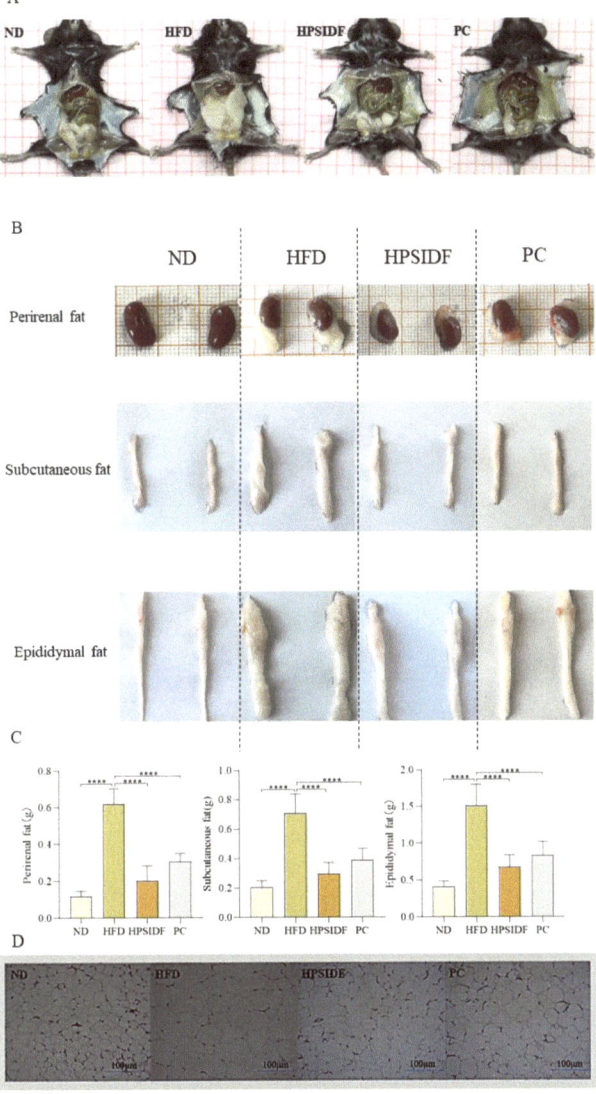

Figure 1. Effects of HPSIDF on fat accumulation in HFD−fed mice. (**A**) Intraperitoneal morphology of mice in each group. (**B,C**) Apparent morphology and weight of white adipose tissues. (**D**) Representative H&E staining images of epididymal fat tissue. ND—normal diet-fed group; HFD—high-fat diet−fed group; HPSIDF—high-fat diet plus HPSIDF (1000 mg/kg) fed group; PC—high-fat diet plus L-carnitine (40 mg/kg) fed group. In contrast to the HFD group, **** $p < 0.0001$.

3.2. Effects of HPSIDF on Serum Biochemical Indicators in HFD-Fed Mice

As shown in Figure 2A–E, serum TC ($p < 0.0001$), TG ($p < 0.01$), LDL-C ($p < 0.0001$), and FFA ($p < 0.05$) contents were memorably elevated in the HFD group in contrast to the ND group. HPSIDF intervention effectively reduced the serum TC ($p < 0.01$), TG ($p < 0.0001$), LDL-C ($p < 0.0001$), and FFA ($p < 0.001$) contents of HFD-fed mice, and there was no considerable difference when compared to the PC group. Furthermore, the HPSIDF and PC groups significantly increased serum HDL-C levels in mice fed with HFD (all $p < 0.0001$). As shown in Figure 2F,G, the levels of 3-OHB ($p < 0.0001$) and ACAC ($p < 0.05$) in the HFD group were observably higher than those of the ND group, and these alterations were effectively reversed by the HPSIDF intervention ($p < 0.05$, $p < 0.01$). Moreover, ACAC levels were dramatically reduced in the PC group as opposed to the HFD group ($p < 0.0001$).

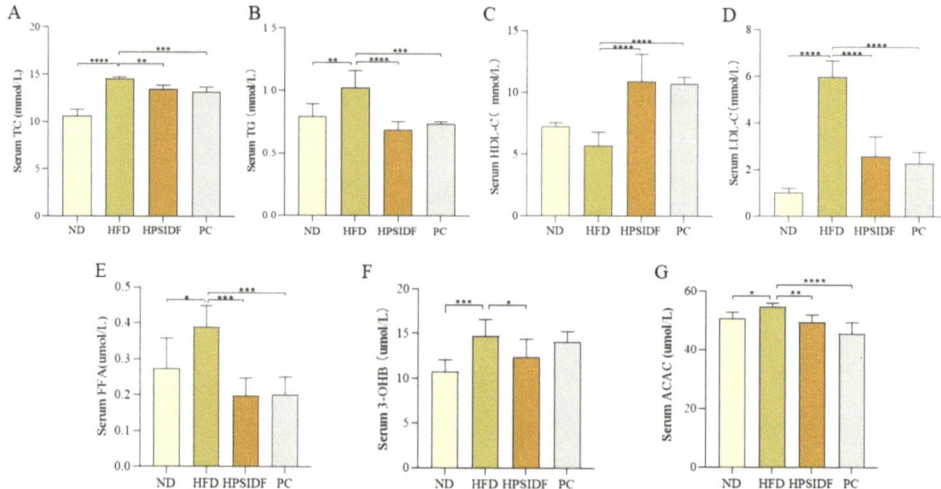

Figure 2. Effects of HPSIDF on serum biochemical factors in HFD–fed mice. (**A–E**) Serum TC, TG, HDL-C, LDL-C, and FFA contents. (**F,G**) Levels of 3-OHB and ACAC. ND—normal diet–fed group; HFD—high–fat diet–fed group; HPSIDF—high-fat diet plus HPSIDF (1000 mg/kg) fed group; PC—high–fat diet plus L–carnitine (40 mg/kg) fed group. Compared with the HFD group, * $p < 0.05$, ** $p < 0.01$, *** $p < 0.001$ and **** $p < 0.0001$.

3.3. Effects of HPSIDF on Hepatic Steatosis in HFD-Fed Mice

The chronic HFD resulted in significantly higher liver TC ($p < 0.001$), TG ($p < 0.0001$), and FFA ($p < 0.0001$) levels than ND (Figure 3A). As expected, the concentrations of TC, TG, and FFA were remarkably reduced in the HPSIDF ($p < 0.01$, $p < 0.001$, $p < 0.001$) and PC groups as opposed to the HFD group ($p < 0.05$, $p < 0.01$, $p < 0.01$). In Figure 3B, increased lipid droplet accumulation with marked steatosis was observed in HFD-induced mice. The degree of steatosis in the hepatocytes was ameliorated in both the HPSIDF and PC groups, with red staining of the hepatocyte cytoplasm and reduced lipid droplets.

3.4. Effects of HPSIDF on the Activity of Enzymes Related to Hepatic Fatty Acid Oxidation and the Production of Intermediate and Final Products in HFD-Fed Mice

We found that ACOX1 ($p < 0.0001$), malonyl CoA ($p < 0.01$), ACS ($p < 0.01$), and ACC ($p < 0.01$) levels were observably enhanced in HFD-fed mice compared to ND-fed mice (Figure 4). However, the levels of ACOX1, malonyl CoA, and ACC were markedly reduced in the HPSIDF ($p < 0.01$, $p < 0.0001$, $p < 0.01$) and PC ($p < 0.05$, $p < 0.01$, $p < 0.001$) groups. Interestingly, CPT-1 and ACS were dramatically increased in the HPSIDF ($p < 0.01$, $p < 0.001$) and PC ($p < 0.05$, $p < 0.001$) groups as opposed to the HFD group. Furthermore, HPSIDF treatment notably promoted the production of SCoA ($p < 0.05$), CS ($p < 0.01$), and A-CoA ($p < 0.001$) and inhibited the synthesis of H_2O_2 ($p < 0.0001$) in the liver of HFD-fed mice.

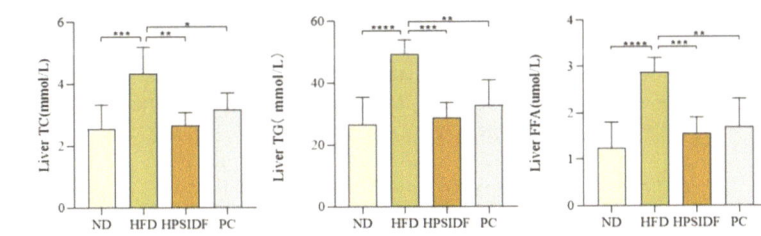

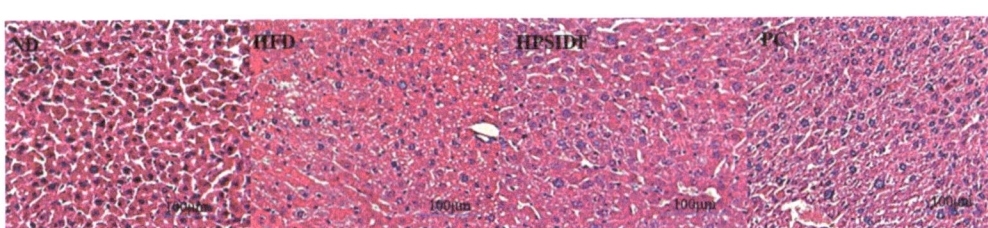

Figure 3. Effects of HPSIDF on hepatic steatosis in mice fed with HFD. (**A**) Levels of hepatic TC, TG and FFA. (**B**) H&E staining of the liver. ND—normal diet–fed group; HFD—high-fat diet–fed group; HPSIDF—high-fat diet plus HPSIDF (1000 mg/kg) fed group; PC—high–fat diet plus L–carnitine (40 mg/kg) fed group. Compared with the HFD group, * $p < 0.05$, ** $p < 0.01$, *** $p < 0.001$, and **** $p < 0.0001$.

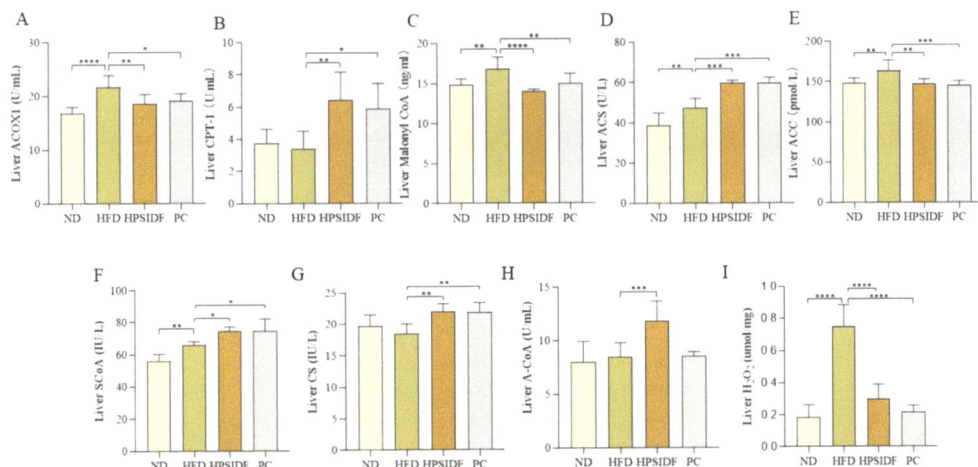

Figure 4. Effects of HPSIDF on the activity of enzymes related to hepatic fatty acid oxidation and the production of intermediate and final products in HFD–fed mice. Determination of ACOX1, CPT-1, Malonyl CoA, ACS, ACC, ScoA, CS, A-CoA, and H_2O_2 in the liver (**A–I**). ND—normal diet-fed group; HFD—high-fat diet–fed group; HPSIDF—high-fat diet plus HPSIDF (1000 mg/kg) fed group; PC—high-fat diet plus L−carnitine (40 mg/kg) fed group. In contrast to the HFD group, * $p < 0.05$, ** $p < 0.01$, *** $p < 0.001$, and **** $p < 0.0001$.

3.5. Effects of HPSIDF on Hepatic Fatty Acid Content and Composition in HFD-Fed Mice

As shown in Figure 5, long term HFD leads to the accumulation of hexanoic acid (C6:0), octanoic acid (C8:0), decanoic acid (C10:0), palmitic acid (C16:0), stearic acid (C18:0), behenic acid (C22:0), tricosanoic acid (C23:0), lignoceric acid (C24:0), cis-10-pentadecenoic acid (C15-1), cis-10-pentadecenoic acid (C18-1n9c), trans-9-octadecenoic acid (C18-1n9t), cis-8,11,14-eicosatrienoic acid (C20-3n6), cis-7,10,13,16,19-docosapentaenoic acid (DPA) (C22-5), cis-4,7,10,13,16,19-docosahexaenoic acid (C22-6n3) and nervonic acid (C24-1) in the liver. After HPSIDF intervention, the contents of hexanoic acid (C6:0), octanoic acid (C8:0), decanoic acid (C10:0), lauric acid (C12:0), myristic acid (C14:0), palmitic acid (C16:0), heptadecanoic acid (C17:0), stearic acid (C18:0), tricosanoic acid (C23:0), lignoceric acid (C24:0), myristoleic acid (C14-1), cis-10-pentadecenoic acid (C15-1), cis-10-heptadecanoic acid (C17-1), linoleic acid (C18-2n6c), γ-linolenic acid (C18-3n6), cis-11-eicosenoic acid (C20-1), trans-11-eicosenoic acid (C20-1T), cis-11,14-eicosadienoic acid (C20-2), cis-11,14,17-eicosatrienoic acid (C20-3n3), cis-8,11,14-eicosatrienoic acid (C20-3n6), cis-5,8,11,14,17-eicosapentaenoic acid(EPA) (C20-5n3), arachidonic acid (C20-4n6), trans-13-docosenoic acid (C22-1T), cis-13,16-docosadienoic acid (C22-2), cis-7,10,13,16,19-docosapentaenoic acid (DPA) (C22-5), nervonic acid (C24-1) were memorably reduced in HFD-fed mice. Thus, the HPSIDF intervention significantly promoted the oxidation of medium- and long-chain fatty acids in HFD-fed mice.

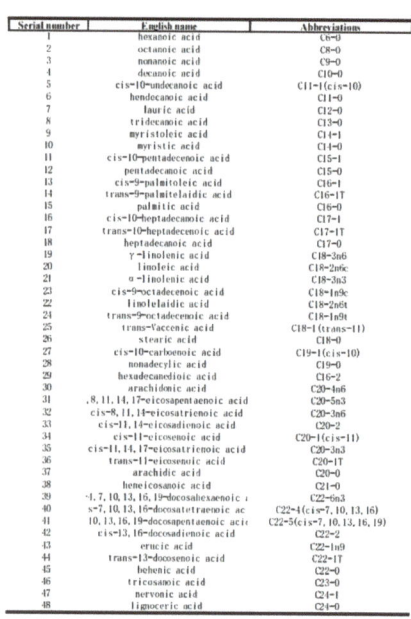
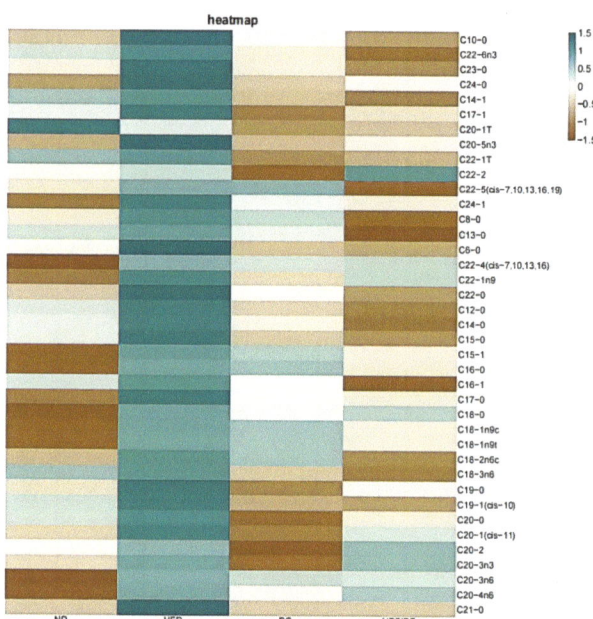

Figure 5. Effects of HPSIDF on hepatic fatty acid composition and content in HFD−fed mice. ND—normal diet−fed group; HFD—high-fat diet−fed group; HPSIDF—high-fat diet plus HPSIDF (1000 mg/kg) fed group; PC—high-fat diet plus L-carnitine (40 mg/kg) fed group.

3.6. Effects of HPSIDF on the Expression Levels of Hepatic Fatty Acid β-Oxidation-Associated Proteins in HFD-Fed Mice

As shown in Figure 6A, several key enzymes for fatty acid β-oxidation were determined in the liver. Long-term HFD markedly upregulated the expression levels of ACSL ($p < 0.01$), ACOX1 ($p < 0.0001$), and SREBP-1c ($p < 0.001$), while downregulating the levels of PPARα ($p < 0.05$) and ACADL ($p < 0.05$) in contrast to the ND group. However, these changes were reversed by HPSIDF intervention, except for the ACSL levels, which were downregulated ($p < 0.0001$). Moreover, HPSIDF treatment observably upregulated the expression levels of CPT-1 ($p < 0.0001$), PGC-1α ($p < 0.0001$), SIRT1 ($p < 0.05$), and pAMPK ($p < 0.001$), and downregulated the expression levels of FAS ($p < 0.05$) in contrast to the HFD group.

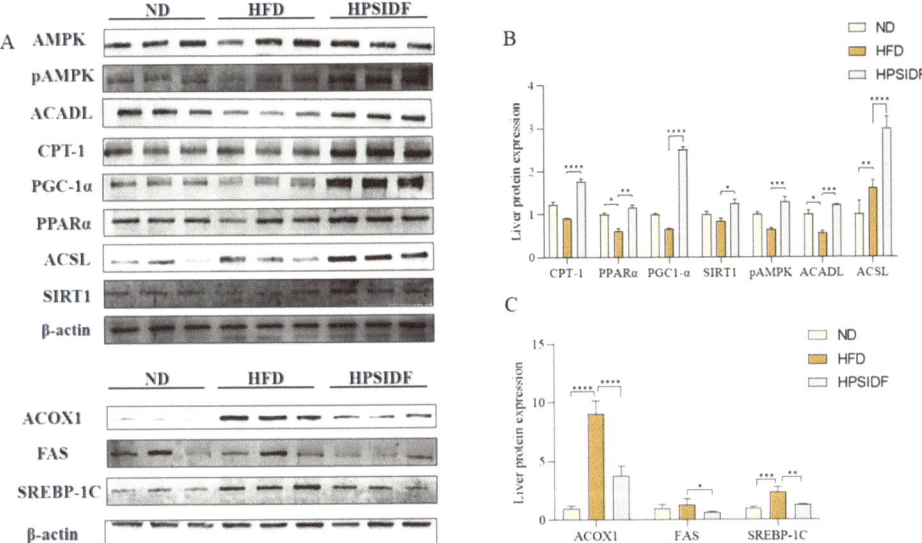

Figure 6. Effects of HPSIDF on the expression levels of hepatic fatty acid oxidation-associated proteins in HFD-fed mice. The levels of CPT-1, PPARα, PGC-1α, SIRT1, pAMPK, ACADL, ACSL, ACOX1, FAS, and SREBP-1c were determined using western blot analysis. The comparative intensities of these protein stripes were analyzed using ImageJ software. β-actin was used as a reference. (**A**) Protein-blotted bands measured. (**B**) CPT-1, PPARα, PGC-1α, SIRT1, pAMPK, ACADL, ACSL protein expression analysis. (**C**) Analysis of ACOX1, FAS, and SREBP-1c protein expression. Values are shown as averages ± SD (n = 10). ND—normal diet-fed group; HFD—high-fat diet-fed group; HPSIDF—high-fat diet plus HPSIDF (1000 mg/kg) fed group. In contrast to the HFD group, * $p < 0.05$, ** $p < 0.01$, *** $p < 0.001$, and **** $p < 0.0001$.

4. Discussion

The majority of nutrition studies over the last few years have emphasized the value of a high fiber intake. The World Health Organization, Food and Agriculture Organization (WHO/FAO), and the European Food Safety Authority (EFSA) recommend dietary fiber intake of not less than 25 g/day [20,21]. Although most of the suggested beneficial effects of fiber intake are attributed to the viscosity of SDF, results from forward-looking cohort studies concordantly suggest that the intake of IDF, but not SDF, is strongly linked to a decreased risk of obesity and overweight [22–24]. Therefore, based on the recommended intake we investigated the effect of different doses of HPSIDF on lipid metabolism in HFD-fed mice in the previous study. It was found that the high-dose group had better effects compared to the low and medium-dose groups. Thus, we chose the high-dose group to explore the effect of HPSIDF on high-fat diet-induced fatty acid oxidation. It is well known that the main feature of obesity is an excessive amount of fat, which leads to a variety of complications, such as dyslipidemia, liver steatosis, insulin resistance, and inflammation [25–27]. In this study, HPSIDF intervention remarkably improved fat accumulation, dyslipidemia, and hepatic steatosis in HFD-fed mice. This is in line with the views of Frank et al., who found that supplementation with suitably fermentable insoluble grain fiber prevented HFD-induced obesity and related metabolic disorders [14]. Furthermore, abnormal fat oxidation can raise ketone body levels above the established cutoff, which would then result in ketosis. Interestingly, supplementing with HPSIDF reversed the HFD-induced spike in ketone body levels and brought them back to normal. On the basis of these results, we further explored the potential mechanism of HPSIDF for obesity prevention by studying fatty acid oxidation-related enzymes and proteins.

The liver is an important site of fatty acid metabolism. Huang et al. reported that fatty acids are generated in a series of enzymatic processes and can be oxidized and metabolized to carbon dioxide and water under an adequate oxygen supply. This process is accompanied by the release of tremendous energy. β-oxidation is the primary type of fatty acid oxidation [28]. Kim et al. reported the existence of two different β-oxidation systems, mitochondria and peroxisomes, in mammals as well as higher animals, including humans [29]. Mitochondria mainly oxidize short- and medium-length chain fatty acids, while peroxisomes oxidize substrates such as very-long-chain fatty acids and long-chain fatty acids [30,31]. Research has shown that the peroxisome plays only a minor role in the oxidation of long-chain fatty acids, most of which are oxidized in the mitochondria [32,33]. In addition, the oxidation of fatty acids in the peroxisome is partial and just a carbon chain-shortening reaction. Very long-chain fatty acids enter the peroxisome to form shorter acyl coenzymes, then undergo β-oxidation in the mitochondria to produce acetyl CoA, and finally enter the tricarboxylic acid cycle to produce carbon dioxide and water [34,35]. Therefore, we closely monitored the effects of HPSIDF intervention on the content of enzymes related to fatty acid oxidation and metabolites during oxidation in the liver of HFD-fed mice. Notably, intake of HPSIDF markedly reduced the levels of ACOX1, Malonyl CoA and ACC and increased the levels of CPT-1 and ACS in the liver of HFD-fed mice. Meanwhile, HPSIDF treatment observably promoted the production of SCoA, CS and A-CoA, inhibited the synthesis of H_2O_2 and diminished the oxidation of peroxisomal fatty acids. It is reported that excessive peroxisomal fatty acid oxidation inhibits mitochondrial fatty acid oxidation, leading to impaired fatty acid oxidation and metabolic disturbances [21]. We speculate that HPSIDF intervention promotes the rate of mitochondrial oxidation. Chen et al. discovered that chronic consumption of high-erucic acid rapeseed oil caused hepatic steatosis in both animals and humans. This may be due to the increased production of hepatic malonyl coenzyme A in rats by peroxides of erucic acid, which inhibit fatty acid oxidation in mitochondria [36]. Therefore, the levels of malonyl CoA and ACC in the liver were measured in this study. Long-term HFD feeding resulted in a significant increase in malonyl CoA and ACC in the liver. The intervention of HPSIDF clearly reversed this situation. These results demonstrated that HPSIDF promotes overall fatty acid oxidation by promoting mitochondrial fatty acid oxidation and offers to a theoretical foundation for further investigation of its mechanism of action at the protein level.

Studies have shown that hepatic fatty acid metabolism is regulated by the AMPK signaling pathway [37,38]. AMPK contains three subunits: -α, -β, and -γ, among which the -α subunit contains a catalytic phosphorylation site at its NH2 terminal (Thr172) [27,39]. Activation of AMPK phosphorylation downregulates the expression of SREBP-1c to inhibit lipid synthesis while stimulating PPARα expression to promote fatty acid oxidation [40]. Meanwhile, the activation of PPARα leads to increased expression of ACSL1 to provide more conjugated acyl coenzymes for use as fuel via the fatty acid oxidation pathway [41]. Gao et al. also explored the conflicting reports on ACSL, concluding that the destiny of long-chain acyl-coenzyme A in cells is based on the positioning of ACSL1 [42]. In this study, we discovered that long-term HFD resulted in a remarkable increase in the expression levels of SREBP-1C, FAS, and ACOX1. Interestingly, the HPSIDF treatment reversed these changes while significantly upregulating the expression levels of pAMPK, PPARα, CPT-1, ACADL, and ACSL. Our findings indicated that HFD inhibits mitochondrial fatty acid oxidation. This is consistent with our previous hypothesis that HPSIDF intervention could effectively promote mitochondrial fatty acid oxidation. In addition to AMPK activation, research suggests that SIRT1 may also be involved in the regulation of PPARα. According to Cohen et al., fasting and dietary restriction activated SIRT1 and PPARα [43]. Furthermore, PGC-1α is a key coactivator of PPARα signaling and a direct substrate of SIRT1 [44,45]. Aparna et al. demonstrated that SIRT1 regulated PPARα signaling mainly through the activation of PGC-1α and that increased levels of SIRT1 stimulated PPARα activity [46–51]. We also determined the protein expression of PGC-1α and SIRT1 in the liver [52–55]. There was no significant difference in the HFD group in contrast to the ND group, and the HP-

SIDF intervention greatly upregulated the expression levels of both proteins. Furthermore, ACSL1 and CPT-1 are key rate-limiting enzymes that catalyze mitochondrial fatty acid oxidation. Briefly, ACSL1 catalyzes the production of lipid acyl-coenzyme A at the outer mitochondrial membrane, which is subsequently transported to the mitochondrial matrix by CPT1 to complete the fatty acid oxidation process. ACADL catalyzes the dehydrogenation of long-chain fatty acyl-coenzyme A in the first step of β-oxidation in mitochondria. The HPSIDF intervention significantly upregulated the expression levels of the above key enzymes, which also provided a reasonable explanation for the decrease in the content of medium- and long-chain fatty acids represented by lauric acid (C12:0), myristic acid (C14:0), palmitic acid (C16:0), heptadecanoic acid (C17:0), stearic acid (C18:0), and tridecanoic acid (C23:0) in the HPSIDF group. These results suggest that HPSIDF intervention promotes hepatic fatty acid β-oxidation in HFD-fed mice by activating AMPK phosphorylation to upregulate the expression levels of SIRT1, PGC-1α, and PPARα, while stimulating the expression of downstream proteins such as CPT-1, ACOX1, ACADL, and ACSL.

5. Conclusions

In summary, our results indicated that HPSIDF supplementation effectively alleviated body weight gain, fat accumulation, dyslipidemia, and hepatic steatosis induced by HFD. Furthermore, HPSIDF treatment promoted medium- and long-chain fatty acid oxidation in hepatic mitochondria by increasing the contents of CPT-1 and ACS and inhibiting the synthesis of ACOX1, malonyl CoA, and ACC. Meanwhile, HPSIDF treatment dramatically regulated the expression levels of hepatic fatty acid oxidation-related proteins. Overall, our findings gave new perspectives to elucidate the intervention mechanisms of HPSIDF on obesity and play an active role in promoting the comprehensive utilization rate and added value of okara.

Author Contributions: Conceptualization, H.Y. and B.L.; software, J.W.; formal analysis, H.G.; investigation, W.L.; resources, Z.Z.; writing—original draft preparation, J.Z.; writing—review and editing, S.W. All authors have read and agreed to the published version of the manuscript.

Funding: This work was supported by the China Agriculture Research System of MOF and MARA (CARS-04), the Young & Middle-Aged Technological Innovation Outstanding Talent (team) Project (Innovation) (20210509015RQ), and the Changbai Mountain Leading Team Project (ZZ202010098810020102).

Data Availability Statement: Raw data can be provided by the corresponding author upon request.

Conflicts of Interest: The authors declare no conflict of interest.

Abbreviations

DF—dietary fiber; CDF—crude soybean dietary fiber; HPSIDF—high purity insoluble dietary fiber from soybean residue; HFD—high-fat diet; TC—total cholesterol; TG—triglyceride; LDL-C—low-density lipoprotein cholesterol—HDL-C—high-density lipoprotein cholesterol; FA—fatty acid; FFA—free fatty acids; AMPK—AMP-activated protein kinase; SREBP-1c—sterol regulatory element-binding protein-1c; PPARα—peroxisome proliferator-activated receptor-α; SIRT1—silent mating type information regulation 2 homolog-1; PGC-1α—proliferator-activated receptor gamma coactivator 1-alpha; CPT-1—carnitine palmitoyl transferase 1; ELISA—Enzyme-linked immunosorbent assay; 3-OHB—3-hydroxybutyric acid; ACAC—acetoacetate; ACOX1—acyl-coa oxidase; ACS—acetyl-coa synthase; ACC—acetyl coenzyme a carboxylase; H_2O_2—hydrogen peroxide content; A-CoA—acetyl-coa; CS—citrate synthase; SCoA—succinyl-coa; FAS—fatty acid synthase; ACADL—long chain acyl-coa dehydrogenase; pAMPK—phosphorylatedadenylate-activated protein kinase; ACSL—long chain acyl coenzyme A synthetase.

References

1. Mattson, M.P. Roles of the Lipid Peroxidation Product 4-Hydroxynonenal in Obesity, the Metabolic Syndrome, and Associated Vascular and Neurodegenerative Disorders. *Exp. Gerontol.* **2009**, *44*, 625–633. [CrossRef] [PubMed]
2. Wang, Y.C.; McPherson, K.; Marsh, T.; Gortmaker, S.L.; Brown, M. Obesity 2 Health and Economic Burden of the Projected Obesity Trends in the USA and the UK. *Lancet* **2011**, *378*, 815–825. [CrossRef] [PubMed]
3. Gauvreau, D.; Villeneuve, N.; Deshaies, Y.; Cianflone, K. Novel adipokines: Links between obesity and atherosclerosis. *Ann. Endocrinol.* **2011**, *72*, 224–231. [CrossRef] [PubMed]
4. Korenblat, K.M.; Fabbrini, E.; Mohammed, B.S.; Klein, S. Liver, Muscle, and Adipose Tissue Insulin Action Is Directly Related to Intrahepatic Triglyceride Content in Obese Subjects. *Gastroenterology* **2008**, *134*, 1369–1375. [CrossRef] [PubMed]
5. Kotronen, A.; Yki-Jarvinen, H.; Sevastianova, K.; Bergholm, R.; Hakkarainen, A.; Pietilainen, K.H.; Juurinen, L.; Lundbom, N.; Sorensen, T.I.A. Comparison of the Relative Contributions of Intra-Abdominal and Liver Fat to Components of the Metabolic Syndrome. *Obesity* **2011**, *19*, 23–28. [CrossRef]
6. Harwood, J. Fatty-Acid Metabolism. *Annu. Rev. Plant Physiol. Plant Mol. Biol.* **1988**, *39*, 101–138. [CrossRef]
7. Habinowski, S.A.; Witters, L.A. The Effects of AICAR on Adipocyte Differentiation of 3T3-L1 Cells. *Biochem. Biophys. Res. Commun.* **2001**, *286*, 852–856. [CrossRef]
8. Lage, R.; Dieguez, C.; Vidal-Puig, A.; Lopez, M. AMPK: A Metabolic Gauge Regulating Whole-Body Energy Homeostasis. *Trends Mol. Med.* **2008**, *14*, 539–549. [CrossRef]
9. Lim, C.T.; Kola, B.; Korbonits, M. AMPK as a Mediator of Hormonal Signalling. *J. Mol. Endocrinol.* **2010**, *44*, 87–97. [CrossRef]
10. Peng, I.-C.; Chen, Z.; Sun, W.; Li, Y.-S.; Marin, T.L.; Hsu, P.-H.; Su, M.-I.; Cui, X.; Pan, S.; Lytle, C.Y.; et al. Glucagon Regulates ACC Activity in Adipocytes through the CAMKK Beta/AMPK Pathway. *Am. J. Physiol.-Endocrinol. Metab.* **2012**, *302*, E1560–E1568. [CrossRef]
11. Ducharme, N.A.; Bickel, P.E. Minireview: Lipid Droplets in Lipogenesis and Lipolysis. *Endocrinology* **2008**, *149*, 942–949. [CrossRef] [PubMed]
12. Szkudelski, T.; Szkudelska, K. Effects of AMPK Activation on Lipolysis in Primary Rat Adipocytes: Studies at Different Glucose Concentrations. *Arch. Physiol. Biochem.* **2017**, *123*, 43–49. [CrossRef]
13. Elgebaly, A.; Radwan, I.A.I.; AboElnas, M.M.; Ibrahim, H.H.; Eltoomy, M.F.M.; Atta, A.A.; Mesalam, H.A.; Sayed, A.A.; Othman, A.A. Resveratrol Supplementation in Patients with Non-Alcoholic Fatty Liver Disease: Systematic Review and Meta-Analysis. *J. Gastrointest. Liver Dis.* **2017**, *26*, 59–67. [CrossRef] [PubMed]
14. Isken, F.; Klaus, S.; Osterhoff, M.; Pfeiffer, A.F.H.; Weickert, M.O. Effects of Long-Term Soluble vs. Insoluble Dietary Fiber Intake on High-Fat Diet-Induced Obesity in C57BL/6J Mice. *J. Nutr. Biochem.* **2010**, *21*, 278–284. [CrossRef]
15. Han, X.; Yang, D.; Zhang, S.; Liu, X.; Zhao, Y.; Song, C.; Sun, Q. Characterization of Insoluble Dietary Fiber from Pleurotus Eryngii and Evaluation of Its Effects on Obesity-Preventing or Relieving Effects via Modulation of Gut Microbiota. *J. Future Foods* **2023**, *3*, 55–66. [CrossRef]
16. Wang, S.; Sun, W.; Swallah, M.S.; Amin, K.; Lyu, B.; Fan, H.; Zhang, Z.; Yu, H. Preparation and Characterization of Soybean Insoluble Dietary Fiber and Its Prebiotic Effect on Dyslipidemia and Hepatic Steatosis in High Fat-Fed C57BL/6J Mice. *Food Funct.* **2021**, *12*, 8760–8773. [CrossRef] [PubMed]
17. Agostoni, C.; Bresson, J.-L.; Fairweather-Tait, S.; Flynn, A.; Golly, I.; Korhonen, H.; Lagiou, P.; Lovik, M.; Marchelli, R.; Martin, A.; et al. Scientific Opinion on Dietary Reference Values for Carbohydrates and Dietary Fibre. *Efsa J.* **2010**, *8*, 1462. [CrossRef]
18. Esmail, M.; Anwar, S.; Kandeil, M.; El-Zanaty, A.M.; Abdel-Gabbar, M. Effect of Nigella Sativa, Atorvastatin, or L-Carnitine on High Fat Diet-Induced Obesity in Adult Male Albino Rats. *Biomed. Pharmacother.* **2021**, *141*, 111818. [CrossRef]
19. Alhasaniah, A.H. L-Carnitine: Nutrition, Pathology, and Health Benefits. *Saudi J. Biol. Sci.* **2023**, *30*, 103555. [CrossRef]
20. Nishida, C.; Uauy, R.; Kumanyika, S.; Shetty, P. The Joint WHO/FAO Expert Consultation on Diet, Nutrition and the Prevention of Chronic Diseases: Process, Product and Policy Implications. *Public Health Nutr.* **2004**, *7*, 245–250. [CrossRef]
21. Ye, S.; Shah, B.R.; Li, J.; Liang, H.; Zhan, F.; Geng, F.; Li, B. A Critical Review on Interplay between Dietary Fibers and Gut Microbiota. *Trends Food Sci. Technol.* **2022**, *124*, 237–249. [CrossRef]
22. Zhao, G.; Zhang, R.; Dong, L.; Huang, F.; Tang, X.; Wei, Z.; Zhang, M. Particle Size of Insoluble Dietary Fiber from Rice Bran Affects Its Phenolic Profile, Bioaccessibility and Functional Properties. *Lwt-Food Sci. Technol.* **2018**, *87*, 450–456. [CrossRef]
23. Kapravelou, G.; Martinez, R.; Andrade, A.M.; Sanchez, C.; Lopez Chaves, C.; Lopez-Jurado, M.; Aranda, P.; Cantarero, S.; Arrebola, F.; Fernandez-Segura, E.; et al. Health Promoting Effects of Lupin (*Lupinus albus* Var. *Multolupa*) Protein Hydrolyzate and Insoluble Fiber in a Diet-Induced Animal Experimental Model of Hypercholesterolemia. *Food Res. Int.* **2013**, *54*, 1471–1481. [CrossRef]
24. Ren, L.; Sun, D.; Zhou, X.; Yang, Y.; Huang, X.; Li, Y.; Wang, C.; Li, Y. Chronic Treatment with the Modified Longdan Xiegan Tang Attenuates Olanzapine-Induced Fatty Liver in Rats by Regulating Hepatic de Novo Lipogenesis and Fatty Acid Beta-Oxidation-Associated Gene Expression Mediated by SREBP-1c, PPAR-Alpha and AMPK-Alpha. *J. Ethnopharmacol.* **2019**, *232*, 176–187. [CrossRef]
25. Song, Y.-B.; An, Y.R.; Kim, S.J.; Park, H.-W.; Jung, J.-W.; Kyung, J.-S.; Hwang, S.Y.; Kim, Y.-S. Lipid Metabolic Effect of Korean Red Ginseng Extract in Mice Fed on a High-Fat Diet. *J. Sci. Food Agric.* **2012**, *92*, 388–396. [CrossRef]

26. Smith, U.; Kahn, B.B. Adipose Tissue Regulates Insulin Sensitivity: Role of Adipogenesis, de Novo Lipogenesis and Novel Lipids. *J. Intern. Med.* **2016**, *280*, 465–475. [CrossRef]
27. Smith, B.K.; Marcinko, K.; Desjardins, E.M.; Lally, J.S.; Ford, R.J.; Steinberg, G.R. Treatment of Nonalcoholic Fatty Liver Disease: Role of AMPK. *Am. J. Physiol.-Endocrinol. Metab.* **2016**, *311*, E730–E740. [CrossRef]
28. Huang, X.; Zhou, Y.; Sun, Y.; Wang, Q. Intestinal Fatty Acid Binding Protein: A Rising Therapeutic Target in Lipid Metabolism. *Prog. Lipid Res.* **2022**, *87*, 101178. [CrossRef]
29. Kim, J.J.P.; Battaile, K.P. Burning Fat: The Structural Basis of Fatty Acid Beta-Oxidation. *Curr. Opin. Struct. Biol.* **2002**, *12*, 721–728. [CrossRef]
30. Reddy, J.K.; Rao, M.S. Lipid Metabolism and Liver Inflammation. II. Fatty Liver Disease and Fatty Acid Oxidation. *Am. J. Physiol.-Gastrointest. Liver Physiol.* **2006**, *290*, G852–G858. [CrossRef]
31. Wanders, R.J.A.; Ferdinandusse, S.; Brites, P.; Kemp, S. Peroxisomes, Lipid Metabolism and Lipotoxicity. *Biochim. Biophys. Acta-Mol. Cell Biol. Lipids* **2010**, *1801*, 272–280. [CrossRef]
32. Adeva-Andany, M.M.; Carneiro-Freire, N.; Seco-Filgueira, M.; Fernandez-Fernandez, C.; Mourino-Bayolo, D. Mitochondrial Beta-Oxidation of Saturated Fatty Acids in Humans. *Mitochondrion* **2019**, *46*, 73–90. [CrossRef]
33. Osmundsen, H.; Bremer, J.; Pedersen, J. Metabolic Aspects of Peroxisomal Beta-Oxidation. *Biochim. Biophys. Acta* **1991**, *1085*, 141–158. [CrossRef] [PubMed]
34. Yao, H.; Wang, Y.; Zhang, X.; Li, P.; Shang, L.; Chen, X.; Zeng, J. Targeting Peroxisomal Fatty Acid Oxidation Improves Hepatic Steatosis and Insulin Resistance in Obese Mice. *J. Biol. Chem.* **2023**, *299*, 102845. [CrossRef]
35. Mannaerts, G.; Van veldhoven, P.; Van broekhoven, A.; Vandebroek, G.; Debeer, L. Evidence That Peroxisomal Acyl-Coa Synthetase Is Located at the Cytoplasmic Side of the Peroxisomal Membrane. *Biochem. J.* **1982**, *204*, 17–23. [CrossRef] [PubMed]
36. Chen, X.; Shang, L.; Deng, S.; Li, P.; Chen, K.; Gao, T.; Zhang, X.; Chen, Z.; Zeng, J. Peroxisomal Oxidation of Erucic Acid Suppresses Mitochondrial Fatty Acid Oxidation by Stimulating Malonyl-CoA Formation in the Rat Liver. *J. Biol. Chem.* **2020**, *295*, 10168–10179. [CrossRef] [PubMed]
37. Burri, L.; Thoresen, G.H.; Berge, R.K. The Role of PPAR Alpha Activation in Liver and Muscle. *PPAR Res.* **2010**, *2010*, 542359. [CrossRef] [PubMed]
38. Glosli, H.; Gudbrandsen, O.A.; Mullen, A.J.; Halvorsen, B.; Rost, T.H.; Wergedahl, H.; Prydz, H.; Aukrust, P.; Berge, R.K. Down-Regulated Expression of PPAR Alpha Target Genes, Reduced Fatty Acid Oxidation and Altered Fatty Acid Composition in the Liver of Mice Transgenic for HTNF Alpha. *Biochim. Biophys. Acta-Mol. Cell Biol. Lipids* **2005**, *1734*, 235–246. [CrossRef]
39. Evans, R.M.; Barish, G.D.; Wang, Y.X. PPARs and the Complex Journey to Obesity. *Nat. Med.* **2004**, *10*, 355–361. [CrossRef]
40. Day, E.A.; Ford, R.J.; Steinberg, G.R. AMPK as a Therapeutic Target for Treating Metabolic Diseases. *Trends Endocrinol. Metab.* **2017**, *28*, 545–560. [CrossRef]
41. Singh, A.B.; Kan, C.F.K.; Dong, B.; Liu, J. SREBP2 Activation Induces Hepatic Long-Chain Acyl-CoA Synthetase 1 (ACSL1) Expression in Vivo and in Vitro through a Sterol Regulatory Element (SRE) Motif of the ACSL1 C-Promoter. *J. Biol. Chem.* **2016**, *291*, 5373–5384. [CrossRef]
42. Gao, J.; Gu, X.; Zhang, M.; Zu, X.; Shen, F.; Hou, X.; Hao, E.; Bai, G. Ferulic Acid Targets ACSL1 to Ameliorate Lipid Metabolic Disorders in Db/Db Mice. *J. Funct. Foods* **2022**, *91*, 105009. [CrossRef]
43. Cohen, H.Y.; Miller, C.; Bitterman, K.J.; Wall, N.R.; Hekking, B.; Kessler, B.; Howitz, K.T.; Gorospe, M.; de Cabo, R.; Sinclair, D.A. Calorie Restriction Promotes Mammalian Cell Survival by Inducing the SIRT1 Deacetylase. *Science* **2004**, *305*, 390–392. [CrossRef] [PubMed]
44. Li, S.; Liu, C.; Li, N.; Hao, T.; Han, T.; Hill, D.E.; Vidal, M.; Lin, J.D. Genome-Wide Coactivation Analysis of PGC-1 Alpha Identifies BAF60a as a Regulator of Hepatic Lipid Metabolism. *Cell Metab.* **2008**, *8*, 105–117. [CrossRef] [PubMed]
45. Rodgers, J.T.; Lerin, C.; Haas, W.; Gygi, S.P.; Spiegelman, B.M.; Puigserver, P. Nutrient Control of Glucose Homeostasis through a Complex of PGC-1 Alpha and SIRT1. *Nature* **2005**, *434*, 113–118. [CrossRef] [PubMed]
46. Purushotham, A.; Schug, T.T.; Xu, Q.; Surapureddi, S.; Guo, X.; Li, X. Hepatocyte-Specific Deletion of SIRT1 Alters Fatty Acid Metabolism and Results in Hepatic Steatosis and Inflammation. *Cell Metab.* **2009**, *9*, 327–338. [CrossRef] [PubMed]
47. Abelson, P.; Kennedy, D. The Obesity Epidemic. *Science* **2004**, *304*, 1413. [CrossRef]
48. Stein, C.J.; Colditz, G.A. The Epidemic of Obesity. *J. Clin. Endocrinol. Metab.* **2004**, *89*, 2522–2525. [CrossRef] [PubMed]
49. Maes, H.H.M.; Neale, M.C.; Eaves, L.J. Genetic and Environmental Factors in Relative Body Weight and Human Adiposity. *Behav. Genet.* **1997**, *27*, 325–351. [CrossRef]
50. Brownlee, I.A. The Physiological Roles of Dietary Fibre. *Food Hydrocoll.* **2011**, *25*, 238–250. [CrossRef]
51. Li, L.; Pan, M.; Pan, S.; Li, W.; Zhong, Y.; Hu, J.; Nie, S. Effects of Insoluble and Soluble Fibers Isolated from Barley on Blood Glucose, Serum Lipids, Liver Function and Caecal Short-Chain Fatty Acids in Type 2 Diabetic and Normal Rats. *Food Chem. Toxicol.* **2020**, *135*, 110937. [CrossRef] [PubMed]
52. Gadde, K.M.; Martin, C.K.; Berthoud, H.-R.; Heymsfield, S.B. Obesity Pathophysiology and Management. *J. Am. Coll. Cardiol.* **2018**, *71*, 69–84. [CrossRef] [PubMed]
53. Gonzalez-Muniesa, P.; Martinez-Gonzalez, M.-A.; Hu, F.B.; Despres, J.-P.; Matsuzawa, Y.; Loos, R.J.F.; Moreno, L.A.; Bray, G.; Alfredo Martinez, J. Obesity. *Nat. Rev. Dis. Primer* **2017**, *3*, 17034. [CrossRef] [PubMed]

54. Sorensen, T.I.A. From Fat Cells through an Obesity Theory. *Eur. J. Clin. Nutr.* **2018**, *72*, 1329–1335. [CrossRef] [PubMed]
55. Weickert, M.O.; Mohlig, M.; Koebnick, C.; Holst, J.J.; Namsolleck, P.; Ristow, M.; Osterhoff, M.; Rochlitz, H.; Rudovich, N.; Spranger, J.; et al. Impact of Cereal Fibre on Glucose-Regulating Factors. *Diabetologia* **2005**, *48*, 2343–2353. [CrossRef]

Disclaimer/Publisher's Note: The statements, opinions and data contained in all publications are solely those of the individual author(s) and contributor(s) and not of MDPI and/or the editor(s). MDPI and/or the editor(s) disclaim responsibility for any injury to people or property resulting from any ideas, methods, instructions or products referred to in the content.

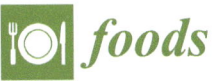 foods

Article

Protective Effect of *Anoectochilus formosanus* Polysaccharide against Cyclophosphamide-Induced Immunosuppression in BALB/c Mice

Anqi Xie [1], Hao Wan [1], Lei Feng [1,*], Boyun Yang [2] and Yiqun Wan [1,3,*]

[1] State Key Laboratory of Food Science and Technology, Nanchang University, Nanchang 330047, China; xieanqi2023@163.com (A.X.); wanhao424@ncu.edu.cn (H.W.)
[2] School of Life Sciences, Nanchang University, Nanchang 330031, China; yangboyun@163.com
[3] Jiangxi Province Key Laboratory of Modern Analytical Science, Nanchang University, Nanchang 330031, China
* Correspondence: fenglei217@163.com (L.F.); wanyiqun@ncu.edu.cn (Y.W.)

Abstract: In this study, *Anoectochilus formosanus* polysaccharide (AFP) was acquired a via water extraction and alcohol precipitation method. The immunoregulatory activity of AFP was first evaluated on cyclophosphamide (Cy)-treated mice. Galacturonic acid, glucose and galactose were confirmed to be the main components of AFP. AFP demonstrated the ability to stimulate the production of TNF-α and IL-6 in RAW 264.7 macrophages. Not surprisingly, the activation of the NF-κB signaling pathway by AFP was validated via Western blot analysis. Furthermore, AFP could alleviate Cy-induced immunosuppression, and significantly enhance the immunity of mice via increasing the thymus index and body weight, stimulating the production of cytokines (IgA, IgG, SIgA, IL-2, IL-6 and IFN-γ). The improvement in the intestinal morphology of immunosuppressed mice showed that AFP could alleviate Cy-induced immune toxicity. These results have raised the possibility that AFP may act as a natural immunomodulator. Overall, the study of AFP was innovative and of great significance for AFP's further application and utilization.

Keywords: *Anoectochilus formosanus*; polysaccharide; immunosuppression; bioactivities

Citation: Xie, A.; Wan, H.; Feng, L.; Yang, B.; Wan, Y. Protective Effect of *Anoectochilus formosanus* Polysaccharide against Cyclophosphamide-Induced Immunosuppression in BALB/c Mice. *Foods* **2023**, *12*, 1910. https://doi.org/10.3390/foods12091910

Academic Editor: Philippe Michaud

Received: 14 March 2023
Revised: 27 April 2023
Accepted: 4 May 2023
Published: 7 May 2023

Copyright: © 2023 by the authors. Licensee MDPI, Basel, Switzerland. This article is an open access article distributed under the terms and conditions of the Creative Commons Attribution (CC BY) license (https://creativecommons.org/licenses/by/4.0/).

1. Introduction

Over the past decade, the burden of cancer in the world has been increasing continuously [1]. Cyclophosphamide (Cy) is an effective anticancer drug commonly used in the clinic [2]. However, the side effects caused by Cy should not be underestimated. The most common clinical symptom is that Cy has a strong immunosuppressive effect on human body [3]. Intestinal mucosal injury is one of the main manifestations of immunosuppression. Cy not only inhibits the secretion of immune cytokines in mice intestinal mucosa, resulting in immune dysfunction and intestinal injury, but also destroys the intestinal mucosal barrier and affects the integrity of the epithelium and neighboring cell–cell junctions, thereby impacting the absorption of food in the intestine [4–7].

Faced with these constraints, people have focused on polysaccharides derived from natural sources. Studies have proven that polysaccharides have extensive biological functions, such as promoting and protecting intestinal health [8], supporting normal bowel function, maintaining the regular state of blood glucose and lipids [9], and enhancing immunity [10]. Moreover, polysaccharides can be used as an anti-tumor and anti-inflammatory drug [11,12]. As an immunomodulator, polysaccharides have no significant side effects on the body [3]. It has been reported that the polysaccharides extracted from yellow pear residue markedly improve the immune function of mice [13].

The genus *Anoectochilus* (Orchidaceae) is a very precious perennial herb with 40 species worldwide, mainly distributed in China, Japan, India, Nepal, Sri Lanka, and other Asian countries. It is regarded as a traditional Chinese medicine and as beneficial to cancer, hypertension, diabetes mellitus, consumption, and nephritis [14–16]. At present, the major research species in China are produced in Fujian, Zhejiang, Jiangxi, and Taiwan [17]. *Anoectochilus formosanus* (AF) is one variety in the *Anoectochilus* family. According to reports, the water extract of AF has been shown to act not only as a protective agent in the liver, but also as an important immunomodulator [18]. In addition, studies have pointed out that the methanol extract of AF shows potential applicative value in the immunochemical prevention/treatment of cancer via the lowering of blood glucose, the scavenging of ROS, and the inhibition of PD-L1 [19]. Polysaccharides extracted from different parts of AF have shown different antidiabetic activity in vivo due to the different M_w and monosaccharide compositions [20]. However, the reports on *Anoectochilus formosanus* polysaccharide (AFP) are relatively superficial. Little is known about the protective effects of AFP against immunosuppression. Therefore, exploring the bioactivity of AFP is of great significance in order to elucidate its function and utilization.

Based on these questions, AFPs were isolated from AF and their chemical properties were further investigated. The protective effect of AFP against the immunosuppression of mice induced by Cy was also invested. Therefore, our study was conducted in order to explore the immunomodulatory activities of AFP and provide a theoretical basis for developing AF.

2. Materials and Methods

2.1. Materials

Anoectochilus formosanus was obtained from Fujian province and verified by Prof. Boyun Yang from the Life Science Center of Nanchang University. It was then dried at 55 °C for 48 h before preparation. The monosaccharide standards used, D-Mannose, L-Arabinose, D-Ribose, etc., were purchased from Merck Co. (Darmstadt, Germany). Levamisole hydrochloride and cyclophosphamide were purchased from Aladdin Industrial Inc. (Shanghai, China). Cytokine (IgA, IgG, SIgA, IL-2, IL-6, IFN-γ, TNF-α) detecting ELISA kits were purchased from Biosharp biological technology Co., Ltd. (Shanghai, China). Lipopolysaccharide (LPS) and PBS buffer powder were purchased from Beijing Solarbio Science & Technology Co., Ltd. (Beijing, China). Commercially available analytical grade reagents were used in this study.

2.2. Extraction of Polysaccharides

Fresh plants were used as raw material and dried at 55 °C in the air-drying oven. After mechanical crushing, the coarse powder was passed through 80-mesh sieves to obtain a fine powder. Fat, pigment and small molecule were removed by soaking the powder in 95% ethanol for 10 h; this was repeated 4 times. After soaking, the powder was centrifuged and dried. The dried powder was extracted 4 times with distilled water at 80 °C with a material-to-liquid ratio of 1:20 (w/v) for 6 h. The supernatant was collected and the condensed solution was obtained by using a rotary evaporator under vacuum at 55 °C. Then, 85% ethanol was used to precipitate the polysaccharides with vigorous stirring; this was then stored at 4 °C overnight. The precipitate was collected after 10 min of centrifugation and washed three times with ethanol and acetone in succession. Finally, the precipitates were solubilized in distilled water and dialyzed (cut-off M_w 3500 Da) for 48 h with distilled water, and then concentrated and lyophilized to obtain the polysaccharide named AFP [21].

2.3. Homogeneity and Molecular Weight Distribution of AFP

An Agilent 1260 Infinity system (Agilent Technologies, Amstelveen, The Netherlands) equipped with a refractive index detector (RID, G1362A) was used to measure the homogeneity and molecular weight of polysaccharide fractions via the method of high-performance gel permeation chromatography (HPGPC), according to a previous study [22,23].

2.4. Determination of Chemical Components

Glucose was treated as the standard in order to verify the neutral sugar content, using the phenol-sulphuric acids method [24]. The meta-hydroxydiphenyl method was performed according to a previous report, but with some modifications, to determine the uronic acid content in AFP. D-galacturonic acid was used as a standard [25]. In addition, protein content was determined using bovine serum albumin as a standard according to the Coomassie Brilliant Blue method [26]. Fat content was analyzed via the Soxhlet method [27].

2.5. Monosaccharide Composition Analysis

AFP monosaccharides were identified according to a published report but with some amendments [28], and the samples were analyzed on an Agilent 1260 Infinity system equipped with a UV detector (250 nm) and a Diamonsil C18 column (4.6 mm i.d. ×250 mm, 5 µm, Dikma, Foothill Ranch, CA, USA). The temperature of the column was maintained at 35 °C. The mobile phase was composed of acetonitrile and 0.1 mol/L PB (pH 6.8) in a ratio of 17:83 (v/v) at a flow rate of 1.0 mL/min. The injection volume was 20 µL, and the time of data collection was 50 min. Briefly, the AFP (5 mg) was hydrolyzed in 4 mL of 3 M TFA at 100 °C for 6 h in a sealed glass tube. After hydrolysis, the products were cooled to room temperature and dried with nitrogen. Diluting them with 1 mL of ultra-pure water, the hydrolysates were then obtained as derivatized, filtrated, loaded samples and monitored with the UV detector at an absorbance of 250 nm.

2.6. Fourier Transform Infrared Spectrum

A Thermo Nicolet 5700 infrared spectrophotometer (Thermo Electron, Madison, WI, USA) was used to characterize the organic functional groups of AFP using the KBr-pellets method, with the range of 400–4000 cm^{-1} [29].

2.7. Cell Culture

The murine macrophage RAW 264.7 cell was cultured in Dulbecco's Modified Eagle's medium (DMEM) medium containing 13% (v/v) fetal bovine serum (FBS). The cells were grown in a humidified incubator at 37 °C with an atmosphere comprising 5% CO_2.

2.7.1. Cell Viability

The Cell Counting Kit-8 (CCK-8) method was used to verify the cell viability. RAW 264.7 cells (2.5×10^5 cells/well, 100 µL) were plated in 96-well plates for 24 h, followed by incubation with 100 µL of AFP (50, 100, 200, and 400 µg/mL) or lipopolysaccharides (LPS) (1 µg/mL) dissolved in DMEM medium for another 24 h. Subsequently, each well was incubated with 100 µL of diluted CCK-8 solution for another 2 h. Using a microplate reader, absorbance was measured at 450 nm. The experiment was carried out in triplicate.

2.7.2. Influence of AFP on TNF-α and IL-6 Production of RAW 264.7

RAW 264.7 macrophage cells were plated into a 96-well plate with a density of approximately 2.5×10^5 cells/mL and stimulated with AFP (100, 200, and 400 µg/mL) and LPS (1 µg/mL). TNF-α and IL-6 were detected in RAW 264.7 cells after 24 h of incubation with a commercial ELISA kit. The experiment was carried out in triplicate.

2.7.3. Western Blot Analysis

RAW 264.7 cells were co-cultured with different concentrations of AFP (100, 200, and 400 µg/mL) and LPS (1 µg/mL) dissolved in DMEM medium for 24 h. The precipitates of the different treated cells were obtained using a centrifuge. The cell protein was prepared by adding 250 µL of Radio Immunoprecipitation Assay Lysis buffer (RIPA) lysate per 10^6 cells. The denatured proteins were transferred by sodium dodecyl sulfate-polyacrylamide gel electrophoresis (SDS-PAGE) electrophoresis onto polyvinylidene fluoride (PVDF) (0.45 µm) membranes pre-activated with methanol and subsequently subjected to immunoreactivity.

The PVDF membranes were treated successively using the primary antibody (anti-p-NF-κB p65, anti-NF-κB p65) and secondary antibody, followed by an elution with Tris Buffered Saline with Tween 20 (TBST) 3 times. Electrochemiluminescence (ELC) was used to visualize the protein band. Finally, the images were sorted and decolored to analyze the optical density values of the target bands.

2.8. Animals' Experiments

2.8.1. Animals and Treatment

SPF female BALB/c mice (20 ± 0.2 g, 6–8-week-old) were purchased from the Hunan Slac Jingda Laboratory Animal Co. Ltd. (Hunan, China), with the certificate number SYXK (Xiang) 2019-0004. All mice were maintained in an appropriate environment with free access to standard rodent chow and water at 22 ± 2 °C, with 60 ± 5% relative humidity, and a 12 h light/12 h dark cycle. The guidelines of Regulations for the Administration of Affairs Concerning Experimental Animals were strictly followed, and the study was approved by the State Council of the People's Republic of China. After one week of acclimatization in the laboratory, all the mice were randomly divided into six groups, as follows: normal control group (denoted as NC group), model control group (denoted as MC group), AFP low-dose group (denoted as AFPL group), AFP medium-dose group (denoted as AFPM group), AFP high-dose group (denoted as AFPH group) and positive control group (denoted as PC group). Each group contained 12 mice, which were weighed every experiment day. The volume of intraperitoneal injection or gavage was one percent of the body weight of mice. For the first three consecutive days, the NC group received normal saline only as a normal control, while the other five groups received an intraperitoneal injection with Cy at a dose of 80 mg·kg^{-1}·d^{-1} to construct a model of immune suppression [10]. The NC and MC groups received only normal saline intragastrically for the next seven days, while the AFPL, AFPM, and AFPH groups were given 50 mg·kg^{-1} BW, 100 mg·kg^{-1} BW, and 200 mg·kg^{-1} BW by gavage, respectively. Levamisole hydrochloride (LH) at 40 mg·kg^{-1} BW was administered by gavage to the PC group.

All mice were weighed and sacrificed 24 h after the last drug administration. The serum was obtained and the intact thymus was isolated via dissection. The small intestine was divided into segments according to the needs of different experiments. All anatomical tissues were frozen at −80 °C for subsequent analysis.

2.8.2. Influence of AFP on Body Weight and Thymus Index

The weight of the mice was recorded every experimental day. After sacrificed, the intact thymus of the mice was harvested, rinsed with normal saline and blotted on filter paper before being weighed. Based on the reference formula, the thymus index was calculated as follows: thymus index = weight of thymus (mg)/weight of the body (g) [30].

2.8.3. Preparation and Staining of Intestinal Section

At this stage, 4–6 cm jejunal tissue was cut and fixed with 10% neutral formalin for over 48 h. The tissues were dehydrated in a graded concentration of ethanol and embedded in paraffin wax afterwards. Samples were sliced into 4 μm thick paraffin sections for further analysis.

For hematoxylin-eosin staining (H&E) staining, paraffin sections were first dewaxed with xylene, absolute ethyl alcohol, and a gradient concentration of ethanol, respectively. Next, the sections were washed with distilled water. Secondly, the nucleus was stained with hematoxylin, and the cytoplasm was stained with Eosin. Thirdly, the sections were made transparent with xylene and then observed for histological changes. The H&E staining results were observed via an optical microscope at a 200-fold field of view. The complete villus and crypts should be present in each random magnified field of view.

For periodic acid schiff and alcian blue stain (AB-PAS) staining, after dewaxing and washing, the tissues were colored via immersion in 1% Alcian blue for 10–20 min, then running water was applied to rinse the tissue for 6 min. Following 10 min of oxidation with 0.5% periodic acid, the tissues were rinsed with running water for 6 min. Afterwards, the tissues were placed in the darkness and dipped in Schiff reagent for 15–30 min. Lastly, the samples were dehydrated, made transparent, fixed, and finally the AB-PAS staining results were observed using an optical microscope at a 200-fold field of view.

2.8.4. Analysis of Serum Immunoglobulin A (IgA) and Immunoglobulin G (IgG) Secretion

The secretion of serum IgA and IgG was determined using ELISA Kits. The manufacturer's instructions were strictly followed during all operating procedures.

2.8.5. Analysis of Small Intestinal Cytokines Level

The production of small intestinal cytokines (secretory immunoglobulin A, SIgA; interleukin-2, IL-2; interleukin 6, IL-6; interferon γ, IFN-γ) was evaluated using ELISA Kits. The manufacturer's instructions were strictly followed during all operating procedures.

2.9. Statistical Analysis

Experimental data were analyzed and expressed as mean ± standard deviation (SD) using SPSS22. IBM SPSS22 (SPSS Inc., Chicago, IL, USA) software was used to assess the statistical differences between groups via one-way analysis of variance (ANOVA) and the Tukey test. $p < 0.05$ indicated that the difference was statistically significant.

3. Results

3.1. Characterization and Identification of Polysaccharide from AF

Hot water extraction and ethanol precipitation were used to extract the AFP. The yield rate of the AFP was designated as approximately 9.20% of the dry weight of raw material. AFP contained 46.70% neutral sugar, 2.98% protein, 25.07% uronic acid, and 0.23% fat. Single and symmetrical elution peaks were acquired using high-performance gel permeation chromatography (Figure 1A), indicating that AFP had relatively homogeneous components. Based on the standard regression equation of dextran and glucose (Figure 1B), AFP had a homogeneous M_w distribution of 16.41 kDa.

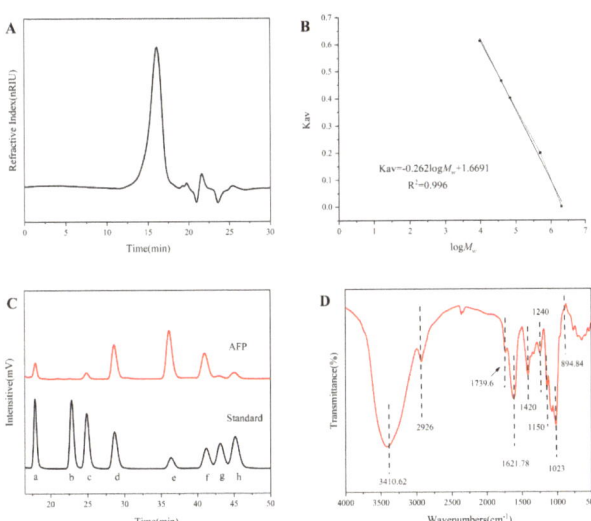

Figure 1. High-performance gel permeation chromatography profiles of AFP (**A**), and the HPGPC calibration curve of dextran standards and glucose (**B**). HPLC chromatogram profiles of monosaccharide composition of AFP (**C**). The monosaccharide standards (a) D-Mannose, (b) D-Ribose, (c) L-Rhamnose, (d) D-Galacturonic acid, Ⓔ D-Glucose, (f) D-Galactose, (g) D-Xylose and (h) L-Arabinose, respectively, were used to qualitatively detect and analyze the samples. FT-IR spectra of AFP (**D**).

3.2. Monosaccharide Composition Analysis

Figure 1C shows the monosaccharide composition of AFP. Based on the retention time of the monosaccharide standard, AFP was mainly composed of D-Mannose, D-Galacturonic acid, D-Glucose, and D-Galactose, accompanied by fewer amounts of L-Rhamnose, D-Xylose, and L-Arabinose. The mole ratios of D-Mannose, L-Rhamnose, D-Galacturonic acid, D-Glucose, D-Galactose, D-Xylose, and L-Arabinose were at 6.69%, 3.73%, 14.51%, 44.19%, 17.63%, 6.07% and 7.16%, respectively.

3.3. Fourier Transform Infrared Spectrum

The FT-IR spectra of AFP are shown in Figure 1D. The stretching vibration of O–H was the broad absorption peak at 3410.62 cm^{-1}. Bands at 2926 cm^{-1} arose from C–H stretching vibrations, and the absorption between 1400~1200 cm^{-1} corresponded to the bending vibrations of C–H [31]. The absorption band of AFP centered at 1739.6 cm^{-1} was caused by an ester carbonyl C=O asymmetric stretching vibration, suggesting the existence of uronic acid [32]. The band at 1621.78 cm^{-1} was attributed to the -OH flexural vibrations of the polysaccharide. Furthermore, the absorption bands centered at 1150 cm^{-1}, 1081 cm^{-1} and 1023 cm^{-1} were assigned to the stretching vibrations of the pyranose ring of the glucosyl residue [29]. In addition, the presence of β-type glycosidic linkages were suggested by the typical absorption at 894.84 cm^{-1} of AFP [33,34].

3.4. In Vitro Immunostimulatory Activities on Macrophages of AFP

To explore the immunoregulatory effects of polysaccharides on macrophages, the ability of macrophages to proliferate in the presence of AFP in various concentrations was first measured. As shown in Figure 2A, the presence of AFP at various doses significantly enhanced the proliferation of macrophages in a dose-related pattern compared to the control group ($p < 0.01$). The highest proliferation ability was found at 400 μg/mL, which was up to 1.8 times the value of that of the control group. With respect to TNF-α, the expression increased with the increment in AFP from 100 to 400 μg/mL, but only notably upregulated TNF-α expression at 400 μg/mL ($p < 0.05$). Compared to the control group, AFP significantly increased IL-6 secretion in a dose-dependent manner ($p < 0.05$). The expression of IL-6 was elevated 8-fold by treatment with 400 μg/mL of AFP in comparison with the control group, and was evidently larger than those in the 100 and 200 μg/mL groups ($p < 0.01$).

3.5. Activation of the NF-κB Signaling Pathway by AFP

The immunomodulatory effect of AFP on RAW 264.7 was assessed by detecting the phosphorylation levels of NF-κB p65 in cells using Western blot analysis. The amount of p-NF-κB p65 was increased in accordance with the concentrations of AFP in a dose-dependent manner, as illustrated in Figure 3A. The phosphorylation level of NF-κB p65 was promoted by 1.41-fold after treatment with 1 μg/mL of LPS, relative to the control group ($p < 0.01$); this indicated that LPS could promote the phosphorylation of the NF-κB signaling pathway proteins markedly. Notably, the AFP group enhanced the amount of phosphorylation in the NF-κB p65 protein of the NF-κB pathway in a surprisingly good dose-dependent manner, in relation to the control group, and was even higher than that in the LPS group; this was responsible for the active inflammatory response. These results suggest that the NF-κB signaling pathway was a key signaling pathway for the immune activity of AFP in the macrophages.

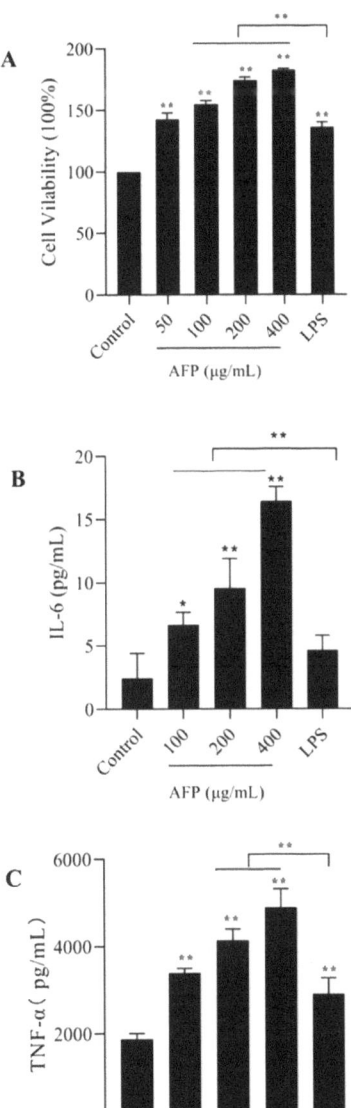

Figure 2. Effect of AFP on RAW 264.7 cells. (**A**) Cell proliferation rate of RAW 264.7 cells pretreated with AFP; (**B**) macrophages IL-6 secretion pretreated with AFP; (**C**) macrophages TNF-α secretion pretreated with AFP. Data are expressed as the mean ± SD (n = 3). * $p < 0.05$, ** $p < 0.01$ compared with the control group (0 μg/mL).

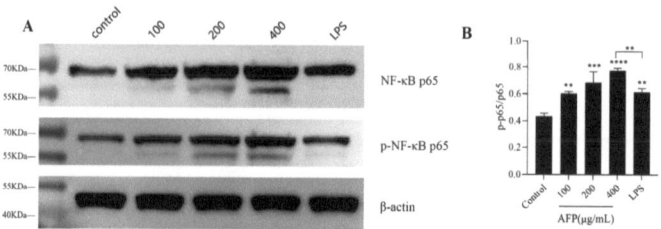

Figure 3. Effects of AFP on NF-κB signaling pathway in RAW 264.7 cells. (**A**) Western blot analysis of NF-κB induced by AFP in RAW264.7 cells. (**B**) Histogram represents the quantification of AFP-stimulated p-p65 in RAW264.7 cells. Data are expressed as the mean ± SD (n = 3). ** $p < 0.01$, *** $p < 0.001$, **** $p < 0.0001$ compared with the control group (0 μg/mL).

3.6. Influence of AFP on Body Weight and Thymus Index

The variation in the body weight of the mice among the six groups was supervised every experimental day and the results are shown in Table 1. In comparison with the first day, the body weight of the Cy-treatment mice decreased dramatically on the fourth day ($p < 0.05$). During the remaining days of the experiment, the mice treated with AFP lost less body weight than those in the MC group. Namely, Cy-treated mice were associated with a risk of weight loss, whereas AFP could effectively reverse the weight loss caused by the Cy treatment.

Table 1. Change in body weight of Cy-exposed mice.

Group	Initial Weight (g)	Weight on the Fourth Day (g)	Final Weight (g)	Weight Gain (g)
NC	18.14 ± 1.31	18.02 ± 0.95 *	18.59 ± 1.00	0.55 ± 0.69
MC	19.28 ± 1.07	17.20 ± 1.02 #	18.56 ± 0.73	−0.72 ± 0.54
AFPL	18.63 ± 1.16	16.63 ± 1.15 #	18.25 ± 0.69	−0.04 ± 0.84
AFPM	18.44 ± 1.02	16.60 ± 1.40 #	17.90 ± 0.82	−0.17 ± 0.61
AFPH	18.63 ± 0.81	16.57 ± 0.93 #	17.81 ± 0.88	−0.48 ± 0.32
PC	19.29 ± 1.12	17.26 ± 0.87 #	18.69 ± 1.04	−0.38 ± 0.52

The values are presented as mean ± SD, n = 10. * $p < 0.05$, compared with MC. # $p < 0.05$, compared with initial weight.

The thymus index is exhibited in Figure 4. The MC group experienced a dramatic decline in the thymus index compared to the NC group ($p < 0.01$), indicating that Cy caused severe damage to the immune system of the mice. The thymus index of the AFP groups was raised significantly, relative to the MC group. The results demonstrated the immunoprotective effect of AFP in Cy-treated mice.

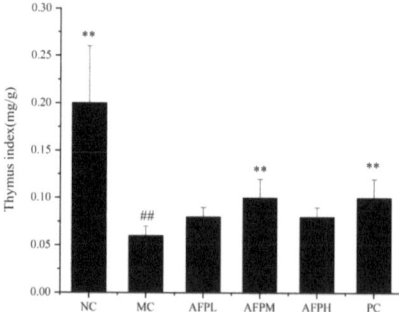

Figure 4. Effect of AFP on the thymus index in mice. Data are expressed as the mean ± SD, n = 10, ** $p < 0.01$ compared with MC; ## $p < 0.01$ compared with NC.

3.7. Effect of AFP on Intestine Tissue

To verify the impact of AFP on the intestinal morphology of Cy-immunosuppressed mice, hematoxylin and eosin (H&E) staining was conducted. In comparison with the NC group, relatively severe intestinal mucosa damage was revealed in the MC group; this was characterized by atrophic and edema villus, a shallower crypt and a disorganized structure. By contrast, the treatment with AFP moderated the damage to the intestinal mucosa caused by Cy, and was associated with a neat and compact villus. As shown in Figure 5A, the villus length of the AFP group was markedly increased compared to that in the MC group ($p < 0.01$). A longer villus could enhance the absorption of nutrients and the resistance ability to bacteria via contacting with intestinal epithelial cells. As Figure 5C indicates, the villus length/crypt ratio was enhanced significantly in the AFP groups compared to the MC group ($p < 0.01$), and was even comparable to the NC group ($p > 0.05$).

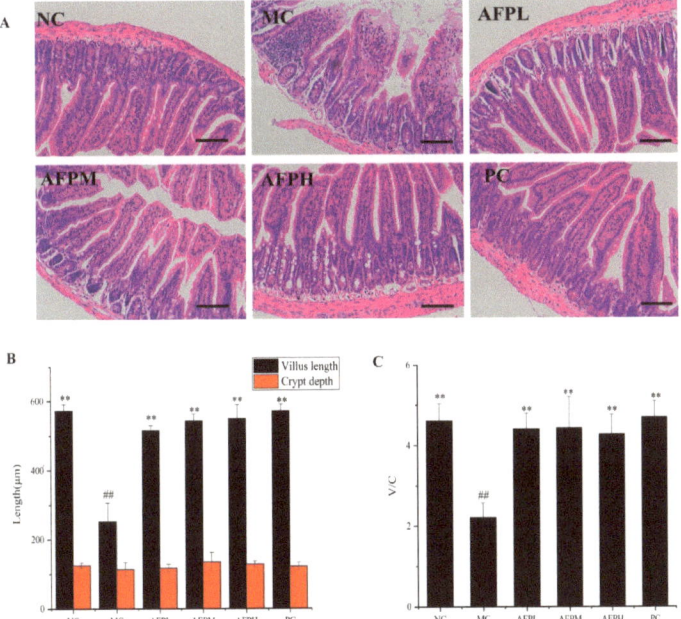

Figure 5. (**A**) Representative images of the small intestine tissue H&E staining sections (200×) among 6 mice, scale bar: 100 μm. (**B**) The villus length and crypt depth. (**C**) The ratio of villus length to crypt depth. Data are expressed as the mean ± SD ($n = 6$). ** $p < 0.01$ compared with MC; ## $p < 0.01$ compared with NC.

3.8. Effect of AFP on the Goblet Cells and PAS-Positive Area

In this study, the state of goblet cells was evaluated using AB-PAS staining. Goblet cells were blue in the staining sections of the small intestine tissue. As exhibited in Figure 6, the numbers of goblet cells in the MC group were obviously inferior to that in the NC group, indicating that Cy caused severe damage to the intestinal mucous cells. In comparison with the MC group, the number of goblet cells was gradually restored after being treated with AFP, but was still lower than the NC group.

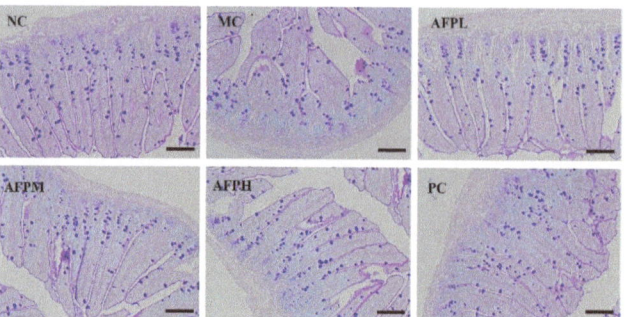

Figure 6. Representative images of the small intestine tissue AB-PAS staining sections (200×) among 6 mice, scale bar: 100 μm.

3.9. Effects of AFP on IgA and IgG Levels in the Serum

As demonstrated in Figure 7, Cy significantly lessened the expression levels of IgA and IgG in serum in comparison to that of normal mice ($p < 0.01$). Inversely, the IgA and IgG content in the serum of mice tended to increase in a dose-dependent manner after being treated with AFP. AFP remarkably upregulated the expression of IgA in serum compared with that of the MC group ($p < 0.01$). The effect of the AFPH group was even similar to that of the PC group. Nevertheless, only the AFPH group was notably different from the MC group regarding the promotion of IgG's expression ($p < 0.01$); meanwhile, the other two groups had no distinct effect on the secretion of IgG.

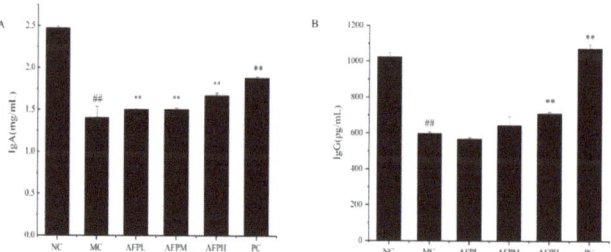

Figure 7. Effect of AFP on the serum IgA (**A**) and IgG (**B**) level in mice. Data are expressed as the mean ± SD ($n = 6$). ** $p < 0.01$ compared with MC; ## $p < 0.01$ compared with NC.

3.10. Effects of AFP on the Cytokine Levels in the Small Intestine

To investigate the change in the small intestinal cytokines in immunosuppressed mice, the secretion of SIgA, IL-2, IL-6, and IFN-γ was determined via an ELISA kit, and the results are revealed in Figure 8. As expected, a sharp decline appeared in four small intestinal cytokines of the MC group, relative to the NC group ($p < 0.01$). This result suggests that the immune system was damaged by Cy in mice. As presented in Figure 8A, compared to the MC group, the AFP-treated groups secreted SIgA at a relatively higher level but did not show a dose-dependent increase ($p < 0.01$). The expression of IL-2 and IL-6 was remarkably enhanced in a dose-dependent manner in comparison with the MC group ($p < 0.01$), especially for the AFPH group (AFPH), the effect of which was equivalent to that of the PC group. In comparison with the MC group, the expression of IFN-γ in the AFPL and AFPM groups was increased to varying degrees without a significant difference; while the AFPH group showed a prominent increase ($p < 0.05$).

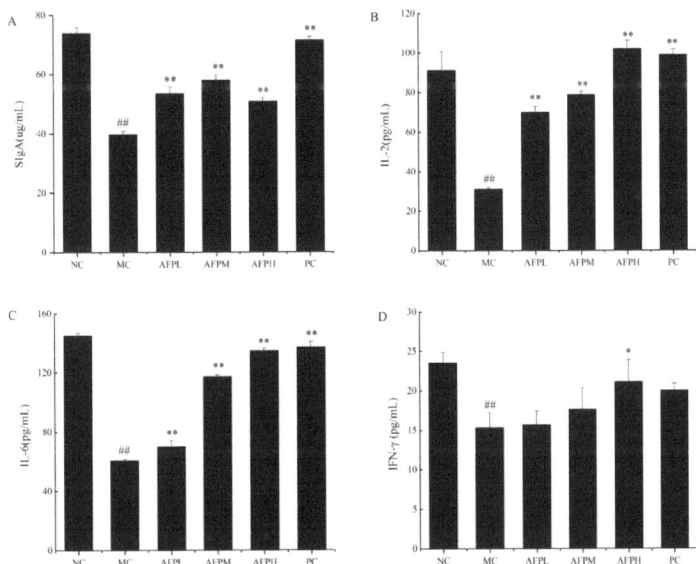

Figure 8. Effect of AFP polysaccharides on the small intestinal cytokine level in mice. (**A**) SIgA, (**B**) IL-2, (**C**) IL-6, (**D**) IFN-γ. Data are expressed as the mean ± SD (n = 6). * p < 0.05, ** p < 0.01 compared with MC; ## p < 0.01 compared with NC.

4. Discussion

As a conventional Chinese remedy, AF has been used for centuries to cure cardiovascular diseases, hypertension, fever, osteoporosis lung disease, and so on [18]. As reported, AFP, the important active component of the AF herb, possesses significant antitumor and antidiabetic activities. Much of the literature on this component focuses on the partial bioactivity of AFP. The immunosuppressive activity of AFP following oral administration is less clear. In this study, the immunosuppressive mice model induced by Cy was used to evaluate the immunomodulatory effect of AFP.

Macrophages are important effector cells of nonspecific immune response and are widely distributed in organisms [35]. Studies have shown that polysaccharides can not only enhance the proliferation of macrophages, but can also activate macrophages to release cytokines to resist or kill pathogens, thereby improving host immunity [36]. In our study, a dose-dependent enhancement of cell proliferation, IL-6, and TNF-α was observed in RAW 264.7 cells treated with 100 to 400 μg/mL doses of AFP. AFP has a significant immunomodulatory effect on macrophages.

Studies have shown that the immunomodulatory effects of polysaccharides on the body are mediated via different intracellular signaling pathways [37]. Therefore, we further explored the potential mechanisms by which AFP regulates the immune activity of the RAW 264.7 NF-κB transcription factor, which has been suggested to be directly associated with the expression of apoptosis, senescence, immunity and inflammation-related genes; it is also an essential signaling pathway that plays a crucial role in the immune system, of which, NF-κB p65 is the most important subunit and is involved in the expression and regulation of many genes as an indicator of activated cells [38]. Therefore, we analyzed the phosphorylation levels of NF-κB p65 in RAW 264.7 cells. In our study, the significantly enhanced phosphorylation expression levels of NF-κB p65 indicted the good activation of the NF-κB signaling pathway after AFP treatment. With an increase in the concentration, the best performance was obtained at the dosage of 400 μg/mL of AFP, which is 1.23-fold higher than the positive control group and 1.78-fold higher than the control group. These results suggest that NF-κB is a key signaling pathway via which AFP can exert immune activity in RAW 264.7 cells, and may account for the AFP-induced cytokine production in RAW 264.7 cells.

Body weight and the thymus index are basic physiological conditions of mice. The loss of body weight indicated that Cy caused a certain degree of damage to the mice, which is in accordance with the previous literature [39]. In addition, the decrease in the thymus index was a typical feature of immunosuppressed mice, on account of the weight of the immune organ correlating with the number of immune cells [40]. After the administration of AFP, the weight and the thymus index were enhanced, which demonstrated that polysaccharides can slow down the damage caused by Cy and restore the immune response.

A complete intestinal morphology is a prerequisite for the normal functioning of the mucosal barrier. The inner wall of the gastrointestinal tract has a layer of mucus that is produced by goblet cells, thus preventing pathogens from invading the mucosa and causing intestinal inflammation [41]. The current study found that the number of goblet cells in the MC group was clearly decreased compared to the NC group, indicating that Cy caused severe damage to intestinal mucous cells. However, the introduction of AFP helps to rebuild the secretion of goblet cells, but there is always room to improve compared with the normal group. Beneath the mucus layer, epithelial cells form another line of defense in the gut, preventing the invasion of pathogenic microorganisms [42]. Intestinal villus is a finger-like small protrusion of the epithelium cell protruding into the intestinal lumen. The length of the intestinal villus is positively correlated with the number of epithelial cells. In this study, the villus length was obviously shorter after treated with Cy, suggesting a decrease in the number of epithelial cells. According to the literature, as the villus becomes shorter, the number of epithelial cells decreases, resulting in the reduced digestion and uptake of nutrients [43]. The base of each villus is surrounded by crypts. The crypt depth reflects the regeneration rate of intestinal epithelial cells [44]. The researchers found that Moringa oleifera polysaccharides restored the villus height and crypt depth in a Cy-induced mice model of intestinal injury [45]. Consistent with previous studies, AFP promoted the regular and compact arrangement of the small intestinal villus, improved the integrity of the physical barrier of the small intestine and enhanced the villus length and the villus length/crypt ratio. Thus, we could confirm that AFP possesses pronounced immunomodulatory activities, and plays an essential role in enhancing the intestinal morphology of the immunological system in vivo.

Cy inhibited the generation of the antibody by mediating B cells. Levels of IgA and IgG were significantly decreased in immunosuppressed mice. However, both the IgA and IgG content in the serum of mice tended to increase in a dose-dependent manner after being treated with AFP. AFP remarkably upregulated the expression of IgA and IgG in serum compared with that of the MC group ($p < 0.01$), which is consistent with the results of a previous study [46]. Once the body was attacked by disease, the IgA and IgG levels became abnormal [47]. An increase in IgA and IgG helps the body to remove harmful antigens. On the basis of the above-mentioned results, it could be concluded that AFP regulates the immune activity of mice from the perspective of humoral immunity.

As the major class of antibody present on intestinal mucosal surfaces [48], SIgA provides an invaluable barrier that limits the access of intestinal antigens to the intestinal mucosa, controls the intestinal microbiota and attenuates pro-inflammatory immune responses. Similar to previous research [49], compared to the MC group, AFP-treated groups displayed a relatively higher secretion of SIgA, but no dose-related increase ($p < 0.01$). The results indicated that AFP could be used as a protective agent in order to alleviate Cy-induced intestinal damage and immune suppression in mice. To further investigate the regulatory effect of AFP on the intestinal mucosal barrier, the secretion of small intestinal cytokine in mice was measured. IL-2 mediates the activation of $CD4^+$ and $CD8^+$ T cells, induces the differentiation of T helper cells and facilitates the proliferation of immunoglobin synthesis by activated B cells [50]; while IL-6 plays a role in activating B-cells and plasma cells, involves in the differentiation into plasma cells, and produces IgG [51]. Our data highlighted that the levels of IL-2 and IL-6 were remarkably heightened compared to the

MC group ($p < 0.01$), especially for the AFPH group, the effect of which was equivalent to that of the PC group. IFN-γ is mainly produced by NK/ILC1 cells and T cells, and plays an important role in the immune response to bacterial infections [52]. The results of this study revealed that, compared to the MC group, the expression of IFN-γ in the AFPL and AFPM groups was increased to varying degrees without a significant difference; this was different from AFPH group, which exhibited a prominent increase. These results indicated that AFP has a good alleviating effect on mice immunosuppressed by Cy.

5. Conclusions

In summary, AFP was extracted from *Anoectochilus formosanus* with a homogeneous M_w distribution of 16.41 kDa using a water extraction and alcohol precipitation method. To the best of our knowledge, this was the first in-depth study of AFP's immunoregulatory activity and its mechanism in immunosuppressed mice. This study confirmed that AFP has an ability to enhance the secretion of TNF-α and IL-6 in RAW 264.7 macrophages, as well as the production of cytokines (IgA, IgG, SIgA, IL-2, IL-6 and IFN-γ) in immunosuppressed mice. The western blot analysis showed that NF-κB signaling pathways were involved in macrophage activation induced by AFP. Moreover, AFP could accelerate the recovery of the thymus index and body weight. Additionally, the repair effects of AFP on the intestinal morphology of Cy-induced immunosuppressed mice demonstrated the ability of AFP to help the mice mitigate the immunotoxicity caused by Cy. Our investigations suggested that AFP might have immunomodulatory effects in vivo and in vitro.

These preliminary investigations will lay the theoretical groundwork for the subsequent study of functional food based on *Anoectochilus formosanus*. However, the interaction between the structure and immune activity of AFP needs further study.

Author Contributions: Conceptualization, Y.W. and B.Y.; methodology, L.F.; software, H.W.; validation, Y.W., L.F. and H.W.; formal analysis, A.X.; investigation, A.X.; resources, B.Y.; data curation, L.F.; writing—original draft preparation, A.X.; writing—review and editing, L.F.; visualization, A.X.; supervision, Y.W.; project administration, Y.W.; funding acquisition, Y.W. All authors have read and agreed to the published version of the manuscript.

Funding: This work was funded by National Key Research and Development Project (2019YFC1604904). Science and Technology Innovation Platform Project of Jiangxi Province (20192BCD40001). Research Program of State Key Laboratory of Food Science and Technology in Nanchang University (SKLF-ZZB-202127).

Institutional Review Board Statement: The animal experimental procedures followed institutional guidelines for animal care of Nanchang University (Nanchang, China) and was approved by the Institutional Animal Care and Use Committee of Nanchang University (SYXK (Gan) 2015-0001).

Informed Consent Statement: Not applicable.

Data Availability Statement: Data is contained within the article.

Conflicts of Interest: The authors declare no conflict of interest.

References

1. Torre, L.A.; Bray, F.; Siegel, R.L.; Ferlay, J.; Lortet-Tieulent, J.; Jemal, A. Global cancer statistics, 2012. *CA Cancer J. Clin.* **2015**, *65*, 87–108. [CrossRef] [PubMed]
2. Ahlmann, M.; Hempel, G. The effect of cyclophosphamide on the immune system: Implications for clinical cancer therapy. *Cancer Chemother. Pharmacol.* **2016**, *78*, 661–671. [CrossRef] [PubMed]
3. Gao, X.; Qu, H.; Gao, Z.; Zeng, D.; Wang, J.; Baranenko, D.; Li, Y.; Lu, W. Protective effects of Ulva pertusa polysaccharide and polysaccharideiron (III) complex on cyclophosphamide induced immunosuppression in mice. *Int. J. Biol. Macromol.* **2019**, *133*, 911–919. [CrossRef] [PubMed]
4. Li, C.; Duan, S.; Li, Y.; Pan, X.; Han, L. Polysaccharides in natural products that repair the damage to intestinal mucosa caused by cyclophosphamide and their mechanisms: A review. *Carbohydr. Polym.* **2021**, *261*, 117876. [CrossRef]
5. Chen, X.; Nie, W.; Fan, S.; Zhang, J.; Wang, Y.; Lu, J.; Jin, L. A polysaccharide from Sargassum fusiforme protects against immunosuppression in cyclophosphamide-treated mice. *Carbohydr. Polym.* **2012**, *90*, 1114–1119. [CrossRef] [PubMed]

6. Zhao, Y.; Yan, Y.M.; Zhou, W.T.; Chen, D.; Huang, K.Y.; Yu, S.J.; Mi, J.; Lu, L.; Zeng, X.X.; Cao, Y.L. Effects of polysaccharides from bee collected pollen of Chinese wolfberry on immune response and gut microbiota composition in cyclophosphamide-treated mice. *J. Funct. Foods* **2020**, *72*, 104057. [CrossRef]
7. Bai, Y.; Huang, F.; Zhang, R.; Dong, L.; Jia, X.; Liu, L.; Yi, Y.; Zhang, M. Longan pulp polysaccharides relieve intestinal injury in vivo and in vitro by promoting tight junction expression. *Carbohydr. Polym.* **2020**, *229*, 115475. [CrossRef] [PubMed]
8. Besednova, N.N.; Zaporozhets, T.S.; Kuznetsova, T.A.; Makarenkova, I.D.; Kryzhanovsky, S.P.; Fedyanina, L.N.; Ermakova, S.P. Extracts and Marine Algae Polysaccharides in Therapy and Prevention of Inflammatory Diseases of the Intestine. *Mar. Drugs* **2020**, *18*, 289. [CrossRef] [PubMed]
9. Bai, Z.; Meng, J.; Huang, X.; Wu, G.; Zuo, S.; Nie, S. Comparative study on antidiabetic function of six legume crude polysaccharides. *Int. J. Biol. Macromol.* **2020**, *154*, 25–30. [CrossRef]
10. Chen, X.; Cai, B.; Wang, J.; Sheng, Z.; Yang, H.; Wang, D.; Chen, J.; Ning, Q. Mulberry leaf-derived polysaccharide modulates the immune response and gut microbiota composition in immunosuppressed mice. *J. Funct. Foods* **2021**, *83*, 104545. [CrossRef]
11. Wen, L.; Sheng, Z.; Wang, J.; Jiang, Y.; Yang, B. Structure of water-soluble polysaccharides in spore of Ganoderma lucidum and their anti-inflammatory activity. *Food Chem.* **2022**, *373*, 131374. [CrossRef] [PubMed]
12. Chen, X.; Xu, X.; Zhang, L.; Zeng, F. Chain conformation and anti-tumor activities of phosphorylated (1→3)-β-d-glucan from Poria cocos. *Carbohydr. Polym.* **2009**, *78*, 581–587. [CrossRef]
13. Chen, S.J.; Li, J.Y.; Zhang, J.M. Extraction of yellow pear residue polysaccharides and effects on immune function and antioxidant activity of immunosuppressed mice. *Int. J. Biol. Macromol.* **2019**, *126*, 1273–1281. [CrossRef]
14. Gao, H.; Ding, L.; Liu, R.; Zheng, X.; Xia, X.; Wang, F.; Qi, J.; Tong, W.; Qiu, Y. Characterization of Anoectochilus roxburghii polysaccharide and its therapeutic effect on type 2 diabetic mice. *Int. J. Biol. Macromol.* **2021**, *179*, 259–269. [CrossRef] [PubMed]
15. Liu, Y.; Tang, T.; Duan, S.; Li, C.; Lin, Q.; Wu, H.; Liu, A.; Hu, B.; Wu, D.; Li, S.; et al. The purification, structural characterization and antidiabetic activity of a polysaccharide from Anoectochilus roxburghii. *Food Funct.* **2020**, *11*, 3730–3740. [CrossRef]
16. Wu, T.; Li, S.; Huang, Y.; He, Z.; Zheng, Y.; Stalin, A.; Shao, Q.; Lin, D. Structure and pharmacological activities of polysaccharides from Anoectochilus roxburghii (Wall.) Lindl. *J. Funct. Foods* **2021**, *87*, 104815. [CrossRef]
17. Wu, Y.; Liu, C.; Jiang, Y.; Bai, B.; He, X.; Wang, H.; Wu, J.; Zheng, C. Structural characterization and hepatoprotective effects of polysaccharides from Anoectochilus zhejiangensis. *Int. J. Biol. Macromol.* **2022**, *198*, 111–118. [CrossRef] [PubMed]
18. Tseng, C.C.; Shang, H.F.; Wang, L.F.; Su, B.; Hsu, C.C.; Kao, H.Y.; Cheng, K.T. Antitumor and immunostimulating effects of Anoectochilus formosanus Hayata. *Phytomedicine* **2006**, *13*, 366–370. [CrossRef]
19. Ho, Y.; Chen, Y.F.; Wang, L.H.; Hsu, K.Y.; Chin, Y.T.; Yang, Y.S.H.; Wang, S.H.; Chen, Y.R.; Shih, Y.J.; Liu, L.F.; et al. Inhibitory Effect of Anoectochilus formosanus Extract on Hyperglycemia-Related PD-L1 Expression and Cancer Proliferation. *Front. Pharmacol.* **2018**, *9*, 807. [CrossRef]
20. Tang, T.; Duan, X.; Ke, Y.; Zhang, L.; Shen, Y.; Hu, B.; Liu, A.; Chen, H.; Li, C.; Wu, W.; et al. Antidiabetic activities of polysaccharides from Anoectochilus roxburghii and Anoectochilus formosanus in STZ-induced diabetic mice. *Int. J. Biol. Macromol.* **2018**, *112*, 882–888. [CrossRef]
21. Zhang, Z.; Guo, L.; Yan, A.; Feng, L.; Wan, Y. Fractionation, structure and conformation characterization of polysaccharides from Anoectochilus roxburghii. *Carbohydr. Polym.* **2020**, *231*, 115688. [CrossRef]
22. Zhang, W.N.; Gong, L.L.; Liu, Y.; Zhou, Z.B.; Wan, C.X.; Xu, J.J.; Wu, Q.X.; Chen, L.; Lu, Y.M.; Chen, Y. Immunoenhancement effect of crude polysaccharides of Helvella leucopus on cyclophosphamide-induced immunosuppressive mice. *J. Funct. Foods* **2020**, *69*, 103942. [CrossRef]
23. Liu, X.; Ren, Z.; Yu, R.; Chen, S.; Zhang, J.; Xu, J.; Meng, Z.; Luo, Y.; Zhang, W.; Huang, Y.; et al. Structural characterization of enzymatic modification of Hericium erinaceus polysaccharide and its immune-enhancement activity. *Int. J. Biol. Macromol.* **2021**, *166*, 1396–1408. [CrossRef] [PubMed]
24. Feng, L.; Yin, J.; Nie, S.; Wan, Y.; Xie, M. Fractionation, physicochemical property and immunological activity of polysaccharides from Cassia obtusifolia. *Int. J. Biol. Macromol.* **2016**, *91*, 946–953. [CrossRef] [PubMed]
25. Blumenkratz, N.; Asboe-Hansen, G. New Method for Quantitative Determination of Uranic Acids. *Anal. Biochem.* **1973**, *54*, 484–489. [CrossRef] [PubMed]
26. Bradford, M.M. A Rapid and Sensitive Method for the Quantitation of Microgram Quantities of Protein Utilizing the Principle of Protein-Dye Binding. *Anal. Biochem.* **1976**, *72*, 248–254. [CrossRef]
27. Zeng, H.; Chen, J.; Zhai, J.; Wang, H.; Xia, W.; Xiong, Y. Reduction of the fat content of battered and breaded fish balls during deep-fat frying using fermented bamboo shoot dietary fiber. *LWT* **2016**, *73*, 425–431. [CrossRef]
28. Li, G.; Chen, P.; Zhao, Y.; Zeng, Q.; Ou, S.; Zhang, Y.; Wang, P.; Chen, N.; Ou, J. Isolation, structural characterization and anti-oxidant activity of a novel polysaccharide from garlic bolt. *Carbohydr. Polym.* **2021**, *267*, 118194. [CrossRef] [PubMed]
29. Liu, N.; Dong, Z.; Zhu, X.; Xu, H.; Zhao, Z. Characterization and protective effect of Polygonatum sibiricum polysaccharide against cyclophosphamide-induced immunosuppression in Balb/c mice. *Int. J. Biol. Macromol.* **2018**, *107*, 796–802. [CrossRef] [PubMed]
30. Chen, S.; Wang, J.; Fang, Q.; Dong, N.; Ie, S. Polysaccharide from natural Cordyceps sinensis ameliorated intestinal injury and enhanced antioxidant activity in immunosuppressed mice. *Food Hydrocoll.* **2019**, *89*, 661–667. [CrossRef]
31. Liu, Y.; Wu, X.; Wang, Y.; Jin, W.; Guo, Y. The immunoenhancement effects of starfish Asterias rollestoni polysaccharides in macrophages and cyclophosphamide-induced immunosuppression mouse models. *Food Funct.* **2020**, *11*, 10700–10708. [CrossRef]

32. Omar-Aziz, M.; Yarmand, M.S.; Khodaiyan, F.; Mousavi, M.; Gharaghani, M.; Kennedy, J.F.; Hosseini, S.S. Chemical modification of pullulan exopolysaccharide by octenyl succinic anhydride: Optimization, physicochemical, structural and functional properties. *Int. J. Biol. Macromol.* **2020**, *164*, 3485–3495. [CrossRef] [PubMed]
33. Chen, Q.; Zhang, S.; Ying, H.; Dai, X.; Li, X.; Yu, C.; Ye, H. Chemical characterization and immunostimulatory effects of a polysaccharide from Polygoni Multiflori Radix Praeparata in cyclophosphamide-induced anemic mice. *Carbohydr. Polym.* **2012**, *88*, 1476–1482. [CrossRef]
34. Xu, Y.; Cai, F.; Yu, Z.; Zhang, L.; Li, X.; Yang, Y.; Liu, G. Optimisation of pressurised water extraction of polysaccharides from blackcurrant and its antioxidant activity. *Food Chem.* **2016**, *194*, 650–658. [CrossRef] [PubMed]
35. Castro-Alves, V.C.; do Nascimento, J.R.O. Polysaccharides from raw and cooked chayote modulate macrophage function. *Food Res. Int.* **2016**, *81*, 171–179. [CrossRef]
36. Yin, M.; Zhang, Y.; Li, H. Advances in Research on Immunoregulation of Macrophages by Plant Polysaccharides. *Front. Immunol.* **2019**, *10*, 145. [CrossRef]
37. Ren, D.; Zhao, Y.; Zheng, Q.; Alim, A.; Yang, X. Immunomodulatory effects of an acidic polysaccharide fraction from herbal Gynostemma pentaphyllum tea in RAW264.7 cells. *Food Funct.* **2019**, *10*, 2186–2197. [CrossRef] [PubMed]
38. He, J.; Lu, J.; Zhan, L.; Zheng, D.; Wang, Y.; Meng, J.; Li, P.; Zhao, J.; Zhang, W. An Alkali-extracted polysaccharide from Poria cocos activates RAW264.7 macrophages via NF-κB signaling pathway. *Arab. J. Chem.* **2023**, *16*, 104592. [CrossRef]
39. Zhang, Q.; Cong, R.; Hu, M.; Zhu, Y.; Yang, X. Immunoenhancement of Edible Fungal Polysaccharides (Lentinan, Tremellan, and Pachymaran) on Cyclophosphamide-Induced Immunosuppression in Mouse Model. *Evid.-Based Complement. Altern. Med.* **2017**, *2017*, 9459156. [CrossRef]
40. Arce-Sillas, A.; Alvarez-Luquin, D.D.; Tamaya-Dominguez, B.; Gomez-Fuentes, S.; Trejo-Garcia, A.; Melo-Salas, M.; Cardenas, G.; Rodriguez-Ramirez, J.; Adalid-Peralta, L. Regulatory T Cells: Molecular Actions on Effector Cells in Immune Regulation. *J. Immunol. Res.* **2016**, *2016*, 12. [CrossRef]
41. Yang, S.; Yu, M. Role of Goblet Cells in Intestinal Barrier and Mucosal Immunity. *J. Inflamm. Res.* **2021**, *14*, 3171–3183. [CrossRef]
42. Tang, C.; Ding, R.; Sun, J.; Liu, J.; Kan, J.; Jin, C. The impacts of natural polysaccharides on intestinal microbiota and immune responses—a review. *Food Funct.* **2019**, *10*, 2290–2312. [CrossRef] [PubMed]
43. Caspary, W.F. Physiology and pathophysiology of intestinal absorption. *Am. J. Clin. Nutr.* **1992**, *55*, 299S–308S. [CrossRef] [PubMed]
44. Nelson, C.M. The mechanics of crypt morphogenesis. *Nat. Cell Biol.* **2021**, *23*, 678–679. [CrossRef]
45. Tian, H.; Liang, Y.; Liu, G.; Li, Y.; Deng, M.; Liu, D.; Guo, Y.; Sun, B. Moringa oleifera polysaccharides regulates caecal microbiota and small intestinal metabolic profile in C57BL/6 mice. *Int. J. Biol. Macromol.* **2021**, *182*, 595–611. [CrossRef]
46. Feng, H.; Fan, J.; Lin, L.; Liu, Y.; Chai, D.; Yang, J. Immunomodulatory Effects of Phosphorylated Radix Cyathulae officinalis Polysaccharides in Immunosuppressed Mice. *Molecules* **2019**, *24*, 4150. [CrossRef] [PubMed]
47. Xiong, L.; Ouyang, K.; Chen, H.; Yang, Z.; Hu, W.; Wang, N.; Liu, X.; Wang, W. Immunomodulatory effect of Cyclocarya paliurus polysaccharide in cyclophosphamide induced immunocompromised mice. *Bioact. Carbohydr. Diet. Fibre* **2020**, *24*, 100224. [CrossRef]
48. Yu, Z.M.; Huang, X.H.; Yan, C.Q.; Gao, J.; Liang, Z.S. Effect of Fuzheng Jiedu granule on immunological function and level of immune-related cytokines in immune-suppressed mice. *J. Integr. Agric.* **2016**, *15*, 650–657. [CrossRef]
49. Fu, Y.P.; Feng, B.; Zhu, Z.K.; Feng, X.; Chen, S.F.; Li, L.X.; Yin, Z.Q.; Huang, C.; Chen, X.F.; Zhang, B.Z.; et al. The Polysaccharides from Codonopsis pilosula Modulates the Immunity and Intestinal Microbiota of Cyclophosphamide-Treated Immunosuppressed Mice. *Molecules* **2018**, *23*, 1801. [CrossRef]
50. Waldmann, T.A. The biology of interleukin-2 and interleukin-15: Implications for cancer therapy and vaccine design. *Nat. Rev. Immunol.* **2006**, *6*, 595–601. [CrossRef]
51. Smith, K.A.; Maizels, R.M. IL-6 controls susceptibility to helminth infection by impeding Th2 responsiveness and altering the Treg phenotype in vivo. *Eur. J. Immunol.* **2014**, *44*, 150–161. [CrossRef] [PubMed]
52. Kim, E.Y.; Ner-Gaon, H.; Varon, J.; Cullen, A.M.; Guo, J.; Choi, J.; Barragan-Bradford, D.; Higuera, A.; Pinilla-Vera, M.; Short, S.A.; et al. Post-sepsis immunosuppression depends on NKT cell regulation of mTOR/IFN-gamma in NK cells. *J. Clin. Investig.* **2020**, *130*, 3238–3252. [CrossRef] [PubMed]

Disclaimer/Publisher's Note: The statements, opinions and data contained in all publications are solely those of the individual author(s) and contributor(s) and not of MDPI and/or the editor(s). MDPI and/or the editor(s) disclaim responsibility for any injury to people or property resulting from any ideas, methods, instructions or products referred to in the content.

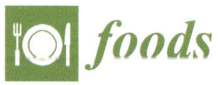

Article

Entanglement between Water Un-Extractable Arabinoxylan and Gliadin or Glutenins Induced a More Fragile and Soft Gluten Network Structure

Fan Li [1], Tingting Li [2], Jiajia Zhao [3], Mingcong Fan [1], Haifeng Qian [1], Yan Li [1] and Li Wang [1,*]

[1] State Key Laboratory of Food Science and Technology, School of Food Science and Technology, National Engineering Research Center for Functional Food, Jiangnan University, 1800 Lihu Avenue, Wuxi 214122, China; 6200112039@stu.jiangnan.edu.cn (F.L.)

[2] Department of Food Science and Engineering, College of Light Industry and Food Engineering, Nanjing Forestry University, 159 Longpan Road, Nanjing 210037, China

[3] College of Cooking Science and Technology, Jiangsu College of Tourism, Yangzhou 225000, China

* Correspondence: wangli@jiangnan.edu.cn

Abstract: This study aimed to investigate the effects of water-unextractable arabinoxylan (WUAX) on the gluten network structure, especially on gliadins and glutenins. The results indicated that the free sulfhydryl (free SH) of gliadins increased by 25.5% with 100 g/kg WUAX, whereas that of glutenins increased by 65.2%, which inhibited the formation of covalent bonds. Furthermore, β-sheets content decreased 5.63% and 4.75% for gliadins and glutenins with 100 g/kg WUAX, respectively, compared with the control. WUAX increased β-turns prevalence for gliadins, while the content of α-helixes and random coils had less fluctuation. In glutenins, the contents of α-helixes and β-sheets decreased and β-turns increased. Moreover, compared with the control, the weight loss rate for gliadins and glutenins increased by 2.49% and 2.04%, respectively, with 60 g/kg WUAX. The dynamic rheological analysis manifested that WUAX impaired the viscoelasticity property of gliadin and glutenin. Overall, WUAX weakened the structure of the gliadins and glutenins, leading to quality deterioration of gluten.

Keywords: water-unextractable arabinoxylan; gliadins; glutenins; chemical interactions

Citation: Li, F.; Li, T.; Zhao, J.; Fan, M.; Qian, H.; Li, Y.; Wang, L. Entanglement between Water Un-Extractable Arabinoxylan and Gliadin or Glutenins Induced a More Fragile and Soft Gluten Network Structure. *Foods* **2023**, *12*, 1800. https://doi.org/10.3390/foods12091800

Academic Editor: Lovedeep Kaur

Received: 13 March 2023
Revised: 12 April 2023
Accepted: 17 April 2023
Published: 26 April 2023

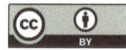

Copyright: © 2023 by the authors. Licensee MDPI, Basel, Switzerland. This article is an open access article distributed under the terms and conditions of the Creative Commons Attribution (CC BY) license (https://creativecommons.org/licenses/by/4.0/).

1. Introduction

Recently, many reports have shown that whole grains decreased the risk of chronic diseases, such as colorectal cancer, cardiovascular disease, and type 2 diabetes mellitus [1]. Thus, whole grain-based products are increasing rapidly for nutritional and health benefits. Compared with refined grains, whole grains have more healthy components, such as dietary fiber, micronutrients, minerals, and polyphenols [2], which are mainly located in the bran or germ. However, these components lead to a rough texture and a poor appearance, significantly affecting consumers' desires. Wheat-based foods are the most widely consumed cereal products globally, among which whole wheat foods are increasingly popular for consumers [3]. Wheat bran, a by-product in the wheat flour processing process, is mainly composed of polysaccharides (56–66%), protein (15–22%), and lignin (4–8%) [4]. Arabinoxylan (AX) is an important component of non-starch polysaccharide (NSP) in wheat bran, accounting for approximately 70% of the NSP of wheat bran [5]. Ferulic acid (FA) is the main phenolic compound present in the bran and attached to arabinose in the AX side chain. In addition, FA has antioxidant, antithrombotic, and anticancer activities [6], which means that AX has a variety of nutritional and health effects, such as moistening the bowel and enabling defecation, reducing cholesterol, regulating blood sugar, anti-oxidation, and immune regulation [7]. According to its solubility in water, AX was classed into water-unextractable AX (WUAX) and water-extractable AX (WEAX).

Many researchers reported that the rough texture of whole wheat foods was due to the AX in wheat bran. Therefore, more and more attention was paid to improving the texture through physical or chemical methods. Reports showed that the viscoelasticity and the thermal aggregation of gluten was improved by WEAX during heating. Thus, it contributed to the dough network's structural compatibility, among which it enlarged the loaf volume and made the textural property of Chinese steamed bread softer [8]. However, the WUAX, which accounted for 90% of total AX in the wheat bran, has significant adverse effects on the gluten network formation, especially weakening the gas holding capacity during heating. Therefore, it results in a rough texture, a lower specific volume, and an undesirable appearance of whole wheat-based products. Wang et al. found that WUAX competed with gluten for water to weaken the attraction between gluten protein molecules, which indirectly interfered with the formation of the gluten network [9]. Arif et al. also found that WUAX weakened the sensory and physical properties of the bread, affecting the quality of the final product [10]. In addition, our previous study reported that the WUAX could damage the viscoelasticity and the thermal properties of gluten, which was attributed to the competition with gluten for water and the disruption of the covalent cross-linking caused by WUAX, making whole wheat-based foods poor [11]. Moreover, Jiang et al. found that WUAX hydrolyzed by pentosanase was beneficial to the formation of uniform and fine crumb structures, leading to the higher volume and lower firmness of wholewheat Chinese steamed bread [12].

In summary, the mechanism of WUAX's action in dough mainly focused on the interaction between WUAX and the main ingredients of flour, such as starch or gluten. However, the detailed mechanism of WUAX on the gluten components, especially on gliadins and glutenins, is still unclear and needs to be further explored regarding the quality deterioration mechanism in whole wheat-based foods. Therefore, in this work, the gluten protein was further separated into gliadins and glutenins. In addition, the interaction between WUAX and gluten protein components was observed by thermal analysis, secondary structure content, rheological behavior, and other methods in order to provide theoretical support for the subsequent improvement of whole wheat-based products.

2. Materials and Methods

2.1. Materials and Chemicals

Gluten (protein content was 70%) and wheat bran were gained from Yihai Kerry Co., Ltd. (Kunshan, China). 5,5'-dithiobis (2-nitrobenzoic acid) (DTNB) were purchased from Yuanye Co., Ltd. (Shanghai, China). The solvents and the remaining chemicals were of analytical quality.

2.2. Exaction of Water-Unextractable Arabinoxylans

The WUAX was obtained according to the method of Si et al. with some modifications [11]. First, wheat bran was defatted with 90% ethanol, and the step was repeated three times. Next, starch and protein in the wheat bran were removed with amylase and protease, followed by heat inactivation of the enzyme (100 °C, 30 min). The pretreated bran was then dried at 45 °C in a low-temperature oven. WUAX was extracted with saturated barium hydroxide at 1:15 (w/w), and the extracted suspension was adjusted to pH 5 with acetic acid in order to precipitate the protein. Subsequently, the supernatant was dialyzed (Mw cut-off 14 kDa) at 4 °C for 72 h to remove small molecular salts, and the crude polysaccharide solution was then concentrated using a vacuum rotary evaporator. It was precipitated with a final ethanol concentration of 65% (v/v) and freeze-dried with a vacuum freezing dryer. Finally, the solid was ground through an 80-mesh sieve, and the obtained AX powder was stored in a desiccator. The WUAX content was 82.01%, as measured by the orcinol-hydrochloric acid method, and its moisture content was 4.10 ± 0.49%.

2.3. Preparation of Wheat Gliadins and Glutenins

Glutenins and gliadins were separated from gluten according to the method of traditional Osborne-Mendel separation. Gluten was defatted with n-hexane, and the step was repeated three times. The defatted gluten (100 g) was added to 2400 mL of 65% ethanol, stirred at 35 °C for 3 h, and centrifuged at 5000× g for 20 min. The ethanol in the supernatant was then removed using a rotary evaporator at 45 °C to obtain the gliadins solution. Glutenins in lower precipitation were extracted with 1200 mL of deionized water using 0.1 M NaOH solution to adjust to pH 10. It was stirred at 50 °C for 3 h, and centrifuged at 5000× g for 20 min. The obtained supernatant was added to a final ethanol concentration of 65% (v/v), and glutenins were obtained by the precipitation method, which used 0.1 M HCl solution to adjust pH at 7. The glutenins were then washed with 400 mL of deionized water and stirred at room temperature for 2 h, followed by centrifugation at 5000× g for 20 min to discard the supernatant. The above step was repeated twice to obtain glutenins. The precipitations of gliadins and glutenins were freeze-dried, ground, and passed through a 60-mesh sieve. The moisture contents of gliadins and glutenins (5.97 ± 0.29% and 6.51 ± 0.44%, respectively) were measured by 44-15A (AACC, 2000). The crude protein contents of gliadins and glutenins (92.54 ± 0.64% and 90.73 ± 0.49% (wet basis, w/w), respectively) were measured by the Kjeldahl method (GB 5009.5-2016).

2.4. Sample Preparation

Gliadins (5.0 g) or glutenins (5.0 g) were separately mixed with different amounts of WUAX (0, 100, 200, 300, 400, and 500 g/kg (protein-based)). 15 mL of deionized water was added to the mixed powder and stirred well. The mixture was stirred at room temperature for 3 h and stored at 4 °C overnight. Subsequently, all samples were lyophilized with a vacuum dryer, ground, and passed through an 80-mesh sieve. The final sample (Gliadins-WUAX and Glutenins-WUAX abbreviated as Glia-W and Glu-W) concentrations of WUAX were 0, 2, 4, 6, 8, and 10% (w/w, wet weight of protein). The lyophilized powder was used to determine chemical interaction, the free sulfhydryl (free SH) content, thermal properties, intrinsic fluorescence spectra, and fourier transform infrared (FTIR) spectroscopy analysis. The sample without WUAX served as the control group (abbreviated as Glia and Glu). Samples with WUAX were abbreviated as glia-W and glu-W.

2.5. Determination of Free SH Content

Based on the method of Feng et al., the free SH content of all samples was determined [13]. The freeze-dried protein powder (30 mg) was added to 5.5 mL Ellman's reagent [250 mmol/L Tris-HCl buffer (pH 8.5), propan-2-ol and 4 g/L DTNB) in ethanol (5/5/1, $v/v/v$)], stirred for 30 min at room temperature in the dark, and centrifuged at 4800× g for 10 min. Spectrophotometer (T9 type, Puchan universal instrument Co., Ltd., Beijing, China) was used to measure the absorbance value of supernatant at 412 nm. Finally, the free SH content was obtained by the following formula:

$$SH_{free} \text{ content} = \frac{A * V}{\varepsilon * b * m}$$

where A is the absorption of the sample at 412 nm; m is sample mass, g; ε is the molar absorption coefficient, $\varepsilon = 13,600$ M^{-1}cm^{-1}; V is the total volume of samples during determining free SH, L; and b is the thickness of the cuvette, $b = 1$ cm.

2.6. Measurement of Intrinsic Fluorescence Spectra

The intrinsic fluorescence spectra were determined, according to the method of Guo et al., with slight modifications [14]. WUAX solutions (2, 4, 6, 8, and 10 g/L) were prepared. Gliadins (500 mg) were dissolved in 650 mL/L ethanol (250 mL), and glutenins (500 mg) were dissolved in 0.1 M NaOH solution (250 mL) and centrifuged. WUAX solution (1 mL) was added to the supernatant (1 mL) and diluted to 10 mL. The protein solution without WUAX was served as the control group. The solution was set at room temperature for 10 min in the dark. Spectrofluorometer (F-7000, Hitachi, Ltd., Tokyo, Japan) was used to measure the intrinsic fluorescence spectra from 300 to 500 nm at room temperature. The emission was excited at 280 nm, and the slits of excitation and emission were set at 5 nm.

2.7. Determination of Gliadins and Glutenins Solubility in Different Solvents

Non-covalent interaction was determined according to Wang et al. with some modifications [15]. Different selective buffer dissolved proteins were used to disrupt ionic, hydrogen bonds or hydrophobic interactions, prepared in phosphate buffer (0.05 M, pH = 7.0) as follows: (PA) 0.05 M NaCl; (PB) 0.6 M NaCl; (PC) 0.6 M NaCl and 1.5 M urea; and (PD) 0.6 M NaCl and 8 M urea. Protein powder (200 mg) was added to each solvent (10 mL) and stirred for 1 h at 25 °C, followed by centrifugation at $10,000 \times g$ for 20 min. The bicinchoninic acid (BCA) protein assay kit was used to measure the protein concentration in the supernatant. A standard was prepared with bovine serum albumin, expressed as g soluble protein/L of supernatant. The difference between soluble gliadins or glutenins in PB and PA, PC and PB, and PD and PC represented ionic bonds, Hydrogen bonds, and Hydrophobic interactions.

2.8. Fourier Transform Infrared Spectroscopy

FTIR was used to research the secondary structure of the protein. 10.0 mg protein was mixed with 1.0 g KBr, ground, and then pressed into a slice. The FTIR spectrometer (Antaris II, Thermo Nicolet Corporation, Madison, WI, USA) was used to obtain the spectrum over the wavelength range of 400 cm^{-1} to 4000 cm^{-1} with 32 scans and at 4 cm^{-1} resolution. Omnic software package (version 8.0) and PeakFit software (version 4.12) was used to analyze the secondary structures of all samples [16]. The amide I region spectra were classified into 1660–1700 cm^{-1}, 1650–1659 cm^{-1}, 1640–1650 cm^{-1}, and 1610–1640 cm^{-1}, corresponding to β-turns, α-helixes, random coil, and β-sheets, respectively [17].

2.9. Dynamic Rheological Measurements

According to the method reported by Wang et al., with slight modifications [15], the rheological properties of gliadins and glutenins were determined by the rotational rheometer (DHR-3, TA Instrument, New Castle, DE, USA). Dynamic rheological measurements were performed using freshly prepared samples of gliadins and glutenins with/without WUAX. First, the linear viscoelastic region of the protein was obtained by stress scanning over frequencies ranging from 0.1 to 100 Hz. Subsequently, the sample was placed between 40 mm steel plates (1 mm gap) and allowed to rest for 20 min to relax the residual stresses. The edge of all samples was covered with a thin layer of silicone oil in order to avert moisture loss during testing. The frequency sweep was measured over the range of frequency 0.1–100 Hz at 25 °C, within the linear viscoelastic region at a constant strain of 0.1%.

2.10. Thermal Properties Analysis

According to the method reported by Feng et al. [13], the thermal properties of glutenins and gliadins were analyzed by thermos-gravimetric analysis (TGA). A Mettler Toledo Star (Mettler Toledo Corp., Greifensee, Switzerland) was used to obtain TGA analysis for all samples (approximately 10 mg), among which a heating rate of nitrogen atmosphere was set from 50 to 600 °C at 10 °C/min. STAR software (version 9.01) was used to analyze the degradation temperature (T_d) and weight loss rate.

2.11. Statistical Analysis

The results were described as a mean of three replicates ± SD (standard deviation) and evaluated for their statistically significant difference with ANOVA using SPSS 26 software, where $p < 0.05$ represented statistical significance. All figures were obtained by origin 2018 software.

3. Results and Discussions

3.1. Free SH Content Analysis

The content of free SH groups can be used to characterize the degree of protein aggregation, and its content is negatively correlated with the degree of gluten protein aggregation [18]. Extra WUAX has obvious modification effects on the free SH contents of gliadins and glutenins, which are summarized in Figure 1. With 10% of WUAX, the SH content of gliadins increased by 25.5% compared with the control (0.98 µmol/g), which demonstrated that WUAX inhibited the formation of SS bonds and loosened the molecular structure of gliadins. The free SH content in glutenins remarkably increased by 65.2% compared with the control group (1.15 µmol/g) in accordance with the variety of gliadins. This trend showed that WUAX prompted the unfolding or denaturation of the structure of glutenins. The addition of WUAX had a more significant effect on the content of free SH in glutenins than that of gliadins. This was due to the intermolecular SS bonds of glutenins being readily damaged by the external environment [19]. Our results of the free SH content for gliadins and glutenins with and without WUAX were consistent with those of Guo et al., whose results suggested that additional inulin restrained the formation of the SS bonds in glutenins and gliadins and loosened the molecular structure of glutenins and gliadins [14]. Therefore, the enhancive free SH content of the gluten protein components caused by WUAX may be related to the large steric hindrance of WUAX. The physical entanglement between WUAX and protein decreased the chance of free SH groups contacting each other and weakened binding interactions between proteins, which hindered the formation of SS bonds [11].

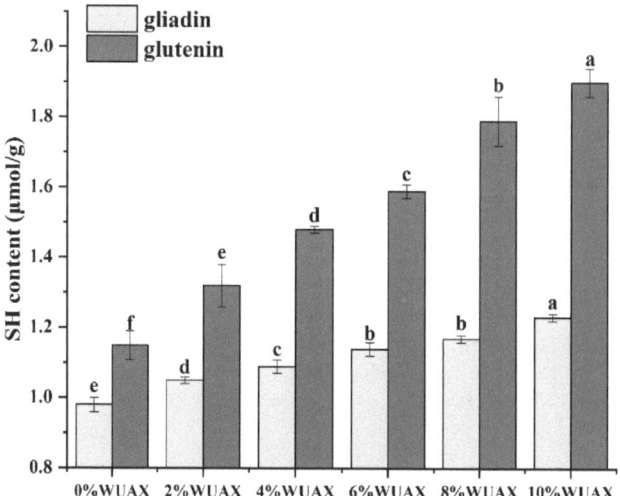

Figure 1. The effect of water un-extractable arabinoxylan (WUAX) on free sulfhydryl (free SH) content of gliadin and glutenin. Data are means of three independent experiments (n = 3) ± SD. Different letters above the bar mean significant differences ($p < 0.05$).

3.2. Intrinsic Fluorescence Spectra Analysis

Intrinsic fluorescence spectrum analysis can be used to characterize the microenvironment changes of a fluorescent amino acid, and it serves as an essential indicator to characterize proteins based on their intermolecular interactions, dynamics and conformation [15].

The effect of WUAX on the intrinsic fluorescence intensity (I_{max}) and maximum fluorescence absorption wavelength (λ_{max}) of gliadins and glutenins is shown in Table 1. Compared with the gliadins group, the λ_{max} of gliadins with WUAX changed slightly, and there was no significant difference. These indicated that WUAX had a weak effect on the microenvironment of tryptophan residues in gliadins, but the addition of WUAX affected the hydration process of gliadins, making the structure of gliadins unfold and loosen. However, the I_{max} of gliadins with WUAX increased, which means that WUAX increased the exposure degree of fluorescent chromophobe groups in gliadins. In particular, the increase in AX content further hindered the aggregation between the subunits of gliadins and aggravated the structural changes of the gliadins.

Table 1. Fluorescence spectra profiles (I_{max} and λ_{max}) of gliadin and glutenin.

Sample	WUAX Content	λ_{max}	I_{max}
Glia-W	0%	339.5 ± 0.3 [a]	1941.0 ± 2.6 [a]
	2%	339.6 ± 1.0 [a]	1969.7 ± 8.0 [b]
	4%	339.7 ± 0.4 [a]	1994.7 ± 6.4 [c]
	6%	340.1 ± 0.9 [a]	2011.7 ± 6.7 [d]
	8%	340.2 ± 0.5 [a]	2069.7 ± 8.0 [e]
	10%	340.5 ± 0.8 [a]	2091.7 ± 12.7 [f]
Glu-W	0%	339.8 ± 1.0 [b]	2190.7 ± 6.4 [a]
	2%	339.3 ± 0.7 [b]	2162.0 ± 15.0 [b]
	4%	339.8 ± 1.4 [b]	2106.3 ± 17.2 [c]
	6%	340.3 ± 1.3 [b]	2024.3 ± 13.5 [d]
	8%	343.7 ± 0.5 [a]	1964.7 ± 12.4 [e]
	10%	343.7 ± 1.9 [a]	1936.3 ± 15.0 [f]

Data are mean ± SD (n = 3). Different lowercase letters in the same column mean significant differences ($p < 0.05$). Glia-W means gliadin-WUAX and Glu-W means glutenin-WUAX (the same below).

For glutenins, when WUAX content was less than <60 g/kg, the λ_{max} of glutenins experienced no significant changes. However, the λ_{max} of glutenins occurred the red shift with the high level of WUAX. This was likely because that the increased concentration of WUAX caused that WUAX to come into contact with amino acids in the hydrophobic core of glutenins, and its hydroxyl group on the side chain increased the polarity of the tryptophan residue microenvironment. After the addition of WUAX, the I_{max} of glutenins with WUAX was the opposite of gliadins. A regular decreasing trend was observed (Table 1) with the increase in WUAX level. However, the change of free SH (Figure 1) showed that WUAX obstructed cross-linking of glutenins, resulting in protein structure unfolding. Therefore, we speculated that WUAX caused the decrease in the I_{max} of glutenins, probably because WUAX interacted with glutenins to form a new complex, which led to an obvious quenching effect of tryptophan groups on the surface of glutenins.

Si et al. reported that the addition of WUAX caused a decrease in the I_{max} and a red shift of gluten protein [11]. As a result, we speculated that the hydrophilicity of WUAX's side chain hydroxyl group altered the polarity of the environment around tryptophan residues in gliadins and glutenins. However, due to the network structure of glutenins, a more specific surface area came into contact with WUAX, which resulted in the decrease in gluten fluorescence intensity. Therefore, we guessed that the addition of WUAX changed the conformation, dynamics, intermolecular interactions, and the microenvironment of glutenins and gliadins, thereby resulting in the gluten protein structure change.

3.3. Non-Covalent Interaction Analysis

Non-covalent interactions between proteins are critical in maintaining the three-dimensional structure and stability of the protein complex. Since different concentrations of solvents (NaCl and urea) have a destructive effect on the ionic bonds, hydrogen bonds, and hydrophobic interactions in protein intramolecular or intermolecular, the solubility of the protein in different solvents indirectly expresses the stabilizing force of the protein (hydrogen bonds, hydrophobic interactions, and ionic bonds).

The effect of WUAX on the non-covalent bond between wheat glutenins and gliadins is shown in Figure 2. Hydrophobic interactions played an critical role in maintaining the conformation of gliadins [20]. However, the main non-covalent forces in glutenins were hydrogen bonds and hydrophobic interactions (Figure 2B). The phenomenon suggested that it was pivotal for maintaining the conformation of gliadins and glutenins [21], resulting from gliadins and glutenins containing abundant non-polar amino acids, and leading to more hydrophobic interactions at hydration [22]. The ionic bond strength of the two proteins was relatively low compared with hydrophobic interactions and hydrogen bonds (Figure 2), which indicated the presence of weak ionic bonds in proteins formed by few ionizable amino acid residues [23]. Due to the large molecular weight of glutenins, the concentration of glutenins dissolved in different solvents was lower than that of gliadins.

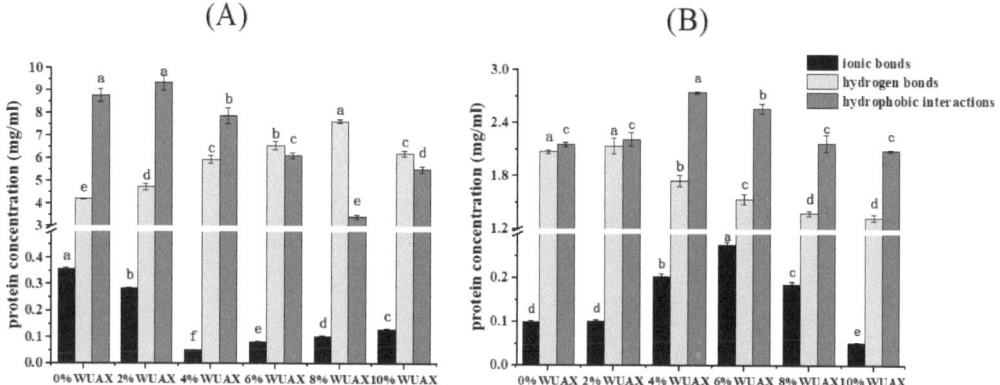

Figure 2. The effect of a different amount of WUAX on the non-covalent interaction of gliadin (**A**) and glutenin (**B**). Note: Data are means of three independent experiments ($n = 3$) ± SD. Different letters above the bar mean significant differences ($p < 0.05$).

After adding WUAX to gliadins, it was observed that the ionic bond strength of gliadins decreased, and 4% WUAX had the lowest strength. The hydrogen bonds between proteins can be broken into low urea concentrations, increasing protein solubility. As the urea concentration increased, the non-covalent interactions were further destroyed, resulting in protein solvation [11]. As the amount of WUAX increased, weaker hydrogen bonds were formed, but the hydrophobic interaction decreased, except for the 10% WUAX. This phenomenon may result from the large steric hindrance of WUAX, which presents a linear structure in an aqueous solution. They can entangle and hinder mutual contact between gliadins, resulting in the reduction of hydrophobic interactions, and this facilitates the formation of hydrogen bonds within gliadin molecules. A study reported by Guo et al. found that inulin with a high molecular weight could hinder the molecular movement of gluten protein and facilitate the formation of weaker hydrogen bonds [14]. However, the high steric hindrance inhibited the formation of ionic bonds and hydrophobic interactions in gluten protein and prevented the aggregation of gluten protein.

After adding WUAX to glutenins (Figure 2B), it was observed that the hydrogen bonds had decreased. However, the hydrophobic interaction increased and then decreased in accordance with the changing trend of the ionic bond of glutenins. Nonetheless, the strength of the ionic bond and the hydrophobic interaction were higher than the control, except for the 10% WUAX. However, the changing trend of glutenins was opposite to that of gliadins. This may be due to the structural differences between glutenins and gliadins. Since the network structure of glutenins was more likely to be broken by WUAX, the addition of WUAX changed the microenvironment of the hydrophobic amino acids inside the protein, so the protein structure would be unfolded. However, due to the larger steric hindrance of WUAX, the higher addition of WUAX entangled to form a physical barrier on the surface of the glutenin molecules, hindering their structure extension and the form of hydrogen bonding between the glutenins. We thus concluded that WUAX mainly destroyed the hydrophobic interactions of gliadins and the hydrogen bonds of glutenins.

Si et al. reported that the effect of adding WUAX on the non-covalent force of gluten protein, which is consistent with the results of glutenins; this indicated that WUAX might affect the network structure of gluten protein mainly by changing the spatial conformation of glutenins, leading to the poor quality of the final product [11].

3.4. Secondary Structure of Protein Analysis

FTIR can quickly analyze the secondary structure content of protein in the amide I band (1600–1700 cm^{-1}). The characteristic absorption peaks of the amide I band are shown in Figure 3, and the secondary structure content is summarized in Table 2. It was observed that the protein's secondary structure in all samples was mainly β-sheets and β-turns structure, and random coils and α-helixes account for a low fraction, which was consistent with the results of Feng et al. [13].

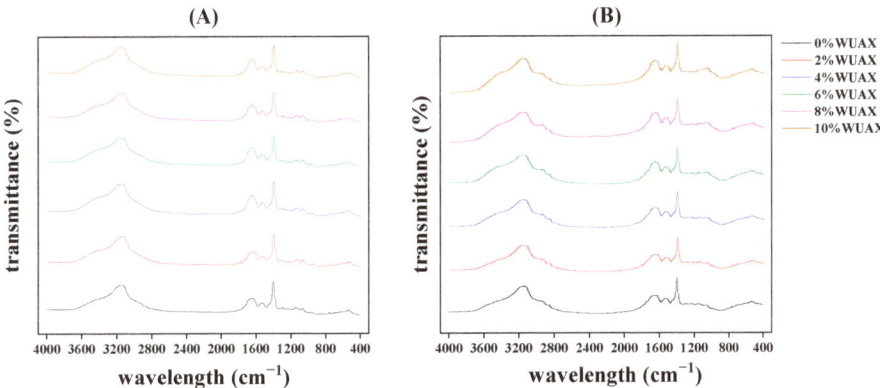

Figure 3. FTIR profiles of gliadin (**A**) and glutenin (**B**) treated with different concentrations of WUAX.

Table 2. Secondary structure of gliadin and glutenin with different amounts of WUAX.

Sample	WUAX Content	β-Sheets	α-Helixes	Random Coils	β-Turns
Glia-W	0%	43.27 ± 0.42 [a]	13.80 ± 0.28 [a]	13.28 ± 0.25 [a]	29.67 ± 0.94 [c]
	2%	42.35 ± 0.48 [a]	12.50 ± 0.32 [b]	12.31 ± 0.01 [c]	32.85 ± 0.79 [b]
	4%	38.93 ± 0.20 [b]	12.68 ± 0.09 [b]	12.97 ± 0.08 [b]	35.43 ± 0.37 [a]
	6%	37.19 ± 0.10 [c]	12.55 ± 0.57 [b]	13.30 ± 0.04 [a]	36.97 ± 0.63 [a]
	8%	37.49 ± 0.06 [c]	12.18 ± 0.09 [b]	13.36 ± 0.08 [a]	36.98 ± 0.04 [a]
	10%	37.64 ± 0.73 [c]	11.98 ± 0.23 [b]	13.37 ± 0.06 [a]	37.02 ± 0.56 [a]
Glu-W	0%	47.42 ± 0.29 [a]	12.32 ± 0.20 [a]	12.09 ± 0.57 [c]	28.17 ± 0.09 [c]
	2%	46.25 ± 0.39 [b]	12.24 ± 0.31 [ab]	12.17 ± 0.38 [c]	29.33 ± 0.33 [bc]
	4%	46.09 ± 0.14 [b]	11.85 ± 0.20 [bc]	12.35 ± 0.03 [bc]	29.71 ± 0.02 [b]
	6%	43.77 ± 0.51 [c]	11.49 ± 0.09 [c]	12.85 ± 0.42 [abc]	31.89 ± 1.02 [a]
	8%	42.88 ± 0.02 [d]	11.40 ± 0.08 [c]	13.34 ± 0.08 [ab]	32.38 ± 0.03 [a]
	10%	42.67 ± 0.25 [d]	11.51 ± 0.03 [c]	13.58 ± 0.59 [a]	32.24 ± 0.87 [a]

Data are mean ± SD (n = 3). Different lowercase letters in the same column mean significant differences (p < 0.05).

Table 2 illustrates that there was a fluctuation within a narrow range in the random coil structure of gliadins after adding WUAX. The β-sheets content and α-helixes decreased, and the β-turns content increased subjected to the WUAX treatment, which indicated that the increasing β-sheets were at the expense of β-turns after the addition of WUAX. Ang et al. reported that β-turns could change the orientation of protein-peptide chains and achieve multiple reversals of protein structure, thereby making gliadins appear as prolate ellipsoidal protein [24]. Guo et al. reported that the lower β-turns in gliadins caused by adding KGM was helpful to the stability of gliadins compared with the control group [14]. In addition, according to the fact that the structure of the β-sheets was the most stable structure [25], our results demonstrated that adding WUAX decreased the stability of gliadins through the change of secondary structure. Interestingly, when the additional amount of WUAX was more than 4%, β-sheets and β-turns contents had little change. This may be due to the mutual entanglement of WUAX to form a larger physical barrier on the surface of gliadins, which also prevented WUAX from destroying the structure of the gliadins, so increasing the amount of WUAX (more than 6%) would not damage the secondary structure of gliadins.

Glutenins presented a fiber structure; thus, the structure of β-sheets played a critical role in maintaining the secondary structure of glutenins [26]. As demonstrated in Table 2, the content of the β-sheets presented a decreased trend; the random coils and α-helixes had a slight increase and decrease, respectively, compared with the control. The changing trend of β-turns was the opposite of β-sheets. Interestingly, changes in all structures were relatively low when the addition of WUAX was more than 6%. This confirmed that the spatial conformation of the conformation change of glutenins caused by WUAX was limited, which accorded with the change of gliadins. Moreover, Liu et al. studied the effects of inulin addition with different degrees of polymerization on the contents of the secondary structure of gliadins and glutenins [27]. With the increase in the degree of inulin polymerization, the β-sheets of gliadins and glutenins increased, while the β-turns trend was the opposite.

Based on the changes of free SH, we thought that WUAX induced protein structural rearrangement at lower levels, reducing the chance of free SH contact between glutenins. With the increase in WUAX content, the changes in the secondary structure of proteins tended to be stable, suggesting that the increase in free SH content was likely because the physical entanglement of WUAX prevented the cross-linking of glutenins.

3.5. Dynamic Rheological Analysis

Gluten protein is composed of glutenins and gliadins, which is a critical component of wheat protein. As we all know, gliadins confer viscosity and extensibility properties, while glutenins impart elasticity and strength properties [28]. Therefore, the dynamic rheological measurement could be used to evaluate the effects of WUAX on the viscoelasticity of the two proteins. Figure 4 provides the elastic modulus (storage modulus G′) and viscous modulus (loss modulus G″) as a function of the frequency for all samples at 25 °C subjected to the WUAX treatment.

As shown in Figure 4, after the addition of WUAX, the viscoelasticity of gliadins and glutenins with WUAX was lower than the control group. However, it was reduced and then increased with the increase in the WUAX. When the WUAX was 4% and 6%, respectively, it reached the lowest point. Unlike the glutenins, the effects of the WUAX amounts on the viscoelasticity of gliadins were not dramatically distinct. In addition, after the addition of WUAX, the tan δ of gliadins was increased, followed by the decrement, but it was higher compared with the control group (Figure 4C), which was consistent with the change of viscosity and elasticity. Therefore, WUAX damaged the elasticity of gliadins more readily and formed the soft and viscous gliadins [8], making the rheological properties of gliadins more liquid-like [20]. The reason may be that WUAX, a hydrophilic macromolecule polysaccharide, had a higher viscosity, which can maintain the viscosity of gliadins. For glutenins (Figure 4F), the tan δ gradually increased with increasing WUAX, which indicated that G′ was close to and just above G″. Thus, the samples with WUAX displayed the typical weak gel properties, which suggested that the weak junction zone can easily be damaged at a low shear rate [29]. The addition of WUAX had a more significant effect on the viscosity of glutenins than on the elasticity from Figure 4D,E. This might be due to the high viscosity of WUAX, which can bring some compensation to the viscosity damage of the protein. In addition, compared with gliadins, the relative solid-like behavior of glutenins via the tan δ analysis, was caused by the intermolecular disulfide bonds in glutenins, which created a strong structure for glutenins [30].

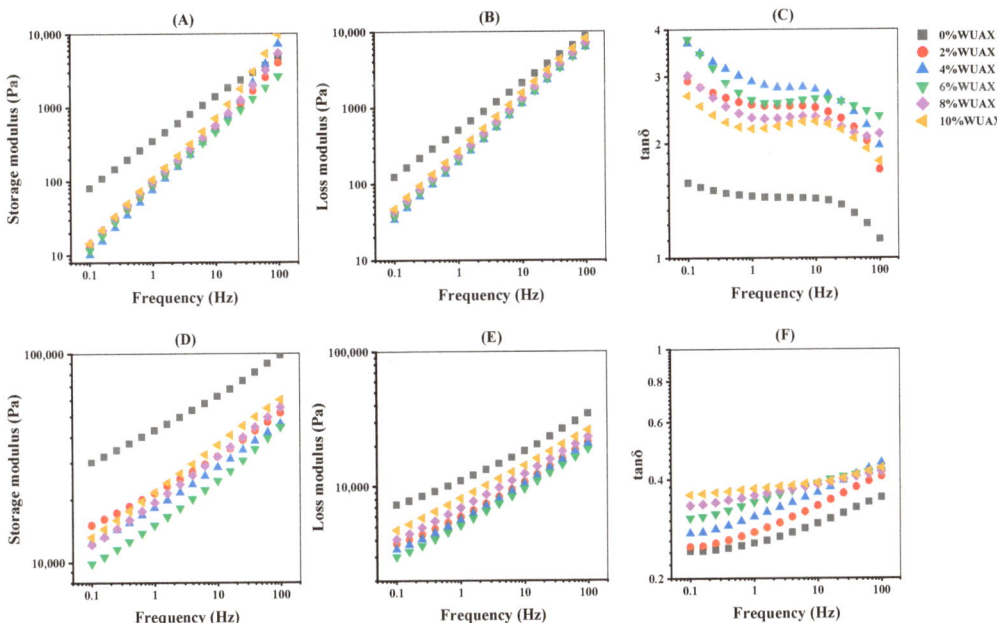

Figure 4. Frequency sweeps of G' (**A,D**), G'' (**B,E**), and tan δ (**C,F**) of gliadin (**A–C**) and glutenin (**D–F**) with different amounts of WUAX. Note: Data are the mean of three independent experiments (*n* = 3).

Compared with gliadins, the WUAX amount obviously influences glutenins, which might be related to the structure of glutenins and gliadins. There were more sites to form non-covalent interactions with WUAX in that glutenins had a larger molecular weight and a certain network structure. The viscoelasticity of both proteins obviously decreased, which is in harmony with the result of free SH content (Figure 1). Moreover, WUAX could interact with gluten via non-covalent bonds (hydrogen bonds and hydrophobic interaction), inhibiting the cross-linking of protein structure, thereby reducing their ductility. On the one hand, it was related to the good water holding capacity of WUAX. WUAX competed with protein for water, limiting the hydration of protein, and it finally resulted in the softening of the protein (lower G' and G'') [31]. On the other hand, longer chains of WUAX made it difficult to establish a cross-link between gliadins/glutenins and polysaccharide polymers. Therefore, it could be used to explain that whole grains would result in a lower specific volume of whole wheat-based foods during the heating process.

3.6. Thermal Properties Analysis

The effects of WUAX additions on the thermal properties of gliadins and glutenins were investigated by TGA analysis. The weight loss profiles of various proteins are shown in Figure 5. The weight loss at 600 °C and the degradation temperature (T_d) obtained from the TGA profile were the main parameters for the characterization of the protein thermal properties, as shown in Table 3. The weight loss of gliadins and glutenins exhibited the condition of the protein structure. The higher weight loss presented the protein network structure as more open and weaker, while a decrease in the weight loss can be related to the formation of a stronger and more compact protein structure [32]. Our results showed that protein weight loss was first increased and then decreased after adding WUAX, but that it was higher than that of the control (except for the gliadins with 10% WUAX). Feng et al. reported that extra wheat bran increased the weight loss of gliadins, glutenins, and GMP, which was consistent with our result [13]. Therefore, the lower amount of WUAX made the structures of the gliadins and glutenins more open and weaker, which might be because the WUAX hindered the covalent interaction (SS bonds), leading to the stability of the two proteins declining. With the increasing WUAX, it can become entangled between proteins, resulting in structure stability recovery, according to the dynamic rheological result (Figure 4A,B,D,E).

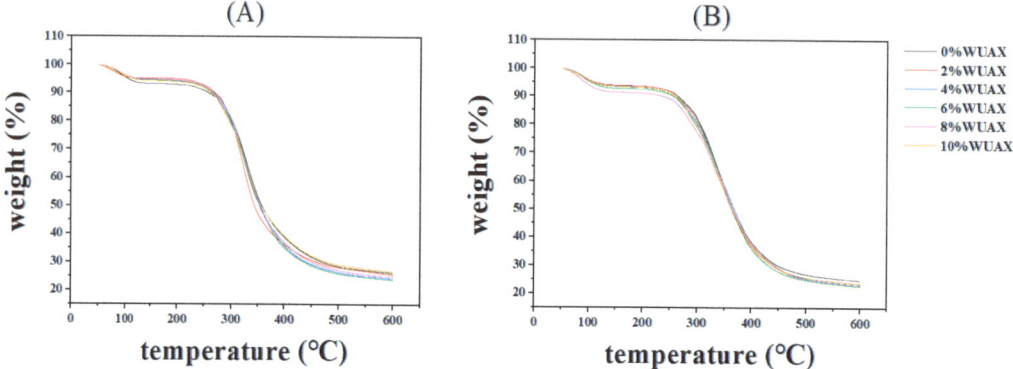

Figure 5. Weight loss profiles of gliadin (**A**) and glutenin (**B**) with different amounts of WUAX.

Table 3. TGA profiles [weight loss at 600 °C and degradation temperature (T_d)].

Sample	WUAX Content (g/kg)	Weight Loss (%)	T_d (°C)
Glia-W	0%	73.74 ± 0.49 [c]	329.7 ± 1.13 [a]
	2%	74.34 ± 0.40 [bc]	328.7 ± 1.56 [ab]
	4%	75.78 ± 0.38 [a]	328.8 ± 2.12 [ab]
	6%	76.23 ± 0.34 [a]	324.8 ± 2.41 [b]
	8%	75.15 ± 0.17 [ab]	327 ± 0.85 [ab]
	10%	73.23 ± 0.27 [c]	331.2 ± 1.83 [a]
Glu-W	0%	75.28 ± 0.36 [b]	333.2 ± 0.71 [a]
	2%	76.80 ± 0.27 [a]	331.3 ± 1.41 [ab]
	4%	76.79 ± 0.21 [a]	328.7 ± 0.99 [b]
	6%	77.24 ± 0.16 [a]	333.2 ± 1.13 [a]
	8%	76.86 ± 0.38 [a]	334.7 ± 2.26 [a]
	10%	76.21 ± 0.23 [a]	334.8 ± 1.69 [a]

Data are mean ± SD (n = 3). Different lowercase letters in the same column mean significant differences ($p < 0.05$).

The TGA profiles of glutenins and gliadins can be divided into two steps (Figure 5): the water evaporation stage at 50–150 °C and the cleavage stage of peptide bonds, disulfide bonds, O-O, and O-N bonds in the protein at 150–600 °C [32]. The T_d of samples from TGA is summarized in Table 3. The result indicated that T_d was decreased and then increased with the addition of WUAX compared with the control group, which was not significant, and which was consistent with the result of Zhao et al. [8]. They reported that both the weight loss rate and the T_d of gluten were not significantly changed when subjected to the WEAX treatment. Similarly, Si et al. also reported that the T_d of gluten with WUAX exhibited a slight variation compared with the control group and did not form new compounds, suggesting that WUAX kept the thermal stability of gluten molecules [11]. Interestingly, our result differed from that of Guo et al., who found that the T_d of wheat gliadins increased after adding inulin, while that of glutenins decreased slightly, which may be related to the changes of disulfide bonds in the protein caused by inulin [33]. Therefore, adding WUAX results in the structures of gliadins and glutenins being more open, but the effect on the stability of the proteins was not significant, which might be related to the non-covalent interaction between gliadins/glutenins and WUAX.

4. Conclusions

The study showed that the free SH content of glutenins and gliadins increased after the addition of WUAX, suggesting that WUAX hindered covalent interaction between proteins resulting in a more fragile and open network structure. However, the changing trend of non-covalent interaction (mainly hydrophobic interactions and hydrogen bonds) between glutenins and gliadins was the opposite when subjected to the WUAX treatment. WUAX might promote the formation of more weakened hydrogen bonds for gliadins, while it adversely influences the formation of hydrogen bonds in glutenins. The rheological results showed that the addition of the WUAX damaged the viscoelasticity of proteins, and the effect of the amount of WUAX on the viscoelastic behavior of the gliadins was lower than that of glutenins, which may be due to the structural differences between the two proteins. Interestingly, the tan δ of the glutenins increased with the increasing amount of WUAX, which was related to the higher viscosity of the WUAX itself. When the WUAX acted alone with glutenins, it partially compensated for the loose structure of the glutenins due to the absence of gliadins as the binding agent of the glutenins. Moreover, the reduction of β-sheets content for gliadins and glutenins weakened the rigid structure. Thermal property analysis suggests that the structure became more open, and the stability of the two proteins decreased after the addition of WUAX. Therefore, we speculated that after the addition of WUAX, a small amount of WUAX has a great impact on the covalent interaction of protein. With increasing WUAX, non-covalent interactions (hydrogen bond and ionic bond) between WUAX and protein played a critical role in the structure of the two proteins. The interactions between WUAX and independent gluten components are a matter of great significance for research into and development of WUAX-gluten gel products; they also provide a theoretical reserve for enhancing the quality of whole wheat-based foods. The effect of WUAX on the nutritional and digestive properties of gliadin and glutenin gels requires further investigation.

Author Contributions: F.L.: Investigation, Formal analysis, Writing—original draft, Methodology. T.L.: Investigation, Software. J.Z.: Investigation, Software. M.F.: Writing—review and editing. H.Q.: Supervision. Y.L.: Investigation, Validation. L.W.: Resources, Supervision, Writing—review and editing. All authors have read and agreed to the published version of the manuscript.

Funding: This research was supported by the National Natural Science Foundation of China (32072254), the National Key Research and Development Program of China (2020YFC1606804), the Research and Development Program of Tianchang (TZY202002), the "Qing Lan Project" of Jiangsu Province, the China Postdoctoral Science Foundation (2021M701462), and the Postdoctoral Research Funding Program of Jiangsu Province (2021K097A).

Data Availability Statement: The datasets generated for this study are available on request to the corresponding author.

Conflicts of Interest: The authors declare no conflict of interest.

References

1. Cheng, W.; Sun, Y.J.; Fan, M.C.; Li, Y.; Wang, L.; Qian, H.F. Wheat bran, as the resource of dietary fiber: A review. *Crit. Rev. Food Sci.* **2022**, *62*, 7269–7281. [CrossRef]
2. Yao, W.; Gong, Y.; Li, L.; Hu, X.; You, L. The effects of dietary fibers from rice bran and wheat bran on gut microbiota: An overview. *Food Chem.* **2022**, *13*, 100252. [CrossRef]
3. Li, Y.; Wang, L.J.; Wang, H.R.; Li, Z.G.; Qiu, J.; Wang, L.L. Correlation of microstructure, pore characteristics and hydration properties of wheat bran modified by airflow impact mill. *Innov. Food Sci. Emerg.* **2022**, *77*, 102977. [CrossRef]
4. Ma, S.; Wang, Z.; Liu, H.M.; Li, L.; Zheng, X.L.; Tian, X.L.; Sun, B.H.; Wang, X.X. Supplementation of wheat flour products with wheat bran dietary fiber: Purpose, mechanisms, and challenges. *Trends Food Sci. Tech.* **2022**, *123*, 281–289. [CrossRef]
5. Anderson, C.; Simsek, S. Mechanical profiles and topographical properties of films made from alkaline extracted arabinoxylans from wheat bran, maize bran, or dried distillers grain. *Food Hydrocolloid* **2019**, *86*, 78–86. [CrossRef]

6. Pazo-Cepeda, M.V.; Aspromonte, S.G.; Alonso, E. Extraction of ferulic acid and feruloylated arabinoxylo-oligosaccharides from wheat bran using pressurized hot water. *Food Biosci.* **2021**, *44*, 101374. [CrossRef]
7. Schupfer, E.; Pak, S.C.; Wang, S.Y.; Micalos, P.S.; Jeffries, T.; Ooi, S.L.; Golombick, T.; Harris, G.; El-Omar, E. The effects and benefits of arabinoxylans on human gut microbiota-A narrative review. *Food Biosci.* **2021**, *43*, 101267. [CrossRef]
8. Zhao, X.H.; Hou, C.D.; Tian, M.Q.; Zhou, Y.L.; Yang, R.Q.; Wang, X.Y.; Gu, Z.X.; Wang, P. Effect of water-extractable arabinoxylan with different molecular weight on the heat-induced aggregation behavior of gluten. *Food Hydrocolloid* **2020**, *99*, 105318. [CrossRef]
9. Wang, M.; Hamer, R.J.; van Vliet, T.; Gruppen, H.; Marseille, H.; Weegels, P.L. Effect of water unextractable solids on gluten formation and properties: Mechanistic considerations. *J. Cereal Sci.* **2003**, *37*, 55–64. [CrossRef]
10. Arif, S.; Ahmed, M.; Chaudhry, Q.; Hasnain, A. Effects of water extractable and unextractable pentosans on dough and bread properties of hard wheat cultivars. *LWT-Food Sci. Technol.* **2018**, *97*, 736–742. [CrossRef]
11. Si, X.J.; Li, T.T.; Zhang, Y.; Zhang, W.H.; Qian, H.F.; Li, Y.; Zhang, H.; Qi, X.G.; Wang, L. Interactions between gluten and water-unextractable arabinoxylan during the thermal treatment. *Food Chem.* **2021**, *345*, 128785. [CrossRef]
12. Jiang, Z.J.; Liu, L.Y.; Yang, W.; Ding, L.; Awais, M.; Wang, L.; Zhou, S.M. Improving the physicochemical properties of whole wheat model dough by modifying the water-unextractable solids. *Food Chem.* **2018**, *259*, 18–24. [CrossRef]
13. Feng, Y.L.; Zhang, H.J.; Fu, B.B.; Iftikhar, M.; Liu, G.Y.; Wang, J. Interactions between dietary fiber and ferulic acid change the aggregation of glutenin, gliadin and glutenin macropolymer in wheat flour system. *J. Sci. Food Agric.* **2021**, *101*, 1979–1988. [CrossRef]
14. Guo, J.Y.; He, Y.J.; Liu, J.J.; Wu, Y.; Wang, P.; Luo, D.L.; Xiang, J.L.; Sun, J.G. Influence of konjac glucomannan on thermal and microscopic properties of frozen wheat gluten, glutenin and gliadin. *Innov. Food Sci. Emerg.* **2021**, *74*, 102866. [CrossRef]
15. Wang, K.Q.; Luo, S.Z.; Zhong, X.Y.; Cai, J.; Jiang, S.T.; Zheng, Z. Changes in chemical interactions and protein conformation during heat-induced wheat gluten gel formation. *Food Chem.* **2017**, *214*, 393–399. [CrossRef]
16. Gao, X.; Liu, T.H.; Yu, J.; Li, L.Q.; Feng, Y.; Li, X.J. Influence of high-molecular-weight glutenin subunit composition at Glu-B1 locus on secondary and micro structures of gluten in wheat (*Triticum aestivum* L.). *Food Chem.* **2016**, *197*, 1184–1190. [CrossRef]
17. Cai, S.; Singh, B.R. Identification of beta-turn and random coil amide III infrared bands for secondary structure estimation of proteins. *Biophys. Chem.* **1999**, *80*, 7–20. [CrossRef]
18. Zhou, Y.; Zhao, D.; Foster, T.J.; Liu, Y.X.; Wang, Y.; Nirasawa, S.; Tatsumi, E.; Cheng, Y.Q. Konjac glucomannan-induced changes in thiol/disulphide exchange and gluten conformation upon dough mixing. *Food Chem.* **2014**, *150*, 164–165. [CrossRef]
19. Ooms, N.; Jansens, K.J.A.; Pareyt, B.; Reyniers, S.; Brijs, K.; Delcour, J.A. The impact of disulfide bond dynamics in wheat gluten protein on the development of fermented pastry crumb. *Food Chem.* **2018**, *242*, 68–74. [CrossRef] [PubMed]
20. Wang, P.; Zou, M.; Liu, K.X.; Gu, Z.X.; Yang, R.Q. Effect of mild thermal treatment on the polymerization behavior, conformation and viscoelasticity of wheat gliadin. *Food Chem.* **2018**, *239*, 984–992. [CrossRef] [PubMed]
21. Li, M.F.; Yue, Q.H.; Liu, C.; Zheng, X.L.; Hong, J.; Wang, N.N.; Bian, K. Interaction between gliadin/glutenin and starch granules in dough during mixing. *LWT-Food Sci. Technol.* **2021**, *148*, 111624. [CrossRef]
22. Veraverbeke, W.S.; Delcour, J.A. Wheat protein composition and properties of wheat glutenin in relation to breadmaking functionality. *Crit. Rev. Food Sci.* **2002**, *42*, 179–208. [CrossRef] [PubMed]
23. Wieser, H. Chemistry of gluten proteins. *Food Microbiol.* **2007**, *24*, 115–119. [CrossRef] [PubMed]
24. Ang, S.; Kogulanathan, J.; Morris, G.A.; Kok, M.S.; Shewry, P.R.; Tatham, A.S.; Adams, G.G.; Rowe, A.J.; Harding, S.E. Structure and heterogeneity of gliadin: A hydrodynamic evaluation. *Eur. Biophys. J.* **2010**, *39*, 255–261. [CrossRef] [PubMed]
25. Ferrer, E.G.; Bosch, A.; Yantorno, O.; Baran, E.J. A spectroscopy approach for the study of the interactions of bioactive vanadium species with bovine serum albumin. *Bioorgan Med. Chem.* **2008**, *16*, 3878–3886. [CrossRef]
26. Thomson, N.H.; Miles, M.J.; Popineau, Y.; Harries, J.; Shewry, P.; Tatham, A.S. Small angle X-ray scattering of wheat seed-storage proteins: Alpha-, gamma- and omega-gliadins and the high molecular weight (HMW) subunits of glutenin. *BBA-Protein Struct. Mol.* **1999**, *1430*, 359–366. [CrossRef] [PubMed]
27. Liu, J.; Luo, D.L.; Li, X.; Xu, B.C.; Zhang, X.Y.; Liu, J.X. Effects of inulin on the structure and emulsifying properties of protein components in dough. *Food Chem.* **2016**, *210*, 235–241. [CrossRef]
28. Wang, P.; Chen, H.Y.; Mohanad, B.; Xu, L.; Ning, Y.W.; Xu, J.; Wu, F.F.; Yang, N.; Jin, Z.Y.; Xu, X.M. Effect of frozen storage on physico-chemistry of wheat gluten proteins: Studies on gluten-, glutenin- and gliadin-rich fractions. *Food Hydrocolloid* **2014**, *39*, 187–194. [CrossRef]
29. Ma, F.Y.; Zhang, Y.; Liu, N.H.; Zhang, J.; Tan, G.X.; Kannan, B.; Liu, X.H.; Bell, A.E. Rheological properties of polysaccharides from Dioscorea opposita Thunb. *Food Chem.* **2017**, *227*, 64–72. [CrossRef]
30. Yazar, G.; Duvarci, O.C.; Tavman, S.; Kokini, J.L. LAOS behavior of the two main gluten fractions: Gliadin and glutenin. *J. Cereal Sci.* **2017**, *77*, 201–210. [CrossRef]
31. Zhu, Y.; Wang, Y.; Li, J.; Li, F.; Teng, C.; Li, X. Effects of Water-Extractable Arabinoxylan on the Physicochemical Properties and Structure of Wheat Gluten by Thermal Treatment. *J. Agric. Food Chem.* **2017**, *65*, 4728–4735. [CrossRef] [PubMed]

32. Khatkar, B.S.; Barak, S.; Mudgil, D. Effects of gliadin addition on the rheological, microscopic and thermal characteristics of wheat gluten. *Int. J. Biol. Macromol.* **2013**, *53*, 38–41. [CrossRef] [PubMed]
33. Guo, Z.H.; Liu, M.; Xiang, X.W.; Wang, Z.R.; Yang, B.; Chen, X.H.; Chen, G.J.; Kan, J.Q. Effects of inulins with various molecular weights and added concentrations on the structural properties and thermal stability of heat-induced gliadin and glutenin gels. *LWT-Food Sci. Technol.* **2021**, *149*, 111891. [CrossRef]

Disclaimer/Publisher's Note: The statements, opinions and data contained in all publications are solely those of the individual author(s) and contributor(s) and not of MDPI and/or the editor(s). MDPI and/or the editor(s) disclaim responsibility for any injury to people or property resulting from any ideas, methods, instructions or products referred to in the content.

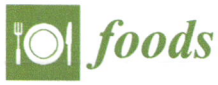

Article

Sulfated Chinese Yam Polysaccharides Alleviate LPS-Induced Acute Inflammation in Mice through Modulating Intestinal Microbiota

Shihua Wu, Xianxiang Chen, Ruixin Cai, Xiaodie Chen, Jian Zhang, Jianhua Xie and Mingyue Shen *

State Key Laboratory of Food Science and Technology, Nanchang University, Nanchang 330047, China; 18222591639@163.com (S.W.); xianxiangchen@email.ncu.edu.cn (X.C.); c18312933692@163.com (R.C.); xdiechen@163.com (X.C.); zj105716@163.com (J.Z.); jhxie@ncu.edu.cn (J.X.)
* Correspondence: shenmingyue1107@163.com

Abstract: This study aimed to test the preventive anti-inflammatory properties of Chinese yam polysaccharides (CYP) and sulfated Chinese yam polysaccharides (SCYP) on LPS-induced systemic acute inflammation in mice and investigate their mechanisms of action. The results showed that SCYP can efficiently reduce plasma TNF-α and IL-6 levels, exhibiting an obvious anti-inflammation ability. Moreover, SCYP reduced hepatic TNF-α, IL-6, and IL-1β secretion more effectively than CYP, and significantly altered intestinal oxidative stress levels. In addition, a 16S rRNA gene sequencing analysis showed that CYP regulated the gut microbiota by decreasing *Desulfovibrio* and *Sutterella* and increasing *Prevotella*. SCYP changed the gut microbiota by decreasing *Desulfovibrio* and increasing *Coprococcus*, which reversed the microbiota dysbiosis caused by LPS. Linear discriminant analysis (LDA) effect size (LEfSe) revealed that treatment with CYP and SCYP can produce more biomarkers of the gut microbiome that can promote the proliferation of polysaccharide-degrading bacteria and facilitate the intestinal de-utilization of polysaccharides. These results suggest that SCYP can differentially regulate intestinal flora, and that they exhibit anti-inflammatory effects, thus providing a new reference to rationalize the exploitation of sulfated yam polysaccharides.

Keywords: yam polysaccharide; sulfation; LPS; anti-inflammation; gut microbiota

Citation: Wu, S.; Chen, X.; Cai, R.; Chen, X.; Zhang, J.; Xie, J.; Shen, M. Sulfated Chinese Yam Polysaccharides Alleviate LPS-Induced Acute Inflammation in Mice through Modulating Intestinal Microbiota. *Foods* 2023, 12, 1772. https://doi.org/10.3390/foods12091772

Academic Editor: Denis Roy

Received: 2 April 2023
Revised: 14 April 2023
Accepted: 19 April 2023
Published: 25 April 2023

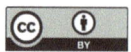

Copyright: © 2023 by the authors. Licensee MDPI, Basel, Switzerland. This article is an open access article distributed under the terms and conditions of the Creative Commons Attribution (CC BY) license (https://creativecommons.org/licenses/by/4.0/).

1. Introduction

Inflammation is a complicated physiological phenomenon which can be triggered by either infectious or non-infectious conditions [1,2]. Cytokines, such as tumor necrosis factor (TNF)-α and interleukin (IL)-6, have been known to play significant roles in inflammatory responses. They are released from cells, which causes the expression of adhesion molecules to recruit lymphocytes, monocytes, and neutrophils, and then move out of vessels to tissues, such as the liver, and induce inflammation and oxidative stress [3]. Lipopolysaccharide, an ideal inflammatory molding agent, derives from the cell wall of gram-negative bacteria and is an important component of the bacterial outer membrane, which can be recognized by the innate immune system [4]. Lipopolysaccharide entering the blood can trigger a systemic inflammatory response and may further cause multi-organ damage and dysfunction in the liver, lungs, intestines, kidneys, and brain, which can lead to clinically identified sepsis [5]. To alleviate inflammation, researchers have tried to find biologically active substances of natural origin. Many plant-derived natural compounds exhibit good biological activities with low toxic effects, and polysaccharides are one of the macromolecules that have received much attention for this reason [6].

Many plant-derived natural compounds exhibit good biological activities with low toxic effects, and polysaccharides are one of the macromolecules that have received much attention for this reason [6–8]. It has been demonstrated that polysaccharides perform a variety of biological activities including antioxidant, anti-inflammatory, antitumor, immunomodulatory, and antiviral activities [9,10], and they can be used in the preparation of new drugs, medicinal materials, and functional foods [9,11]. As a traditional medicinal food homologous plant, Chinese yam (*Dioscorea opposita* Thunb.) is rich in a variety of nutrients and bioactive components, such as polysaccharides, allantoin, saponins, and glycoproteins, which perform various biological activities and have various pharmacological effects [12]. The polysaccharides in yams are usually divided into starch and non-starch polysaccharides, and the yam polysaccharides used in this study were mucilage polysaccharides (non-starch polysaccharides) [13]. The different biological activities of polysaccharides are related to their different molecular weights, molecular structures, and three-dimensional structures, and these can be changed by structural modifications to alter their original active effects [6,14]. Sulfated polysaccharides are polysaccharides containing sulfate groups on the polysaccharide units. Some polysaccharides are naturally sulfated polysaccharides, and some polysaccharides do not originally have sulfate groups, though these can be prepared by chemical modification of sulfation sites [14]. Because of their own characteristics, sulfated polysaccharides perform many biological activities, such as anticoagulant, hypolipidemic, antiviral, antitumor, and antioxidant activities [15–18]. In recent years, synthetic sulfated polysaccharides have attracted attention for their structural modifications, by which their biological activities may be enhanced [19]. Aside from the Wolfrom method and the concentrated sulfuric acid and sulfur trioxide-pyridine method, some researchers prepare arabinogalactan sulfates with sulfur content up to 11.3% using ammonium sulfamate as a sulfating reagent [15]. In addition, few of the non-starch polysaccharides are digested by the mammalian intestine and reach the colon intact to serve as an energy source for the intestinal flora, stimulating their growth and producing healthy metabolites [20,21].

The gut microbiota is a diverse ecosystem which exists in symbiosis with the human body and plays relevant roles in human health, impacting the pathogenesis of many diseases [22]. Certain bacteria can increase intestinal permeability, and their structural components can enter the organism and trigger a cytokine cascade response to inflammation [23,24]. Other bacteria can exert effects on the regulatory cells of the immune system, suppressing inflammation or indirectly performing anti-inflammatory functions through their metabolites [24]. When the intestinal barrier is damaged and intestinal permeability increases, some substances that are not supposed to cross the intestinal wall, which is a component of the cell wall of gram-negative bacteria, escape from the intestinal lumen into the body's circulation [22]. Bacterial translocation in the gut can cause damage to other tissues and organs, including the liver. The colonization of beneficial intestinal bacteria facilitates the alleviation of liver disease, and the health and homeostasis of the gut are important for liver health [22,24].

Our previous studies have demonstrated that sulfated derivatives of yam polysaccharides can regulate immune effects in RAW264.7 cells [25]. However, how sulfated derivatives of yam polysaccharides affect body inflammation and changes in the gut microbiota in mice is not well understood. In this study, the anti-inflammatory activities of CYP and SCYP were investigated by establishing an LPS-induced acute inflammation model in mice. The alleviating effects of both polysaccharides on the systemic inflammatory response, including blood circulation, in the liver and at intestinal sites, as well as the modulating effect on intestinal flora, were the main focuses. This research can provide a reference for the application of yam polysaccharides in food and medicine.

2. Materials and Methods

2.1. Materials

Lipopolysaccharide (LPS) derived from *E. coli* 055: B5 was purchased from Sigma-Aldrich (St. Louis, MO, USA). Acetylsalicylic acid (aspirin) was bought from Aladdin Bio-Chem Technology Co., Ltd. (Shanghai, China). Enzyme-linked immunosorbent assay (ELISA) kits were purchased from Boster Biological Technology Co., Ltd. (Wuhan, China). Total protein contents (BCA), superoxidase dismutase (SOD), catalase (CAT), and malondialdehyde (MDA) were purchased from Beyotime Biotechnology Co., Ltd. (Shanghai, China).

Yams were purchased from Ruichang (Jiangxi, China) and prepared as yam powder by crushing. The yam powder was depigmented, water was extracted, alcohol was precipitated, starch and protein were removed, it was dialyzed, alcohol was again precipitated, and it was redissolved and lyophilized to obtain CYP [19]. Referring to our previous study, SCYP was obtained by further sulfation modification of CYP using the chlorosulfonic acid pyridine method. The ratio of chlorosulfonic acid to pyridine was 1:5 and the degree of substitution (DS) was 0.44 [25]. The two polysaccharides were mainly composed of galacturonic acid, galactose, glucose, xylose, arabinose, and rhamnose. The CYP had a molar ratio of 2.77:1.41:0.98:0.91:0.27:0.18, and the SCYP had a molar ratio of 1.99:2.82:0.65:1.97:0.76:0.12 [25].

2.2. Animals and Experimental Design

Male C57BL/6J mice (7–8 weeks old, 22 ± 2 g body weight) were supplied by the Hunan Slac Jingda Laboratory Animal Co., Ltd. (Changsha, China, certificate number: SCXK (Xiang) 2016-0002). All the mice were kept at the animal laboratory of the State Key Laboratory of Food at Nanchang University. Before the experiments began, the mice underwent a 7-day adaptation period during which they were housed at a temperature of 18–22 °C, 55% relative humidity, and under a 12/12 h light–dark cycle with ad libitum access to a standard diet and water. The thirty mice were randomized into 5 treatment groups (6 mice per group): the normal saline contrast group (N), the LPS model group (M), the aspirin positive contrast group (P), the CYP group (CYP), and the SCYP group (SCYP). The specific treatment was as follows: the N and M groups were gavaged with an equivalent volume of normal saline, the P group was gavaged with aspirin (15 mg/kg BW), and the polysaccharide groups were gavaged with CYP and SCYP 100 mg/kg BW (body weight) once a day for 14 days. At the end of 14 days, the N group was injected with normal saline intraperitoneally, and the rest of the groups were injected with LPS (5 mg/kg BW) intraperitoneally for 12 h. After recording their weights, the mice were sacrificed by cervical dislocation.

All the animal experimental operations were carried out in accordance with the National Institutes of Health (NIH Publication No. 8023, 1978) guidelines for the care and use of laboratory animals, and all the experimental procedures were approved by Nanchang University Animal Ethic Review Committee (license No: SYXK (gan) 2015–0001).

2.3. General Indicators

After the mice were sacrificed, the thymus, spleen, and liver were removed and cleaned with 0.9% NaCl, and the excess solution was aspirated with filter paper and weighed, and the organ index was calculated. Organ index (mg/g) = organ weight (mg)/body weight (g).

2.4. Determination of Plasma Inflammatory Factors

Blood was collected from the eyes of the mice and centrifuged at 3000 rpm for 10 min at 4 °C. The supernatant was collected as plasma, aliquoted, and stored at -80 °C, and the assay was conducted according to the ELISA kit instructions.

2.5. Determination of Liver Inflammatory Factors

The liver was isolated from each mouse and cut into small pieces with scissors. Approximately 30 mg liver tissue was collected to make 10% (m/v) tissue homogenate with pre-cooled PBS, and the supernatant was collected by centrifugation at $12,000\times g$ for 10 min at 4 °C and detected according to the ELISA kit instructions.

2.6. Oxidative Stress Factors and Jejunal Inflammatory Factors

The small intestine was isolated from each mouse, the middle jejunal part was intercepted, and the contents were removed. Approximately 30 mg jejunal tissue was collected to make homogenate, and the centrifugal collection of supernatants was conducted in the same way outlined in Section 2.5. The protein concentrations in the collected supernatants were determined using a BCA kit, and SOD, CAT, MDA, and IL-1β levels were measured according to the kit instructions.

2.7. 16S rRNA High-Throughput Sequencing

After the mice were sacrificed, the colon of each mouse was isolated, the colonic contents were packed in EP tubes by extruding them with forceps, and these were stored in a −80 °C freezer. Total DNA was extracted from the colon contents according to the DNA extraction kit instructions. The extracted DNA was subjected to 0.8% agarose gel electrophoresis for molecular size determination and was quantified using a UV spectrophotometer. Bacterial 16S rRNA V3-V4 region-specific primers were used for PCR amplification. The primers were 338F: 5′-ACTCCTACGGGAGGCAGCA-3′ and 806R: 5′-GGACTACHVGGGTWTCTAAT-3′. The PCR products were purified using 2% gel electrophoresis, quantified using the Quant-iT PicoGreen dsDNA Assay Kit, and mixed according to the amount of data required for each sample. Library construction was performed using the Illumina's TruSeq Nano DNA LT Library Prep Kit. The libraries were quality-checked on Agilent Bioanalyzer using the Agilent High Sensitivity DNA Kit and quantified on Promega QuantiFluor using the Quant-iT PicoGreen dsDNA Assay Kit. For qualified libraries with concentrations above 2 nM, 2×250 bp double-end sequencing was performed on a MiSeq machine using the MiSeq Reagent Kit V3 (600 cycles).

2.8. Statistical Analysis

Data were shown as the means ± standard deviation (SD). IBM SPSS statistical software 20 was used for statistical analysis. A data significance analysis was performed using one-way ANOVA and Duncan's multiple range test. $p < 0.05$ or $p < 0.01$ was considered as significant.

3. Results

3.1. Body Weight and Organ Index

Throughout the entire experiment, changes in the body weight of the mice in each group were monitored (Figure 1A,B). After the intraperitoneal injection with LPS, a 9% weight loss was observed in the M group compared with the N group ($p < 0.05$). Compared with the M group, neither aspirin nor CYP treatment restored the weight loss caused by LPS. However, the SCYP group exhibited a significant ($p < 0.05$) improvement in body weight compared with the M group, indicating that the administration of SCYP could dramatically inhibit LPS-induced weight loss.

According to the results of the spleen index calculation, the spleens of the mice in group M were significantly enlarged by the intraperitoneal injection of LPS compared with those of the normal group ($p < 0.05$). This result is similar to that obtained in [26], in which it was found that the and spleen indices increased in the LPS-treated group compared with the untreated group. The spleen is the largest lymphatic organ and its functions include blood storage, the removal of aging red blood cells, and immune response, and it can therefore reflect the body's inflammatory condition. Thus, the result revealed that the spleen was swollen, and the body was inflamed. Interestingly, this enlargement was not reduced by gavage with CYP, but with SCYP ($p < 0.05$). The liver index was significantly reduced in the M group compared with the normal group ($p < 0.05$). The CYP and SCYP were able to restore the hepatic index to a normal level compared with the model group ($p < 0.05$) (Table 1).

3.2. Plasma Inflammatory Cytokines

The results of the plasma pro-inflammatory cytokine changes in the mice are presented in Figure 1B,C. In normal mouse plasma, low levels of TNF-α and very low levels of IL-6 are typically detected. After LPS stimulation, TNF-α and IL-6 levels were significantly increased compared with those of the normal mice ($p < 0.01$). Compared with those of the M group, the TNF-α and IL-6 levels showed an extremely significant decrease in both the CYP-treated group and the SCYP-treated group ($p < 0.01$). The CYP group showed a stronger reduction plasma TNF-α and IL-6 levels than the SCYP group ($p < 0.05$). Overall, CYP and SCYP were effective in reducing both plasma TNF-α and IL-6 pro-inflammatory factors (Figure 1C,D).

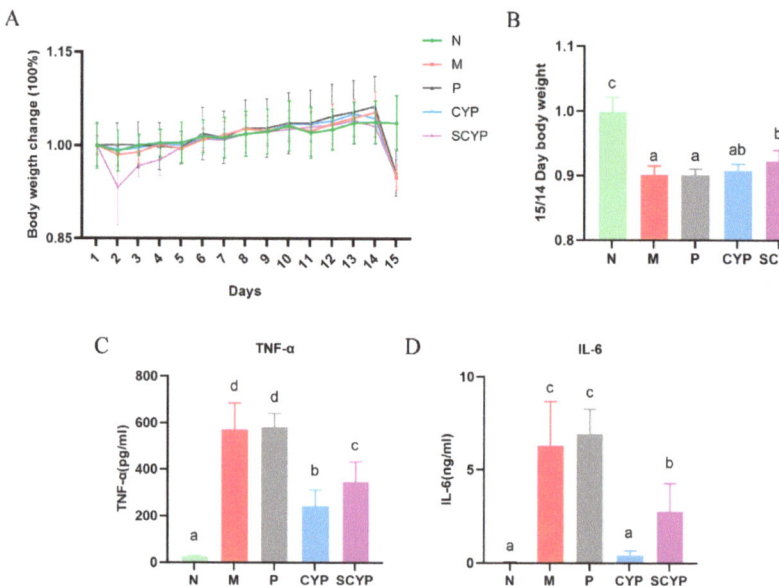

Figure 1. Percentage change in body weight compared with day 1 for each group (**A**). Body weight ratio of day 14/15 for each group (**B**). Levels of pro-inflammatory cytokines TNF-α (**C**) and IL-6 (**D**) in the plasma. Values are expressed as means ± SD. (n = 6 for **A**,**B** and n = 5 for **C**,**D**). Different letters represent significant differences between different groups ($p < 0.05$).

Table 1. The organ indices of the LPS-induced mice.

	Spleen Index	Thymus Index	Liver Index
N	2.64 ± 0.16 a	1.57 ± 0.07 a	30.42 ± 0.89 b
M	4.02 ± 0.23 c	1.33 ± 0.19 a	28.09 ± 1.07 a
P	4.06 ± 0.30 c	1.33 ± 0.24 a	31.19 ± 0.46 b
CYP	3.92 ± 0.10 c	1.36 ± 0.26 a	30.23 ± 0.60 b
SCYP	3.61 ± 0.27 b	1.35 ± 0.08 a	30.33 ± 2.27 b

Values are expressed as means ± standard deviation (SD). Different lowercase letters represent significant differences between different groups ($p < 0.05$) (n = 5).

3.3. Liver Inflammatory Cytokines

Compared with that of the N group, there was a significant increase in the level of TNF-α in the livers of the mice after LPS stimulation ($p < 0.05$) (Figure 2A). Compared with that of the M group, the CYP group showed a slight reduction in TNF-α level. However, the pre-administration of SCYP caused a significant reduction ($p < 0.05$). The IL-6 level was significantly increased in the model group compared with the N group ($p < 0.05$). Interestingly, pre-treatment with SCYP resulted in a significant recovery, and even a return to normal levels (Figure 2B). The level of IL-1β was significantly higher in the M group compared with the normal group ($p < 0.05$). CYP and SCYP had comparable effects; they both significantly reduced the level of IL-1β ($p < 0.05$) (Figure 2C). In general, CYP and SCYP both exhibited a great anti-inflammatory effect by decreasing the production of proinflammatory cytokines, and SCYP showed the better effect than CYP.

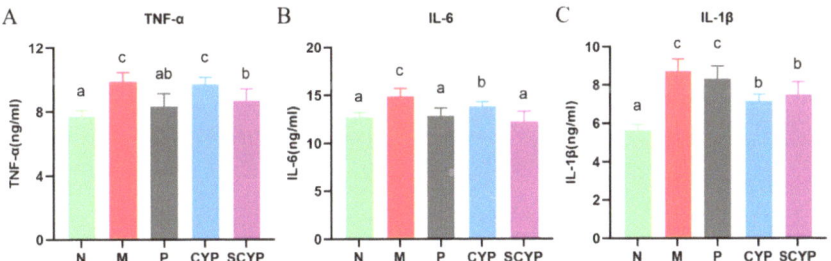

Figure 2. Influence of CYP and SCYP on pro-inflammatory cytokines TNF-α (**A**), IL-6 (**B**) and IL-1β (**C**) in the livers of LPS-induced mice. Values are expressed as means ± SD. (n = 6). Different letters represent significant differences between different groups ($p < 0.05$).

3.4. Jejunal Oxidative Stress Factors and Inflammatory Factors

Indicators related to oxidative stress in the jejunal segment of the small intestine were tested. For both of the antioxidant enzymes SOD and CAT, the model group showed a significant decrease compared with the N group ($p < 0.05$) (Figure 3A,B). The polysaccharide-treated groups had higher levels of both enzymes than the M group. For the lipid oxidation hazard MDA, the model group presented a significant elevation compared with the normal control group ($p < 0.05$) (Figure 3C). A slight reduction in MDA was found in the polysaccharide-treated group compared with the M group. A significant difference in the inflammatory factor IL-1β was not observed in any group (Figure 3D).

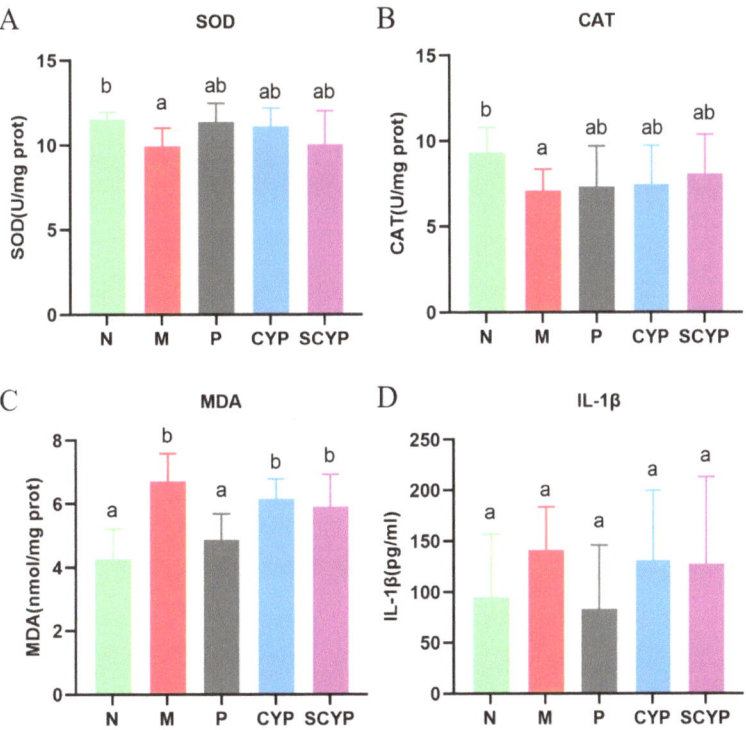

Figure 3. Oxidative stress in jejunal tissue evaluated in terms of SOD (**A**), CAT (**B**), and MDA (**C**). Levels of pro-inflammatory cytokines IL-1β (**D**) in jejunal tissue. Values are expressed as means ± SD. (n = 6 for **A** and n = 5 for **B**,**C**). Different letters represent significant differences between different groups ($p < 0.05$).

3.5. α-Diversity and β-Diversity Analysis of Colon Microbiota

Alpha diversity refers to the indicator of richness, diversity, and evenness of species, and larger Shannon–Simpson, Chao1, and observed indices represent higher within-habitat diversity. Four indices were used to evaluate the effect of LPS modeling and CYP and SCYP on the α-diversity of the intestinal microflora (Figure 4A). Compared with the N group, increases in the Shannon–Simpson, Chao1, and observed species indices ($p < 0.05$) of the intestinal microflora were observed in the CYP and SCYP groups. No significant difference in Simpson index was observed in any of the groups. This indicates that CYP could increase richness and evenness of the gut microorganisms.

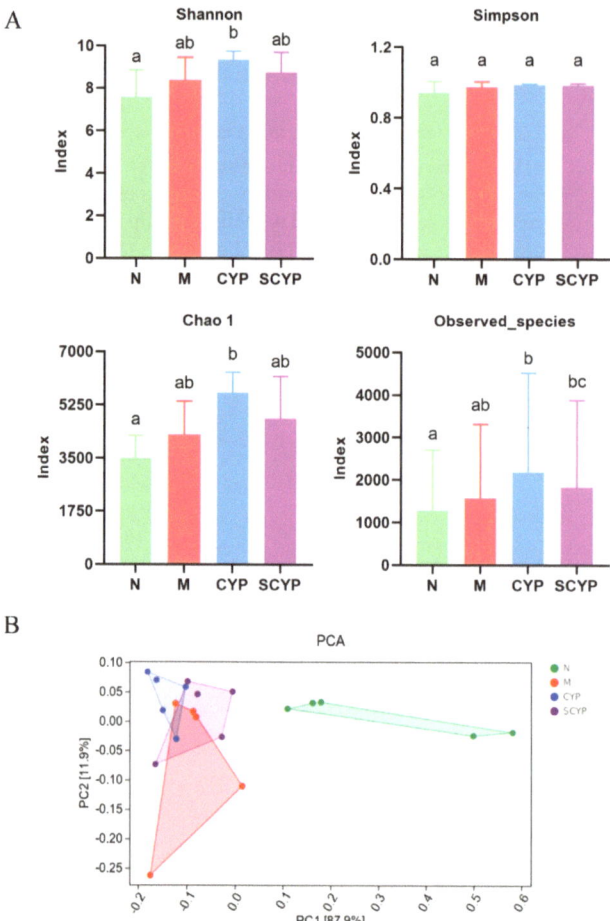

Figure 4. α-diversity evaluated using Shannon, Simpson, Chao1, and observed_species indices (**A**). β-diversity evaluated according to the PCA (**B**). (n = 5). Different letters represent significant differences between different groups ($p < 0.05$).

A β-diversity analysis was used to evaluate the structural changes in the intestinal flora. A principal component analysis (PCA) based on Euclidean distance showed that the individuals in each experimental group exhibited significantly different differential clustering (Figure 4B). The N group was completely separated from the M, CYP, and SCYP groups on the x-axis (87.9%), indicating that LPS treatment greatly altered the intestinal structure of the mice. The CYP and SCYP groups were mostly separate from the M group and mostly overlapped with the N group on the y-axis (11.9%). This suggests that CYP and SCYP treatment affords partial resistance to LPS-induced alterations in gut microflora structure, and these groups increasingly resembled the normal group. This result was similar to the aforementioned results in which pre-treatment with polysaccharides decreased proinflammatory factors when the compared with the absence of such treatment. This might be because the intestinal flora was not seriously damaged by LPS.

3.6. Microbial Community Composition

According to the phylum-level species composition diagram (Figure 5A), the top four represented bacteria were *Bacteroidetes*, *Firmicutes*, *Proteobacteria*, and *TM7* (in that order). The specific relative abundance values of each phylum in each group are shown in Figure 5B–E. The relative abundance of *Bacteroidetes* was significantly increased in the M, CYP, and SCYP groups compared with the N group ($p < 0.05$). The relative abundance of *Proteobacteria* increased significantly in the LPS group compared with the N group ($p < 0.05$). However, the relative abundance was decreased by the polysaccharide treatment. A significant decrease in the relative abundance of *Firmicutes* and *TM7* was observed in the LPS group compared with the N group ($p < 0.05$). Interestingly, polysaccharide treatment can reverse the change in gut microbiota caused by LPS.

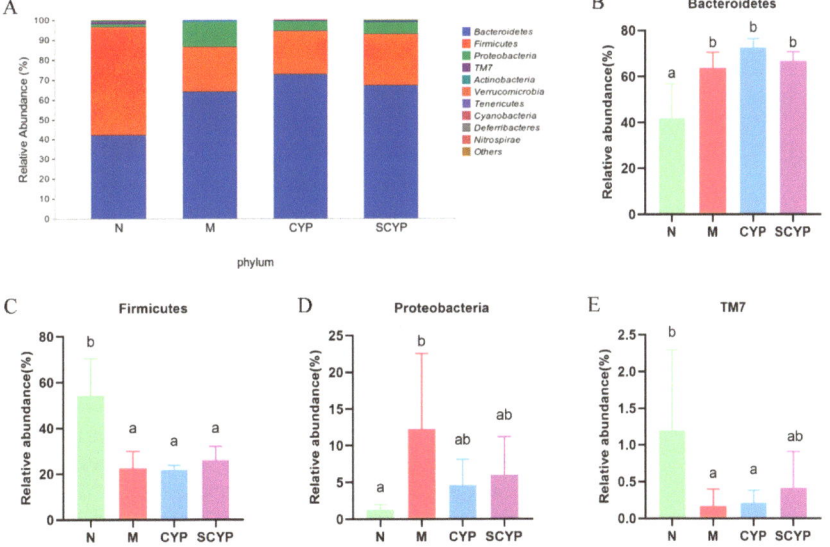

Figure 5. Species composition of colon microbiota at the phylum level (**A**). Relative abundance of colon microbiota at the phylum level (**B–E**). Values are expressed as means ± SD. (n = 5). Different letters represent significant differences between different groups ($p < 0.05$).

The overall species composition of the top 20 bacteria at the genus level is shown in Figure 6A, and the specific relative abundance values for each genus are shown in Figure 6B–G. The relative abundance of *Lactobacilllus* was significantly reduced in the LPS group compared with the N group ($p < 0.05$), and preventive administration of both polysaccharides did not restore the relative abundance. The relative abundances of *Shigella*, *Desulfovibrio*, and *Sutterella* were significantly elevated in the LPS group compared with the N group ($p < 0.05$). Compared with group M, shigella was less abundant in the CYP and SCYP groups, but the difference was not significant. *Desulfovibrio* was significantly reduced in both the CYP and SCYP groups, in which it reached the level of group N ($p < 0.05$). Moreover, the relative abundance of *Sutterella* was significantly reduced in the CYP group ($p < 0.05$). There was no significant difference in *Prevotella* in the N, M, and SCYP groups, though a significant elevation was observed in the CYP group compared with these ($p < 0.05$). There was no significant difference in the relative abundance of *Coprococcus* in the N, M, and CYP groups, though a significant elevation was observed in the SCYP group compared with these ($p < 0.05$).

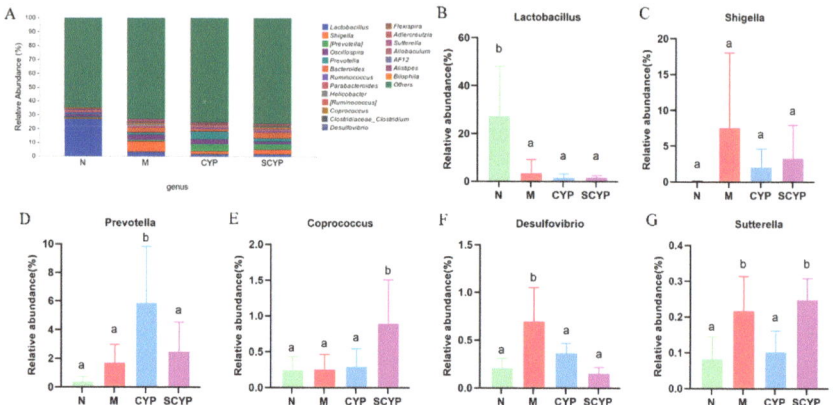

Figure 6. Species composition of colon microbiota at the genus level (**A**). Relative abundance of colon microbiota at the genus level (**B–G**). Values are expressed as means ± SD. (n = 5). Different letters represent significant differences between different groups ($p < 0.05$).

3.7. Biomarker Bacteria

A linear discriminant analysis effect size (LEfSe) combining the rank sum test and a discriminant analysis was used to identify significantly changed microbial taxa. The cladogram demonstrates the taxonomic hierarchical distribution of marker species in each group of samples, with larger solid nodes representing more significant enrichment (Figure 7A). Setting 4 as the LDA score threshold, the histogram shows the biomarker bacteria and their significance, with longer bar lengths representing more significant differences (Figure 7B). In group N, p_*Firmicutes*, f_*Lactobacillaceae*, o_*Lactobacillales*, c_*Bacilli*, g_*Lactobacillus*, and f_*Rikenellaceae* were specific. p_*Proteobacteria*, c_*Gammaproteobacteria*, f_*Enterobacterianceae*, o_*Enterobacteriales*, and g_*Shigella* were the biomarkers in group M. The CYP group was enriched with p_*Bacteroidetes*, c_*Bacteroidia*, o_*Bacteroidales*, f_*Prevotellaceae*, g_*Prevotella*, f_*Flavobacteriaceas*, o_*Flavobacteriales*, and c_*Flavobacteriia*. The SCYP group was enriched with f_*Bacteroidaceae*, g_*Bacteroides*, and g_*Pasteurella*.

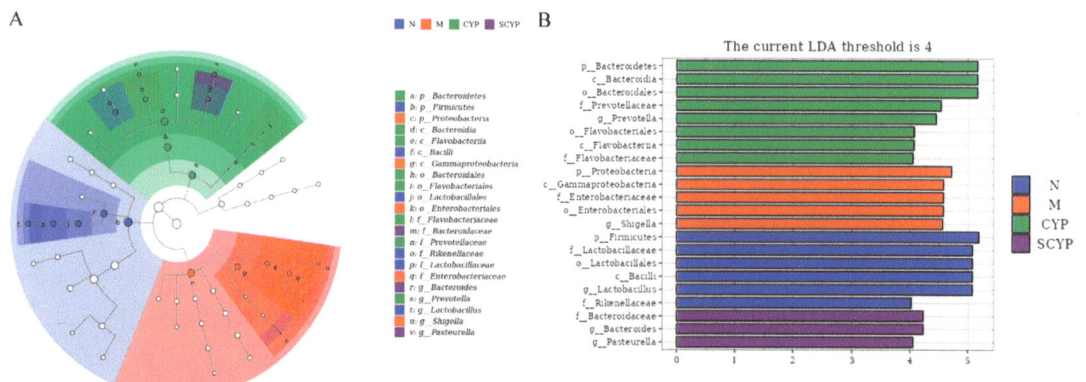

Figure 7. Taxonomic cladogram of the LEfSe analysis (**A**). Distribution histogram of the LEfSe analysis (**B**). The LDA threshold is 4. (n = 5).

4. Discussion

Inflammation is part of a protective reaction against damage caused by invading microorganisms. It is essential to trim or adjust it to avoid any increasing morbidity or shortening of life resulting from its excessive interactions. Chinese yam, a traditional Chinese medicinal and edible plant, has immunoregulatory functions. SCYP, a complex polysaccharide obtained from Chinese yam, was used to explore its effect on inflammation. In the present study, the administration of SCYP was found to alleviate inflammation by changing the composition of the gut microbiota. In order to simulate systemic inflammation induced by infectious injury, an intraperitoneal injection of LPS was used to establish the disease model. This model can be used to identify bioactive substances that can effectively prevent and alleviate inflammation in various parts of the organism. The body and organs have their normal weight ranges, and abnormal changes are associated with abnormal body conditions. Lipopolysaccharides can cause abnormal weight loss, possibly due to increased leptin levels [27]. Previous studies have shown that LPS causes the atrophy of the thymus and the enlargement of the spleen [26,28]. Splenomegaly is a common symptom of immune disorders and infectious inflammation, and this study found that SCYP can alleviate splenomegaly by establishing that SCYP can reduce the spleen index in cy-induced immunosuppressed mice [19]. Abnormal liver weight is a very obvious sign of the development of liver disease, and LPS not only causes the enlargement of the liver, but also its atrophy [29]. In the present study, liver weight was reduced after LPS damage, but was effectively prevented by both CYP and SCYP (Table 1).

In a study by Guo et al., LPS stimulation for 4 h was found to induce 5- to 10-fold increases in TNF-α and IL-6 in the blood, numbers that were even higher in this study after stimulation for 12 h [30]. Increased inflammatory cytokines in the blood, especially TNF-α and IL-6, are the main features of LPS-induced acute inflammation in mice [30]. TNF-α is a multifunctional cytokine that increases vascular permeability, induces fever, has potent pro-inflammatory effects, and plays a role in the induction of other inflammatory factors [31,32]. TNF-α is positively associated with a variety of inflammatory diseases, such as rheumatoid arthritis, acute liver injury, and lung cancer [30]. IL-6 is a more complex cytokine because it can be produced by immune and non-immune cells in multiple organ systems and act on multiple organ systems [31,33]. IL-6 has proinflammatory and pyrogenic functions, and overproduction exacerbates local or systemic inflammation [30]. IL-6 and TNF-α are always present together, showing the same trends, and are likewise positively correlated with various inflammatory diseases. SCYP can effectively reduce the concentration of TNF-α and IL-6 in the blood, indicating that both polysaccharides can inhibit the secretion of systemic pro-inflammatory factors and exert an anti-inflammatory effect (Figure 2).

Intraperitoneal injection of LPS can cause very typical acute liver injury and inflammation in mice. LPS, a typical pathogen-associated molecular pattern (PAMP), binds to pattern-recognition receptors (PRRs) on hepatic immune cells to initiate inflammatory responses after transport to the liver via portal blood [34]. In the response process, the lipopolysaccharide stimulates the immune cells to release a variety of inflammatory factors and chemokines which accelerate the recruitment of neutrophils, macrophages, and other immune cells, resulting in the release of more pro-inflammatory factors, including TNF-α, IL-6, and IL-1β [35–37]. Variations in IL-1β concentrations are associated with pathophysiological changes in different disease states and can be used to monitor disease progression [36,38]. In the present study, stimulation of LPS greatly increased the release of pro-inflammatory cytokines from the liver. Although CYP did not decrease the secretion of TNF-α in the liver, it successfully reduced the production of IL-6 and IL-1β. SCYP effectively reduced the production of three pro-inflammatory factors and was more effective than CYP. One study showed that 50 mg/kg sulfated *Cyclocarya paliurus* polysaccharides reduced IL-6 to normal levels in the liver, and in this study, 100 mg/kg SCYP also reduced IL-6 to normal levels (12 ng/mL). Sulfated polysaccharides were more effective than natural polysaccharides in both studies [29]. Overall, both CYP and SCYP could alleviate the inflammatory response of the liver caused by LPS, and the effectiveness of SCYP is superior (Figure 3).

The α-diversity analysis revealed that the LPS treatment did not cause a difference between the mice in the LPS group and those in the normal group (Figure 4), a result which is consistent with those of other studies [39]. CYP increased three indices, indicating its ability to increase the diversity of the microbial community, and SCYP did not show this effect. In the β-diversity analysis, it was seen that treatment with both yam polysaccharides could partially change the community structure, distinguishing it from the model group (Figure 4).

At the phylum level, *Bacteroidetes* and *Firmicutes* are the two most abundant bacteria in the normal intestine [40], and the ratio of *Bacteroidetes* to *Firmicutes* increased after LPS treatment, indicating that the homeostasis of the organism's intestinal environment was disrupted, resulting in an imbalance [41]. The addition of polysaccharides slightly reversed this imbalance. The abundance of *Proteobacteria* increased after LPS treatment. Most *Proteobacteria* are pathogenic gram-negative bacteria, and as markers of dysbiosis in the intestinal flora, their abnormally elevated levels are associated with inflammatory diseases [39]. There was a tendency for *Proteobacteria* to decrease after treatment with yam polysaccharides (Figure 5). Sulfated *Cyclocarya paliurus* polysaccharides reduced the relative abundance of *Proteobacteria* to 5% in one study, and SCYP was similarly reduced to 5% in this study [40].

At the genus level, two yam polysaccharides have the effect of altering the relative abundance of certain genera. *Shigella* is a kind of pathogenic bacteria belonging to the *Enterobacteriaceae* family which is positively correlated with metabolic endotoxin levels and the severity of systemic inflammation, and its increase may lead to intestinal barrier damage and increased permeability, exacerbating bacterial invasion and translocation [42,43]. *Desulfovibrio*, a kind of gram-negative conditional pathogenic bacteria, is classified as a genus of pro-inflammatory bacteria because of its high endotoxin content [44]. *Desulfovibrio* can reduce sulfate to produce H_2S, which can trigger epithelial apoptosis and intestinal barrier damage, and is associated with obesity and inflammation [45,46]. *Sutterella* is an important kind of commensal bacteria found in the intestinal tract, and changes in its levels have been associated with diseases including autism, depression, Down syndrome, obesity, and inflammatory bowel disease [47–50]. *Sutterella*, a member of the *Proteobacteria* classification, is abnormally increased in intestinal flora disorders [49]. Numerous studies have shown that intraperitoneal injection of LPS causes an increase in the genera *Shigella*, *Desulfovibrio*, and *Sutterella*, and the results of the present study are consistent with this observation [51]. Pretreatment with both polysaccharides had a tendency to reduce *Shigella*. Both CYP and SCYP were effective in reducing *Desulfovibrio* to normal levels, and SCYP showed better effects. Additionally, CYP effectively inhibited *Sutterella*. The above results indicate that both polysaccharides inhibit the growth of harmful bacteria with different strengths.

Prevotella is a dominant genus of bacteria in the human intestine which is associated with plant-based diets rich in carbohydrates and fiber, and which helps to break down polysaccharides [52,53]. *Prevotella* can produce propionic acid, which has the effect of preventing obesity and reducing the risk of diabetes [53,54]. CYP increased *Prevotella*, indicating that CYP effectively changed the mouse enterotype so that the mouse intestine could better utilize polysaccharides to produce SCFAs. *Coprococcus* can synthesize acetate and butyrate. Acetate may be a source of energy for endurance exercise, and butyrate is not only the main source of energy for colonic cells but can also play an anti-inflammatory role [20,55–57]. The experimental results suggest that SCYP may have a beneficial effect on intestinal health by increasing the proportion of *Coprococcus* in the intestine. These results suggest that the two polysaccharides regulate the intestinal flora by promoting the growth of different beneficial bacteria.

The LEfSe analysis revealed that, in the LPS group, *Proteobacteria*, *Gammaproteobacteria*, *Enterobacterianceae*, *Enterobacteriales*, and *Shigella* were the dominant species, and most of these are pathogenic or conditionally pathogenic bacteria [39,42]. *Bacteroidia*, *Bacteroidales*,

Prevotellaceae, Prevotella, Flavobacteriaceas, Flavobacteriales, and *Flavobacteriia* were biomarkers of CYP and are associated with the degradation of biopolymers [58,59]. This indicates that CYP promoted the proliferation of polysaccharide-degrading bacteria and facilitated the intestinal de-utilization of polysaccharides. *Bacteroidaceae, Bacteroides,* and *Pasteurella* became SCYP biomarkers. *Bacteroidaceae* was the dominant bacterial family, indicating that SCYP promoted the proliferation of polysaccharide-utilizing bacteria. *Pasteurella* appeared somewhat anomalously, as was the case in a cactus polysaccharide study in which *Pasteurella* became the dominant bacterium in the polysaccharide group [60].

Substrate specificity is a key facet of the microbial response to complex carbohydrates. Thus, polysaccharides with different structures will be fermented with different kinds of microbiota, resulting in a new component of the gut microbiota. The present study revealed that the two polysaccharides selectively modulated the composition of the gut microbiota, among which SCYP produced different regulatory effects on the gut microbiota and exerted different anti-inflammatory effects from those of CYP, possibly because of its higher number of sulfate groups, higher galactose content, and larger Mw [25]. The effect of the intestinal flora was mediated via the gut–liver axis, where SCYP had a better prophylactic and anti-inflammatory effect than CYP, probably because SCYP was better able to indirectly act on the hepatic receptors to produce a response. The intestinal flora results showed that, overall, CYP was more able than SCYP to promote beneficial bacteria to become the dominant bacteria, a result consistent with the better effect of CYP on alleviating inflammation in the blood circulation. Our previous study showed that sulfation modification could enhance the immunomodulatory activity of yam polysaccharides [19,25], and this present study has shown that sulfation modification can improve the anti-inflammatory activity of yam polysaccharides in certain organs, supporting the notion that chemical modification has different effects on different biological activities. To clarify the differential effects of CYP and SCYP, further research on the anti-inflammatory molecular mechanisms of both should be studied.

5. Conclusions

The present study has demonstrated that sulfated yam polysaccharide has preventive alleviating effects on LPS-induced systemic acute inflammation, including the restoration of body weight and organ index and the reduction of inflammatory factors (TNF-α, IL-6, and IL-1β) released in the blood and liver, which may be associated with maintaining normal intestinal flora and reversing intestinal flora imbalance. CYP and SCYP reduced pathogenic bacteria; CYP increased *Prevotella*, and SCYP increased *Coprococcus*. CYP and SCYP have different effects on the regulation of the intestinal flora and have different advantageous anti-inflammatory effects on different organ systems, which can be attributed to the changes in molecular structure after sulfated modification. This study also showed that both polysaccharides, as natural and modified active substances, can be expected to improve the health of the body when used as prebiotics, and that they may also have the potential to be used as prophylactic agents for the treatment of inflammatory diseases. The molecular mechanisms involved in the sulfated yam polysaccharides can be further researched.

Author Contributions: Conceptualization, S.W.; data curation, S.W.; formal analysis, S.W and R.C.; funding acquisition, M.S. and J.X.; investigation, S.W., X.C. (Xianxiang Chen), R.C., J.Z., X.C. (Xiaodie Chen), M.S. and J.X.; methodology, J.Z. and S.W.; project administration, J.X. and M.S.; supervision, M.S.; validation, X.C. (Xiaodie Chen); visualization, X.C. (Xianxiang Chen); writing—original draft preparation, S.W. and X.C. (Xianxiang Chen); writing—review and editing, M.S. and J.X. All authors have read and agreed to the published version of the manuscript.

Funding: This research work was financially supported by the National Natural Science Foundation of China (81960708) and the Program for Talents in Scientific and Technological Innovation in Jiangxi Province (jxsq2019201092).

Data Availability Statement: The datasets generated for this study are available on request to the corresponding author.

Conflicts of Interest: The authors declare no conflict of interest.

References

1. Furman, D.; Campisi, J.; Verdin, E.; Carrera-Bastos, P.; Targ, S.; Franceschi, C.; Ferrucci, L.; Gilroy, D.W.; Fasano, A.; Miller, G.W.; et al. Chronic inflammation in the etiology of disease across the life span. *Nat. Med.* **2019**, *25*, 1822–1832. [CrossRef] [PubMed]
2. Hotchkiss, R.S.; Monneret, G.; Payen, D. Sepsis-induced immunosuppression: From cellular dysfunctions to immunotherapy. *Nat. Rev. Immunol.* **2013**, *13*, 862–874. [CrossRef] [PubMed]
3. Medzhitov, R. The spectrum of inflammatory responses. *Science* **2021**, *374*, 1070–1075. [CrossRef] [PubMed]
4. Page, M.J.; Kell, D.B.; Pretorius, E. The Role of Lipopolysaccharide-Induced Cell Signalling in Chronic Inflammation. *Chronic Stress* **2022**, *6*, 24705470221076390. [CrossRef] [PubMed]
5. Fujishima, S. Organ dysfunction as a new standard for defining sepsis. *Inflamm. Regen.* **2016**, *36*, 24. [CrossRef]
6. Xie, L.; Shen, M.; Hong, Y.; Ye, H.; Huang, L.; Xie, J. Chemical modifications of polysaccharides and their anti-tumor activities. *Carbohydr. Polym.* **2020**, *229*, 115436. [CrossRef]
7. Guru, P.R.; Kar, R.K.; Nayak, A.K.; Mohapatra, S. A comprehensive review on pharmaceutical uses of plant-derived biopolysaccharides. *Int. J. Biol. Macromol.* **2023**, *233*, 123454. [CrossRef]
8. Kuang, S.D.; Liu, L.M.; Hu, Z.R.; Luo, M.; Fu, X.Y.; Lin, C.X.; He, Q.H. A review focusing on the benefits of plant-derived polysaccharides for osteoarthritis. *Int. J. Biol. Macromol.* **2023**, *228*, 582–593. [CrossRef]
9. Yu, Y.; Shen, M.; Song, Q.; Xie, J. Biological activities and pharmaceutical applications of polysaccharide from natural resources: A review. *Carbohydr. Polym.* **2018**, *183*, 91–101. [CrossRef]
10. Wang, Z.; Xie, J.; Shen, M.; Nie, S.; Xie, M. Sulfated modification of polysaccharides: Synthesis, characterization and bioactivities. *Trends Food Sci. Technol.* **2018**, *74*, 147–157. [CrossRef]
11. Phimolsiripol, Y.; Seesuriyachan, P. Polysaccharides as active ingredients, nutraceuticals and functional foods. *Int. J. Food Sci. Technol.* **2021**, *57*, 1–3. [CrossRef]
12. Ma, F.; Zhang, Y.; Liu, N.; Zhang, J.; Tan, G.; Kannan, B.; Liu, X.; Bell, A.E. Rheological properties of polysaccharides from Dioscorea opposita Thunb. *Food Chem.* **2017**, *227*, 64–72. [CrossRef]
13. Huang, R.; Xie, J.; Yu, Y.; Shen, M. Recent progress in the research of yam mucilage polysaccharides: Isolation, structure and bioactivities. *Int. J. Biol. Macromol.* **2020**, *155*, 1262–1269. [CrossRef]
14. Lu, Y.; Wang, D.; Hu, Y.; Huang, X.; Wang, J. Sulfated modification of epimedium polysaccharide and effects of the modifiers on cellular infectivity of IBDV. *Carbohydr. Polym.* **2008**, *71*, 180–186. [CrossRef]
15. Kazachenko, A.S.; Vasilieva, N.Y.; Malyar, Y.N.; Karacharov, A.A.; Kondrasenko, A.A.; Levdanskiy, A.V.; Borovkova, V.S.; Miroshnikova, A.V.; Issaoui, N.; Kazachenko, A.S.; et al. Sulfation of arabinogalactan with ammonium sulfamate. *Biomass Convers. Biorefinery* **2022**. [CrossRef]
16. Li, S.; Li, J.; Zhi, Z.; Wei, C.; Wang, W.; Ding, T.; Ye, X.; Hu, Y.; Linhardt, R.J.; Chen, S. Macromolecular properties and hypolipidemic effects of four sulfated polysaccharides from sea cucumbers. *Carbohydr. Polym.* **2017**, *173*, 330–337. [CrossRef]
17. Yoshida, O.; Nakashima, H.; Yoshida, T.; Kaneko, Y.; Yamamoto, I.; Matsuzaki, K.; Uryu, T.; Yamamoto, N. Sulfation of the immunomodulating polysaccharide lentinan: A novel strategy for antivirals to human immunodeficiency virus (HIV). *Biochem. Pharmacol.* **1988**, *37*, 2887–2891. [CrossRef]
18. Xie, J.-H.; Wang, Z.-J.; Shen, M.-Y.; Nie, S.-P.; Gong, B.; Li, H.-S.; Zhao, Q.; Li, W.-J.; Xie, M.-Y. Sulfated modification, characterization and antioxidant activities of polysaccharide from Cyclocarya paliurus. *Food Hydrocoll.* **2016**, *53*, 7–15. [CrossRef]
19. Huang, R.; Shen, M.; Yu, Y.; Liu, X.; Xie, J. Physicochemical characterization and immunomodulatory activity of sulfated Chinese yam polysaccharide. *Int. J. Biol. Macromol.* **2020**, *165 Pt A*, 635–644. [CrossRef]
20. Fernández, J.; Redondo-Blanco, S.; Gutiérrez-del-Río, I.; Miguélez, E.M.; Villar, C.J.; Lombó, F. Colon microbiota fermentation of dietary prebiotics towards short-chain fatty acids and their roles as anti-inflammatory and antitumour agents: A review. *J. Funct. Foods* **2016**, *25*, 511–522. [CrossRef]
21. Flint, H.J.; Scott, K.P.; Duncan, S.H.; Louis, P.; Forano, E. Microbial degradation of complex carbohydrates in the gut. *Gut Microbes* **2012**, *3*, 289–306. [CrossRef] [PubMed]
22. Milosevic, I.; Vujovic, A.; Barac, A.; Djelic, M.; Korac, M.; Radovanovic Spurnic, A.; Gmizic, I.; Stevanovic, O.; Djordjevic, V.; Lekic, N.; et al. Gut-Liver Axis, Gut Microbiota, and Its Modulation in the Management of Liver Diseases: A Review of the Literature. *Int. J. Mol. Sci.* **2019**, *20*, 395. [CrossRef] [PubMed]
23. Al Bander, Z.; Nitert, M.D.; Mousa, A.; Naderpoor, N. The Gut Microbiota and Inflammation: An Overview. *Int. J. Environ. Res. Public Health* **2020**, *17*, 7618. [CrossRef] [PubMed]
24. Hakansson, A.; Molin, G. Gut microbiota and inflammation. *Nutrients* **2011**, *3*, 637–682. [CrossRef] [PubMed]
25. Liu, X.; Chen, X.; Xie, L.; Xie, J.; Shen, M. Sulfated Chinese yam polysaccharide enhances the immunomodulatory activity of RAW 264.7 cells via the TLR4-MAPK/NF-kappaB signaling pathway. *Food Funct.* **2022**, *13*, 1316–1326. [CrossRef]
26. Zhang, X.; Zhang, L.; Zhang, H.; Cai, Z.; Wang, P. Optimization Extraction of Crassostrea gigas Polysaccharides and its Antioxidant Activity and Hepatoprotective Against BCG-LPS-Induced Hepatic Injury in Mice. *J. Food Process. Preserv.* **2016**, *40*, 1391–1399. [CrossRef]

27. Sarraf, P.; Frederich, R.; Turner, E. Multiple Cytokines and Acute Inflammation Raise Mouse Leptin Levels Potential Role in Inflammatory Anorexia. *J. Exp. Med.* **1997**, *185*, 171–175. [CrossRef]
28. Deng, D.; Tan, H.; Shangguan, Y.; Wu, D.; Geng, L.; Liu, G.; Chen, J. Effects of pinecone of Pinus yunnanensis on inflammation and oxidative stress of rats with LPS-induced acute lung injury. *Chin. Tradit. Pat. Med.* **2021**, *43*, 1721–1726.
29. Wang, Z.; Xie, J.; Yang, Y.; Zhang, F.; Wang, S.; Wu, T.; Shen, M.; Xie, M. Sulfated Cyclocarya paliurus polysaccharides markedly attenuates inflammation and oxidative damage in lipopolysaccharide-treated macrophage cells and mice. *Sci. Rep.* **2017**, *7*, 40402. [CrossRef]
30. Guo, W.; Xiang, Q.; Mao, B.; Tang, X.; Cui, S.; Li, X.; Zhao, J.; Zhang, H.; Chen, W. Protective Effects of Microbiome-Derived Inosine on Lipopolysaccharide-Induced Acute Liver Damage and Inflammation in Mice via Mediating the TLR4/NF-kappaB Pathway. *J. Agric. Food Chem.* **2021**, *69*, 7619–7628. [CrossRef]
31. Fajgenbaum, D.C.; June, C.H. Cytokine Storm. *N. Engl. J. Med.* **2020**, *383*, 2255–2273. [CrossRef]
32. Zelova, H.; Hosek, J. TNF-alpha signalling and inflammation: Interactions between old acquaintances. *Inflamm. Res.* **2013**, *62*, 641–651. [CrossRef]
33. Taniguchi, K.; Karin, M. IL-6 and related cytokines as the critical lynchpins between inflammation and cancer. *Semin. Immunol.* **2014**, *26*, 54–74. [CrossRef]
34. Szabo, G.; Petrasek, J. Inflammasome activation and function in liver disease. *Nat. Rev. Gastroenterol. Hepatol.* **2015**, *12*, 387–400. [CrossRef]
35. Lim, J.Y.; Lee, J.H.; Yun, D.H.; Lee, Y.M.; Kim, D.K. Inhibitory effects of nodakenin on inflammation and cell death in lipopolysaccharide-induced liver injury mice. *Phytomedicine* **2021**, *81*, 153411. [CrossRef]
36. Ge, Y.; Huang, M.; Yao, Y.M. Recent advances in the biology of IL-1 family cytokines and their potential roles in development of sepsis. *Cytokine Growth Factor Rev.* **2019**, *45*, 24–34. [CrossRef]
37. Nepali, S.; Ki, H.H.; Lee, J.H.; Lee, H.Y.; Kim, D.K.; Lee, Y.M. Wheatgrass-Derived Polysaccharide Has Antiinflammatory, Anti-Oxidative and Anti-Apoptotic Effects on LPS-Induced Hepatic Injury in Mice. *Phytother. Res.* **2017**, *31*, 1107–1116. [CrossRef]
38. Ren, K.; Torres, R. Role of interleukin-1beta during pain and inflammation. *Brain Res. Rev.* **2009**, *60*, 57–64. [CrossRef]
39. Kong, Y.; Yan, T.; Tong, Y.; Deng, H.; Tan, C.; Wan, M.; Wang, M.; Meng, X.; Wang, Y. Gut Microbiota Modulation by Polyphenols from Aronia melanocarpa of LPS-Induced Liver Diseases in Rats. *J. Agric. Food Chem.* **2021**, *69*, 3312–3325. [CrossRef]
40. Yu, Y.; Zhu, H.; Shen, M.; Yu, Q.; Chen, Y.; Xie, J. Sulfation modification enhances the intestinal regulation of Cyclocarya paliurus polysaccharides in cyclophosphamide-treated mice via restoring intestinal mucosal barrier function and modulating gut microbiota. *Food Funct.* **2021**, *12*, 12278–12290. [CrossRef]
41. Wang, P.; Feng, Z.; Sang, X.; Chen, W.; Zhang, X.; Xiao, J.; Chen, Y.; Chen, Q.; Yang, M.; Su, J. Kombucha ameliorates LPS-induced sepsis in a mouse model. *Food Funct.* **2021**, *12*, 10263–10280. [CrossRef] [PubMed]
42. Wang, Y.; Lin, J.; Cheng, Z.; Wang, T.; Chen, J.; Long, M. Bacillus coagulans TL3 Inhibits LPS-Induced Caecum Damage in Rat by Regulating the TLR4/MyD88/NF-kappaB and Nrf2 Signal Pathways and Modulating Intestinal Microflora. *Oxid. Med. Cell. Longev.* **2022**, *2022*, 5463290. [PubMed]
43. Sansonetti, P.J. Rupture, invasion and inflammatory destruction of the intestinal barrier by Shigella: The yin and yang of innate immunity. *Can. J. Infect. Dis. Med. Microbiol.* **2006**, *17*, 117–119. [CrossRef] [PubMed]
44. Zhu, Z.; Huang, R.; Huang, A.; Wang, J.; Liu, W.; Wu, S.; Chen, M.; Chen, M.; Xie, Y.; Jiao, C.; et al. Polysaccharide from Agrocybe cylindracea prevents diet-induced obesity through inhibiting inflammation mediated by gut microbiota and associated metabolites. *Int. J. Biol. Macromol.* **2022**, *209 Pt A*, 1430–1438. [CrossRef]
45. Wang, R.; Wang, L.; Wu, H.; Zhang, L.; Hu, X.; Li, C.; Liu, S. Noni (*Morinda citrifolia* L.) fruit phenolic extract supplementation ameliorates NAFLD by modulating insulin resistance, oxidative stress, inflammation, liver metabolism and gut microbiota. *Food Res. Int.* **2022**, *160*, 111732. [CrossRef]
46. Zhao, Z.; Chen, L.; Zhao, Y.; Wang, C.; Duan, C.; Yang, G.; Niu, C.; Li, S. Lactobacillus plantarum NA136 ameliorates nonalcoholic fatty liver disease by modulating gut microbiota, improving intestinal barrier integrity, and attenuating inflammation. *Appl. Microbiol. Biotechnol.* **2020**, *104*, 5273–5282. [CrossRef]
47. Xiao, Q.; Shu, R.; Wu, C.; Tong, Y.; Xiong, Z.; Zhou, J.; Yu, C.; Xie, X.; Fu, Z. Crocin-I alleviates the depression-like behaviors probably via modulating "microbiota-gut-brain" axis in mice exposed to chronic restraint stress. *J. Affect. Disord.* **2020**, *276*, 476–486. [CrossRef]
48. Sen, T.; Cawthon, C.R.; Ihde, B.T.; Hajnal, A.; DiLorenzo, P.M.; de La Serre, C.B.; Czaja, K. Diet-driven microbiota dysbiosis is associated with vagal remodeling and obesity. *Physiol. Behav.* **2017**, *173*, 305–317. [CrossRef]
49. Hiippala, K.; Kainulainen, V.; Kalliomaki, M.; Arkkila, P.; Satokari, R. Mucosal Prevalence and Interactions with the Epithelium Indicate Commensalism of Sutterella spp. *Front. Microbiol.* **2016**, *7*, 1706. [CrossRef]
50. Xie, M.G.; Fei, Y.Q.; Wang, Y.; Wang, W.Y.; Wang, Z. Chlorogenic Acid Alleviates Colon Mucosal Damage Induced by a High-Fat Diet via Gut Microflora Adjustment to Increase Short-Chain Fatty Acid Accumulation in Rats. *Oxid. Med. Cell. Longev.* **2021**, *2021*, 3456542. [CrossRef]
51. Wang, X.; Xiao, K.; Yu, C.; Wang, L.; Liang, T.; Zhu, H.; Xu, X.; Liu, Y. Xylooligosaccharide attenuates lipopolysaccharide-induced intestinal injury in piglets via suppressing inflammation and modulating cecal microbial communities. *Anim. Nutr.* **2021**, *7*, 609–620. [CrossRef]

52. Galvez, E.J.C.; Iljazovic, A.; Amend, L.; Lesker, T.R.; Renault, T.; Thiemann, S.; Hao, L.; Roy, U.; Gronow, A.; Charpentier, E.; et al. Distinct Polysaccharide Utilization Determines Interspecies Competition between Intestinal Prevotella spp. *Cell Host Microbe* **2020**, *28*, 838–852.e6. [CrossRef]
53. Precup, G.; Vodnar, D.C. Gut Prevotella as a possible biomarker of diet and its eubiotic versus dysbiotic roles: A comprehensive literature review. *Br. J. Nutr.* **2019**, *122*, 131–140. [CrossRef]
54. Yuan, D.; Li, C.; You, L.; Dong, H.; Fu, X. Changes of digestive and fermentation properties of Sargassum pallidum polysaccharide after ultrasonic degradation and its impacts on gut microbiota. *Int. J. Biol. Macromol.* **2020**, *164*, 1443–1450. [CrossRef]
55. Zhang, H.; Jiang, F.; Zhang, J.; Wang, W.; Li, L.; Yan, J. Modulatory effects of polysaccharides from plants, marine algae and edible mushrooms on gut microbiota and related health benefits: A review. *Int. J. Biol. Macromol.* **2022**, *204*, 169–192. [CrossRef]
56. Cui, M.; Zhang, M.; Wu, J.; Han, P.; Lv, M.; Dong, L.; Liu, K. Marine polysaccharides from Gelidium pacificum Okamura and Cereus sinensis reveal prebiotic functions. *Int. J. Biol. Macromol.* **2020**, *164*, 4381–4390. [CrossRef]
57. Zhang, D.; Liu, J.; Cheng, H.; Wang, H.; Tan, Y.; Feng, W.; Peng, C. Interactions between polysaccharides and gut microbiota: A metabolomic and microbial review. *Food Res. Int.* **2022**, *160*, 111653. [CrossRef]
58. Ye, M.; Yu, J.; Shi, X.; Zhu, J.; Gao, X.; Liu, W. Polysaccharides catabolism by the human gut bacterium -Bacteroides thetaiotaomicron: Advances and perspectives. *Crit. Rev. Food Sci. Nutr.* **2021**, *61*, 3569–3588. [CrossRef]
59. Flint, H.J. Polysaccharide breakdown by anaerobic microorganisms inhabiting the mammalian gut. *Adv. Appl. Microbiol.* **2004**, *56*, 89–120.
60. Liu, Z.; Zhang, J.; Zhao, Q.; Wen, A.; Li, L.; Zhang, Y. The regulating effect of Tibet Opuntia ficus-indica (Linn.) Mill. polysaccharides on the intestinal flora of cyclophosphamide-induced immunocompromised mice. *Int. J. Biol. Macromol.* **2022**, *207*, 570–579. [CrossRef]

Disclaimer/Publisher's Note: The statements, opinions and data contained in all publications are solely those of the individual author(s) and contributor(s) and not of MDPI and/or the editor(s). MDPI and/or the editor(s) disclaim responsibility for any injury to people or property resulting from any ideas, methods, instructions or products referred to in the content.

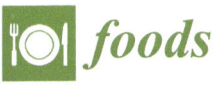

Article

Effects of Soybean Trypsin Inhibitor on Pancreatic Oxidative Damage of Mice at Different Growth Periods

Chunmei Gu [1,2,†], Qiuping Yang [2,3,†], Shujun Li [4], Linlin Zhao [1,5], Bo Lyu [1,2], Yingnan Wang [3,*] and Hansong Yu [1,2,*]

[1] College of Food Science and Engineering, Jilin Agricultural University, Changchun 130118, China; jjnong2008@126.com (C.G.); zhaoll89@163.com (L.Z.); michael_lvbo@163.com (B.L.)
[2] Division of Soybean Processing, Soybean Research & Development Center, Chinese Agricultural Research System, Changchun 130000, China; virginiay@163.com
[3] Heilongjiang Green Food Science Research Institute, Northeast Agricultural University, Harbin 150030, China
[4] Department of Agriculture and Resources Environment, Qinghai Higher Vocational and Technical College, Haidong 810799, China; lishujun1026@163.com
[5] College of Tourism and Culinary Science, College of Food Science and Engineering, Yangzhou University, Yangzhou 225127, China
* Correspondence: wynan@neau.edu.cn (Y.W.); yuhansong@jlau.edu.cn (H.Y.)
† These authors contributed equally to this work.

Abstract: The bioactive components in soybeans have significant physiological functions. However, the intake of soybean trypsin inhibitor (STI) may cause metabolic disorders. To investigate the effect of STI intake on pancreatic injury and its mechanism of action, a five-week animal experiment was conducted, meanwhile, a weekly monitor on the degree of oxidation and antioxidant indexes in the serum and pancreas of the animals was carried out. The results showed that the intake of STI had irreversible damage to the pancreas, according to the analysis of the histological section. Malondialdehyde (MDA) in the pancreatic mitochondria of Group STI increased significantly and reached a maximum (15.7 nmol/mg prot) in the third week. Meanwhile, the antioxidant enzymes superoxide dismutase (SOD), glutathione peroxidase (GSH-Px), trypsin (TPS), and somatostatin (SST) were decreased and reached minimum values (10 U/mg prot, 87 U/mg prot, 2.1 U/mg prot, 10 pg/mg prot) compared with the Group Control. The RT-PCR results of the expression of SOD, GSH-Px, TPS, and SST genes were consistent with the above. This study demonstrates that STI causes oxidative structural damage and pancreatic dysfunction by inducing oxidative stress in the pancreas, which could increase with time.

Keywords: soybean trypsin inhibitor; pancreas; oxidative damage; genetic expression

1. Introduction

The anti-nutritional factors in soybeans can inhibit the growth of animals by interfering with digestion, absorption, and utilization of nutrients [1,2], which limits the application of soybeans in foodstuff and animal feeding because of the necessity of heat treatment and temperature control in this process. As one of the main soybean anti-nutritional factors, soybean trypsin inhibitors (STI) is a polypeptide composed of 72–197 amino acid residues [2], which may cause some physiological reactions, such as pancreatic hypertrophy and even pancreatic cancer [3,4]. The ingestion of diets containing STI by animals can result in the formation of a complex between trypsin and chymotrypsin with the STI in the intestinal tract. This complex can then be excreted, leading to a reduction in enzyme activity. Consequently, the pancreas may attempt to compensate for the reduced enzyme activity by increasing its secretion and synthesis of trypsin [4,5]. In addition, the synthesis of DNA, mRNA, and enzymes require ATP for purine and pyrimidine synthesis, as well as the activation of amino acids. However, the production of ATP also generates free

radicals. Similarly, a large amount of ATP is required by the STI-stimulated pancreas for trypsin synthesis. As a result, consuming STIs may also result in elevated levels of oxygen free radicals.

The excess free radicals, regardless of whether they are generated by the mitochondrial respiratory chain or NAD(p)H, can cause oxidative stress, which has a direct impact on cells. This can result in cell damage and eventually various diseases [6–9], such as cardiovascular diseases, cancer, neurological disorders, diabetes, ischemia/reperfusion, and aging [10–17], which is also one of the risks of STI intake. In vivo, Vitamin C (VC) can react with oxygen free radicals through redox reactions, thereby neutralizing them and safeguarding the body against their damaging effects. Therefore, VC is widely recognized as an antioxidant that can effectively prevent oxidative damage to the pancreas.

While STIs were initially developed as drugs, their potential side effects on the body from daily consumption were not thoroughly understood. This study was conducted to examine the impact of STI consumption on the pancreas, including its effects on pancreatic structure, function, and gene expression in mice with varying growth cycles. Additionally, it investigated the effects of STI on free radical levels during different stages of growth and the degree of oxidative damage to the mouse pancreas, which the potential mechanism was studied, and explored whether the intake of antioxidants can reduce pancreatic oxidative damage. This work offered a theoretical foundation for identifying endogenous strategies to prevent pancreatic injury resulting from the intake of STIs.

2. Material and Methods

2.1. Main Reagents and Reasons for Selection

Soybean trypsin inhibitors (STI), the most common enzyme inhibitors in soybeans, are the most significantly damaging to the pancreas by their ingestion. Additionally, as a strong antioxidant, Vitamin C (VC) has a theoretical potential to mitigate oxidative damage to the pancreas. Therefore, both were chosen to conduct this study.

STI, in which the activity was identified as 4600 BAEE U/mg, was provided by the College of Food Science and Engineering, Jilin Agricultural University. Vitamin C (Ascorbic acid, A8100) was provided by Beijing Solarbio Science & Technology Co., Ltd. (Beijing, China).

2.2. Animals and Diets

Four- to six-week-old KM male mice were purchased from Changchun Yisi Experimental Animal Technology Co., Ltd. (Changchun, China). All animals were housed under a controlled condition in individual cages at 23 ± 2 °C and $50 \pm 10\%$ relative humidity with a 12 h light/dark cycle in a specific pathogen-free environment and were allowed free access to food and water.

After one week of acclimatization, the mice were divided into three groups randomly: the control group (control diet, $n = 10$), Group STI (control diet containing 2.0 mg/g STI, $n = 10$), Group STI + VC (STI diet supplemented with 1500 mg/kg VC, $n = 10$). A total of five intergroup parallels were set up for each group for the weekly sacrifice of animals (Total: 150 mice). All the mice were sacrificed after a 5-week feeding. All the animal experiments were approved by the Institutional Animal Care and Use Committees of Jilin Agricultural University (Protocol code No.20130530001, May 2013), following the National Research Council Guidelines. The composition of the control diet is shown in Table 1.

Table 1. Composition of the control diet [a].

	Ingredient	Diet (g/kg)
Protein	Casein	200
Carbohydrates	Corn starch	660
Fat	Soybean oil (without STI)	50
Fiber	Cellulose powder	30
Others	Mineral mixture [b]	50
	Vitamin mixture [c]	10

Note: The control group chow diet in pellet form (standard chow diet) was provided by the Changchun Yisi Experimental Animal Technology Co., Ltd., Jilin, China. The chow diets of the STI group and the STI + VC group were prepared by adding STI (2.0 mg/g) and VC (1500 mg/kg) into the standard chow diet, respectively, and then pelleted (prepared by the Agricultural Products Processing and Storage Engineering Laboratory of Jilin Agricultural University). [a] The diets were semi-purified (added mineral and vitamin complex additives), and isoenergetic was calculated according to China national standard GB14924.1-2001 (group I 16.3 MJ/kg, group II 15.7 MJ/kg, group III 15.5 MJ/kg). [b] The mineral mixture provides the following amounts (g/kg diet): Ca, 4; K, 2.4; Na, 1.6; Mg, 0.4; Fe, 0.12; trace elements (mg/kg diet): Mn, 32; Cu, 5; Zn, 18; Co, 0.04; I, 0.02. [c] The vitamin mixture provides the following amounts (mg/kg diet): retinol, 12; cholecalciferol, 0.125; thiamin, 40; riboflavin, 30; pantothenic acid, 140; pyridoxine, 20; inositol, 300; cyanobalamine, 0.1; ascorbic acid, 1600; (dL) α-tocopherol, 340; menadione, 80; nicotinic acid, 200; para-aminobenzoic acid, 100; folic acid, 10; biotin, 0.6; choline, 2720.

2.3. Sample Preparation

At the end of each week, the mice that were to be sacrificed were fasted for 12 h but had free access to deionized water. Blood was obtained from the eyeballs of mice and centrifuged at $4000 \times g$ for 3 min at 4 °C using a high-speed desktop refrigerated centrifuge (TGL-16G, Shanghai Anting Scientific Instrument Factory, Shanghai, China), and serum was separated and stored at −20 °C for a maximum of 16 weeks. Then mice were sacrificed by decapitation, and the pancreas was quickly removed, gently rinsed in ice-cold PBS (Wuhan Punuosai Life Technology Co., Ltd., Wuhan, China), and cut into 50–100 mg/100 g body weight, frozen in liquid nitrogen and stored at −80 °C for the follow-up experiments. After thawing at 4 °C, tissue samples were homogenized using a MagNALyser instrument (Roche Diagnostics, Mannheim, Germany) at $4000 \times g$ for 50 s twice, and then diluted with 9 volumes ice-cold 0.9% NaCl solution, then centrifuged at $4000 \times g$ for 15 min at 4 °C. Functional compounds, oxidative, and antioxidant activity were analyzed using the supernatants collected from the samples. All operations were done at 4 °C. Protein content was measured using the method of Lowry (Lowry et al., 1951) with bovine serum albumin as a standard, assuming it to be 100% pure. Protein content was expressed as BSA equivalents.

2.4. Analytical Methods

2.4.1. Determination of Oxidation and Antioxidant Parameters

The malondialdehyde (MDA) content was measured using the TBA reaction method of Koca et al. [18]. After the preparation, according to the kit used (A003-1-1, Nanjing Jiancheng Bioengineering Institute, Nanjing, China), samples were incubated in a 95 °C water bath for 40 min and centrifuged at $3500 \times g$ for 10 min. The absorbance of the supernatant was measured with a double beam UV-Vis spectrophotometer (T6 New Century, Beijing General Instrument Co., Ltd., Beijing, China) at 532 nm, which was attributed so that the MDA could be condensed with TBA to form a red product with the maximum absorption peak at 532 nm. Results were expressed as units nmol/mg of protein for pancreas samples, and nmol/mL for serum samples. The activity of superoxide dismutase (SOD) was measured using the method of Beauchamp & Fridovich [19]. The samples were prepared according to the instructions of the kit (A001-1-1, Nanjing Jiancheng Bioengineering Institute, Nanjing, China) and then placed in a water bath at 37 °C for 40 min. In the process, $O_2^-·$ was produced by the reaction system of xanthine and xanthine oxidase and could oxidize hydroxylamine to form nitrite. Under the action of a chromogenic agent, nitrite could appear purple-red and have a maximum absorption peak at 550 nm, and results were expressed as units U/mg of protein for pancreas samples and U/mL for serum samples. Glutathione peroxidase (GSH-Px) activity was measured according to the method of Sabuncu et al. [20], and results were shown as units U/mg of protein for pancreas samples and U/mL for serum samples.

2.4.2. Determination of Trypsin Activity and Hormone Levels

The trypsin (TPS) activities in serum and tissue samples were assayed at 410 nm using the substrate N-benzoyl-DL-arginine p-nitroaniline hydrochloride (BAPNA) (A080-2-2, Nanjing Jiancheng Bioengineering Institute, Nanjing, Jiangsu, China) according to the manufacturer's instructions [21]. TPS could react with BAPNA to release p-nitroaniline with a maximum absorption peak at 410 nm. Somatostatin (SST) of serum samples and pancreas tissue samples were measured using a radio-immunoassay method (bs-1132R, Anti-Somatostatin/GR, Beijing Huaying Bioengineering Institute, Beijing, China) [22]. The specific antibodies were bound to a solid-phase carrier to form a solid-phase antibody and then combined with the corresponding antigen in the samples to form an immune complex. Then the enzyme-labeled antibody was bound to the antigen in the immune complex to form an enzyme-labeled antibody-antigen-solid phase antibody complex. This complex could be colored by adding a substrate and was with a maximum absorption peak of 450 nm.

2.4.3. Transmission Electron Microscopy (TEM) of the Pancreas

Pancreas tissues that had been fixed with 2.5% glutaraldehyde (Sigma Aldrich Co., St. Louis, MO, USA) were removed from the glutaraldehyde and treated as follows: Samples were post-fixed with 1% osmic acid at 4 °C for 2 h, dehydrated with gradient concentrations of acetone (once with 50%, 70%, and 90% acetone and three times with 100% acetone for 15 min each), and embedded in Epon812 (Beijing Zhongjing Keyi Technology Co., Ltd., Beijing, China) at room temperature (22–25 °C) overnight. The samples were sliced into 5 μm sections with a rotary microtome (Leica Microsystems (Shanghai) Trading Co., Ltd., Shanghai, China), counterstained with 2% (w/v) uranyl acetate and lead citrate (SPI-CHEM, West Chester, PA, USA), and then observed using TEM at 80 kV and a magnification of 12,000× (Hitachi High-tech (Shanghai) International Trade Co., Ltd., Shanghai, China).

2.4.4. RNA Extraction and Real-Time PCR

Total RNA was obtained from the pancreas samples using an RNeasy Minikit (Qiagen, Hilden, Germany). The pancreas sample was fully ground, then 20 mg was taken out, 350 μL of lysate was added, and RNA extraction was performed according to the instructions of the kit and resuspended in 50 μL RNase-free water (included with the kit). Synthesis of cDNA was primed by oligo d (T) using a PrimeScript RT Enzyme (Takara, Beijing, China) according to the Power SYBR Green PCR Master Mix (Life Technologies, Beijing, China) instructions. The primers were synthesized by Shanghai Biological Engineering Design Services Ltd. (Shanghai, China). The reaction system for the synthesis of the first strand of cDNA was 5× PrimeScript buffer 4 μL, Template RNA 1 μL, PrimeScript RT Enzyme Mix I 1 μL, Oligo dT primer 1 μL, RNase-free dH2O 12 μL, and Random 6 mers 1 μL, total reaction volume 20 μL. Before adding the reverse transcriptase, the mixed solution was first dried at 700 °C for 3 min. After taking it out, the temperature inside and outside the tube was the same, then reverse transcriptase was added, and the 37 °C water bath was used for 15 min. Immediately after it taking out, it was put in a dry bath at 85 °C for 5 s to obtain cDNA solution and stored at −80 °C until used. The reactions were done in a thermocycler StepOne™ Real-Time PCR System. The master mix prepared for analysis of each gene was composed of 0.5 μL forward primer, 0.5 μL reverse primer, 10 μL of 2× SYBR premix, and 1 μL cDNA in a total volume of 20 μL. Each sample was analyzed in triplicate. RT-PCR was done using the following conditions: reverse transcription at 50 °C for 2 min, PCR activation at 95 °C for 10 min followed by 40 cycles of denaturation at 95 °C for 15 s, annealing at 60 °C for 1 min, and a final extension at 72 °C for 10 min. β-Actin was the internal reference gene. Sequences of primers are shown in Table 2 (Designed by Shanghai Biotech Biotechnology Co., Ltd., Shanghai, China).

Table 2. The sequence of primers designed for the RT-PCR studies.

Gene Product	Primer Sequence	T (°C)	PCR (bp)
Glutathione Peroxidase (GSH-Px)	5′-TGGCATTGGCTTGGTGATTACTGG-3′(F) 5′-GGTGGAAAGGCATCGGGAATGG-3′(R)	59 60	150
Superoxide Dismutase (SOD)	5′-CCTTGTGACTGGCATCCCTTAGC-3′(F) 5′-AGGCAGACTGTTAGATGGCTTGTTC-3′(R)	58 59	105
Somatostatin (SST)	5′-CCTCTCCCATTCCTCCCTTTTGTTC-3′(F) 5′-GGGCATCATTCTCTGTCTGGTTGG-3′(R)	59 58	108
Somatostatin Receptor 5 (SSTR5)	5′-CGTCTGTGCTGGGCTTCTTTGG-3′(F) 5′-ATGCGAGTCACCTTGCGTTCTG-3′(R)	60 58	136
Trypsin (TPS)	5′-TCCTCATCTCTACCCACAACATTGC-3′(F) 5′-CACTTCCGAACCATAACCGTAGGC-3′(R)	60 58	96

2.5. Statistical Analysis

Data were reported as mean ± SD, $n = 10$ (per week). Differences between mean values were determined using a one-way ANOVA followed by comparisons using the Newman-Keuls multiple range test. Differences with $p < 0.05$ were considered significant. Statistical analyses were done using the Statistical Program for the Social Sciences, SPSS software (Version 22.0, SPSS Inc., Chicago, IL, USA).

3. Results

3.1. The Pancreas Index, Oxidative and Antioxidant Parameters in Serum and Pancreas of Mice

As shown in Table 3, the pancreas weight of the STI group and STI + VC group showed a trend of first increasing and then decreasing, as compared to the control group. However, due to significant individual differences, there was no significant difference except for the first week.

Table 3. Effect of different diets on the ratio of Pancreas/body weight in mice.

Treatment	1 Wk	2 Wk	3 Wk	4 Wk	5 Wk
Control	0.09 ± 0.01	0.09 ± 0.01	0.09 ± 0.02	0.09 ± 0.01	0.08 ± 0.01
STI	0.11 ± 0.01 *	0.10 ± 0.02	0.12 ± 0.02	0.11 ± 0.02	0.10 ± 0.01
STI + VC	0.10 ± 0.02	0.10 ± 0.01	0.11 ± 0.01	0.09 ± 0.02	0.09 ± 0.02

*: Represents the significant difference compared to the control group ($p < 0.05$, $n = 10$).

The levels of MDA in the serum and pancreas increased and subsequently decreased in both the STI and STI + VC groups, with the maximum levels observed during the 3rd week. (Table 4). Mice fed STI and STI + VC showed a significant increase ($p < 0.05$) in the serum MDA content compared with the control group in the first 4 weeks and showed no differences in the 5th week. The addition of VC caused a significant decrease ($p < 0.05$) of the MDA level in the serum than mice in the STI group, except in the 2nd and 5th weeks.

In the pancreas, it showed a significant increase ($p < 0.05$) in MDA content in the STI group and STI + VC group in comparison with those of the control mice, except in the 5th week. MDA content of the STI + VC group was significantly decreased ($p < 0.05$) when compared with those in the STI group in the 3rd, 4th, and 5th weeks.

Table 4. MDA content in serum and pancreas.

	Treatment	1 Wk	2 Wk	3 Wk	4 Wk	5 Wk
Serum (nmol/mL)	Control	2.5 ± 0.3	3.4 ± 0.2	3.8 ± 0.2	4.1 ± 0.2	4.5 ± 0.3
	STI	4.4 ± 0.2 *	4.7 ± 0.1 *	7.6 ± 0.2 *	5.6 ± 0.1 *	4.9 ± 0.1
	STI + VC	3.2 ± 0.1 #	4.6 ± 0.4 *	5.9 ± 0.2 #	4.6 ± 0.3 *	4.8 ± 0.1
Pancreas (nmol/mg prot)	Control	4.2 ± 0.2	4.9 ± 0.3	5.5 ± 0.3	7.4 ± 0.2	8.1 ± 0.3
	STI	6.3 ± 0.1 *	8.3 ± 0.2 *	15.7 ± 0.4 *	11.7 ± 0.4 *	9.6 ± 0.3 *
	STI + VC	6.1 ± 0.1 *	8.1 ± 0.2 *	13.7 ± 0.3 #	9.6 ± 0.4 #	8.6 ± 0.3

*: Represents the significant difference compared to the control group ($p < 0.05$, $n = 10$). #: Represents the significant difference compared to the STI group ($p < 0.05$, $n = 10$).

As shown in Tables 5 and 6, as the feeding periods increased, SOD and GSH-Px activities of the three groups in both the serum and pancreas decreased and then increased and, in the 3rd week, reached a minimum. Compared with the control animals during the whole time, mice fed STI and STI + VC showed a significant decrease ($p < 0.05$) in SOD and GSH-Px activities. Meanwhile, the activities of SOD and GSH-Px in the STI + VC group were significantly higher ($p < 0.05$) than those in the STI group for the majority of the time. Therefore, STI can significantly reduce the level of SOD and GSH-Px in mice, and STI + VC can slightly increase the level of SOD and GSH-Px compared with the STI group.

Table 5. SOD activity in serum and pancreas.

	Treatment	1 Wk	2 Wk	3 Wk	4 Wk	5 Wk
Serum (U/mL)	Control	174 ± 3.2	162 ± 4.5	135 ± 3.5	147 ± 3.8	117 ± 3.5
	STI	150 ± 2.8 *	120 ± 10 *	62 ± 1.8 *	83 ± 0.4 *	92 ± 1.9 *
	STI + VC	162 ± 1.1 #	133 ± 3.0 *	77 ± 1.7 #	94 ± 2.2 #	106 ± 4.0 #
Pancreas (U/mg prot)	Control	81 ± 4.7	68 ± 1.3	50 ± 1.0	39 ± 1.5	22 ± 1.8
	STI	49 ± 3.5 *	38 ± 2.8 *	10 ± 1.7 *	18 ± 0.3 *	16 ± 0.2 *
	STI + VC	55 ± 3.5 *	47 ± 1.3 #	18 ± 0.4 #	23 ± 1.2 #	18 ± 1.7 #

*: Represents the significant difference compared to the control group ($p < 0.05$, $n = 10$). #: Represents the significant difference compared to the STI group ($p < 0.05$, $n = 10$).

Table 6. GSH-Px activity in the serum and pancreas.

	Treatment	1 Wk	2 Wk	3 Wk	4 Wk	5 Wk
Serum (U/mL)	Control	693 ± 33	359 ± 28	260 ± 10	496 ± 35	1380 ± 30
	STI	481 ± 32 *	315 ± 57 *	165 ± 31 *	410 ± 10 *	577 ± 45 *
	STI + VC	540 ± 28 #	345 ± 41 #	240 ± 10 #	456 ± 44 #	640 ± 30 *
Pancreas (U/mg prot)	Control	287 ± 12	190 ± 10	180 ± 10	240 ± 10	384 ± 1.7
	STI	134 ± 14 *	96 ± 4.5 *	87 ± 4.8 *	108 ± 5.5 *	143 ± 4.5 *
	STI + VC	176 ± 20 #	143 ± 5.0 #	138 ± 5.0 #	180 ± 10 #	230 ± 10 #

*: Represents the significant difference compared to the control group ($p < 0.05$, $n = 10$). #: Represents the significant difference compared to the STI group ($p < 0.05$, $n = 10$).

3.2. Trypsin Activity and Hormone Levels

The activities of TPS are summarized in Table 7. As the time increased, the TPS activity of the STI group and STI + VC group in both the serum and pancreas decreased initially and then increased and, in 3rd week, reached a maximum. Mice fed STI and STI + VC showed significant decreases in TPS activity when compared with the control animals during the whole period. Whereas the TPS activity in the STI + VC group was significantly higher ($p < 0.05$) than those in the STI group in the majority of the whole periods.

Table 7. Change of TPS activity in serum and pancreas.

	Treatment	1 Wk	2 Wk	3 Wk	4 Wk	5 Wk
Serum (U/mL)	Control	84 ± 3	92 ± 3	95 ± 3	97 ± 1	98 ± 1
	STI	44 ± 3 *	39 ± 2 *	25 ± 2 *	35 ± 3 *	44 ± 2 *
	STI + VC	68 ± 5 #	62 ± 3 #	48 ± 5 #	63 ± 2 #	69 ± 1 #
Pancreas (U/mg prot)	Control	7.0 ± 0.1	7.8 ± 0.2	8.5 ± 0.3	9.1 ± 0.1	9.0 ± 0.2
	STI	3.5 ± 0.2 *	3.3 ± 0.2 *	2.1 ± 0.1 *	3.1 ± 0.1 *	3.6 ± 0.2 *
	STI + VC	5.2 ± 0.3 #	4.3 ± 0.1 #	3.7 ± 0.1 #	4.3 ± 0.1 #	5.2 ± 0.1 #

*: Represents the significant difference compared to the control group ($p < 0.05$, $n = 10$). #: Represents the significant difference compared to the STI group ($p < 0.05$, $n = 10$).

The contents of SST are summarized in Table 8. With the increase in feeding periods, the SST contents of three groups in both the serum and pancreas were decreased and then increased and, in the 3rd week, reached a minimum. Mice fed STI and STI + VC showed a significant decrease ($p < 0.05$) in SST content when compared with the control animals during the whole period except for that in the serum for the 2nd and 3rd week and the pancreas for the 3rd week. Meanwhile, the SST content in the STI + VC group was higher ($p < 0.05$) than that in the STI group for the majority of the whole period.

Table 8. Change of SST levels in serum and pancreas.

	Treatment	1 Wk	2 Wk	3 Wk	4 Wk	5 Wk
Serum (pg/mL)	Control	50 ± 10	20 ± 5.7	20 ± 10	45 ± 4.3	50 ± 10
	STI	27 ± 3.5 *	16 ± 4.2	14 ± 0.3	19 ± 3.7 *	23 ± 2.8 *
	STI + VC	30 ± 10 *	21 ± 5.1	16 ± 5.6	30 ± 10 *	30 ± 10 *
Pancreas (pg/mg prot)	Control	29 ± 1.2	25 ± 1.5	12 ± 0.4	29 ± 2.0	98 ± 1.7
	STI	21 ± 1.8 *	19 ± 1.7 *	10 ± 0.2	20 ± 1.5 *	38 ± 0.5 *
	STI + VC	24 ± 2.3 #	22 ± 0.1 #	10 ± 0.1	22 ± 1.1 *	87 ± 1.6 #

*: Represents the significant difference compared to the control group ($p < 0.05$, $n = 10$). #: Represents the significant difference compared to the STI group ($p < 0.05$, $n = 10$).

3.3. Analysis of Relative Gene Expression

Five relative genes: GSH-Px, SOD, TPS, SST, and SSTR5, were analyzed using RT-PCR (Figure 1). The transcription levels of GSH-Px, SOD, TPS, SST, and SSTR5 genes in the three groups exhibited a decreasing trend during the initial 3 weeks, reaching a minimum in the 3rd week, followed by a subsequent increase during the next 2 weeks. During the whole experimental period, there was a significant decrease ($p < 0.05$) in the transcription levels of GSH-Px, SOD, TPS, and SST genes in the mice of the STI group compared to the control group. Mice in the STI + VC group exhibited significantly higher transcription levels ($p < 0.05$) of SOD, GSH Px, TPS, and SSTR5 genes, as compared to those in the STI group, although still lower than the control group.

3.4. TEM of Pancreas Tissue

Figure 2 shows the ultrastructure changes in the pancreas of three groups of mice. The analysis of the pancreas showed no pathological alterations in control mice. The nuclear envelope, nucleus, mitochondria, and endoplasmic reticulum were normal. Zymogen granules were diffusely distributed in the cytoplasm (Figure 2a). Since the oxidative damage was less pronounced in the STI group during the first week, the electron micrographs exhibited similarity to those of the control group. Observable damage appeared in the 3rd week, with micrographs of the pancreas of the STI group displaying mitochondrial vacuolization, swelling, and dilatation of the endoplasmic reticulum. The zymogen granules of STI-diet mice were significantly fewer than that of control mice (Figure 2b,d,f,h,j). The protective effect of VC in mice was evident in the form of a moderate increase in zymogen granules, as well as normal mitochondria and endoplasmic reticulum. Mild swelling of the endoplasmic reticulum and mitochondria were also observed, indicating the efficacy of VC in preventing damage caused by STI, as compared to the STI group (Figure 2c,e,g,i,k).

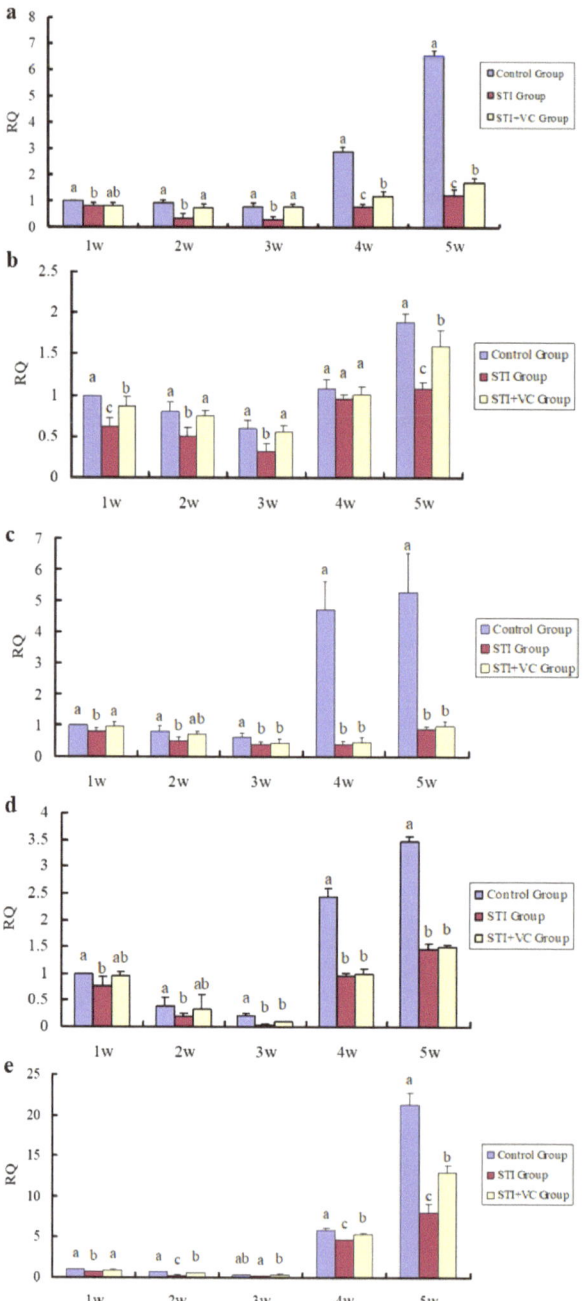

Figure 1. RT-PCR gene expression analysis of relative gene expression. (**a**) SOD; (**b**) GSH-Px; (**c**) TPS; (**d**) SST; (**e**) SSTR5; Different letters indicate significant differences between the groups ($p < 0.05$, $n = 10$).

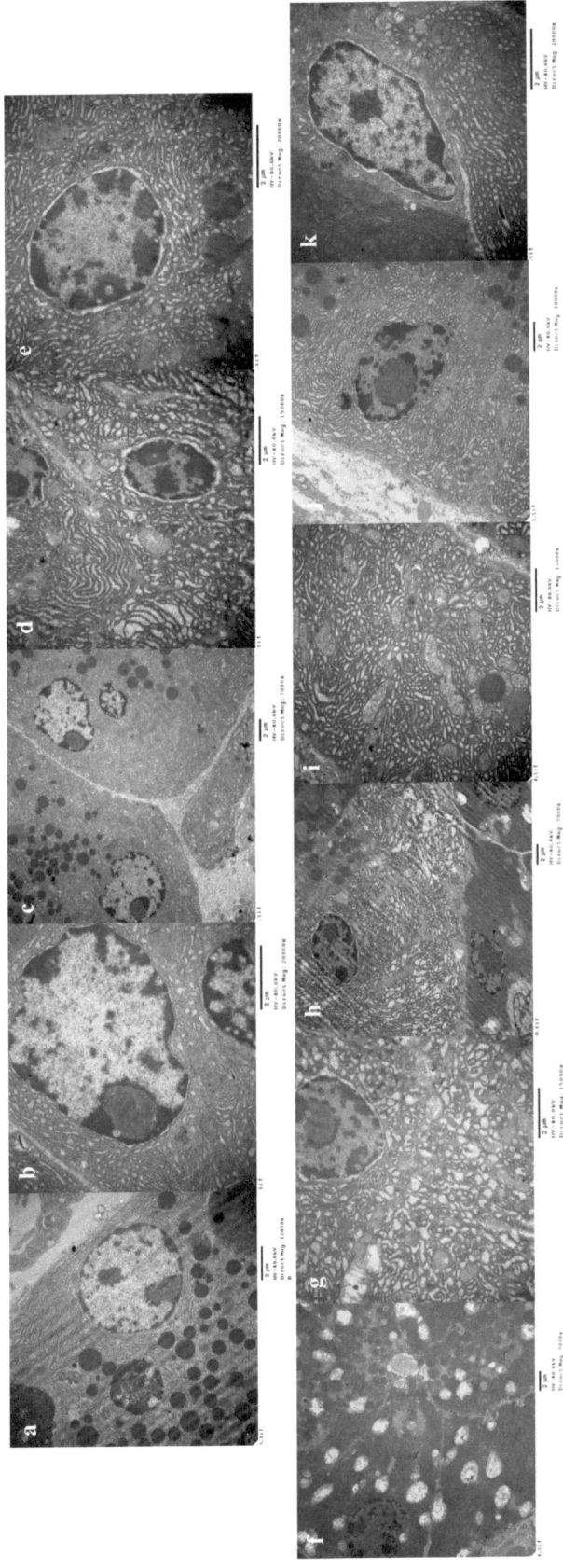

Figure 2. Electron micrographs of mice pancreas. (**a**) Pancreatic ultrastructure of the control group; (**b**,**d**,**f**,**h**,**j**) Ultrastructure of the pancreas in STI group at 1–5 weeks; (**c**,**e**,**g**,**i**,**k**) Ultrastructure of the pancreas in STI + VC group at 1–5 weeks.

4. Discussion

The lipid peroxidation process is initiated by reactive oxygen species in the phospholipids present in biofilms, triggering a free radical chain reaction [23]. As MDA is the result of lipid peroxidation, its concentration can be used as an indicator to measure the extent of lipid peroxidation. The results indicated a significant rise in the MDA level in the serum and pancreas of the STI group when compared to the control group. These results indicated that STI induced a significant increase in lipid peroxidation, indirectly indicating a rise in the levels of free radicals in the pancreas of mice. As the feeding time increased, it was observed that MDA levels in the STI group increased significantly, reaching their peak in the 3rd week. Studies have shown that in the myocardial ischemia and hyperlipidemia animal model [24,25], the level of MDA will rise first and then decline, which was consistent with the findings of this study. The results indicated that MDA levels exhibit periodic fluctuations and are influenced by feeding time, consistent with the pattern observed for free radicals in the experiment. This further demonstrated that the growth cycle of mice influences the level of free radicals affected by STI, with the highest level reached in the 3rd week. TEM analysis of the pancreas also revealed that oxidative damage to the pancreas was most severe in the 3rd week.

As a free radical scavenging system, superoxide dismutase (SOD) and glutathione peroxidase (GSH) exist in all oxygen-metabolizing cells, which can prevent free radical damage to cells and provide an oxidative membrane component of repair mechanism [14], reflecting the capacity of the non-enzymatic antioxidant defense system. Therefore, the aforementioned parameters were utilized to evaluate alterations in the antioxidant status of the pancreas. The findings showed a decrease in the antioxidant indices of both the serum and pancreas in the STI group, which was caused by the STI increasing the level of oxygen free radicals. To maintain the balance between oxidation and antioxidants, the body requires a significant amount of antioxidants. However, this high demand results in damage to the antioxidant defense system, leading to a weakened antioxidant capacity within the body. The activity of SOD in both the serum and pancreas displayed a pattern of initially decreasing, followed by increasing and subsequently reaching the lowest level during the third week. However, the activity of GSH-Px showed an opposite trend. RT-PCR results indicated the down-regulation of transcription levels of SOD and GSH-Px genes in the STI group when compared to the control group. This is due to the STI leading to an increase in free radicals.

The expression of SOD and GSH-Px genes can be inhibited by free radicals, leading to a significant reduction in the activity of SOD and GSH-Px [26]. These results provide more insight into the alteration in antioxidant capacity following oxidative stress, which could be associated with the level of oxygen-free radicals and the developmental stage of the organism.

It was observed that the TPS of the STI group and STI + VC group exhibited a decreasing trend, followed by an increasing trend as the feeding time increased, which reached their minimum value in the third week. TPS, produced in the pancreas, is an endopeptidase that binds to trypsin inhibitors to create a complex of enzymes and inhibitors. During the last two weeks, as oxidative damage decreased, the activity of TPS increased, which led to the formation of these complexes that can be excreted in feces, causing a decrease in trypsin levels.

SST is a natural, ubiquitous neurohormone found in the central nervous system and most major peripheral organs, including the salivary glands, stomach, pancreas, and intestine [27]. It is believed that this peptide has negative effects on various physiological functions. The action of SST is mediated by the 5-somatostatin receptor subtype, known as SSTR1-5. The levels of SSTR5 in the pancreas were higher than those of the other four receptors. SST inhibits the secretion of both insulin and glucagon, which is mediated through distinct SST receptors [28]. In addition, SST has the ability to not only directly impact islet secretion function but also modulate islet function by influencing the responsiveness of islet cells to physiological or pharmacological stimuli [29,30]. Recent studies have shown that various factors that stimulate the release of SST from cells can also trigger the production of intracellular ROS. Wenger's study concluded that the SST analog octreotide impacted oxygen-free radical metabolism by reducing liver re LPO, increasing GSH-Px and SOD activity [31]. The results of this experiment showed that the SST content in the STI group first increased, then decreased, and peaked during the 3rd week. However, RT-PCR results indicated that the transcription levels of SST and SSTR5 genes in the STI group exhibited an inverse correlation. This may be due to the inhibition of the expression of the SST gene and the SSTR5 gene during transcription due to the production of free radicals. The possible reason for the increase in SST content is the autocrine and paracrine factors of SST. In other experimental conditions, SST has demonstrated its effectiveness as an inhibitor of insulin secretion [32]. While promoting SST production, insulin secretion is suppressed. However, in our study, we observed an opposite trend between insulin and SST levels.

VC is involved in metabolic processes in the body and acts as a potent antioxidant by directly or indirectly neutralizing free radicals to prevent cellular damage and immune system disorders [33]. The results of this study suggest that VC may alleviate the oxidative stress caused by STI, thus mitigating the oxidative damage caused by reactive oxygen species.

5. Conclusions

The current research indicates that STI exhibits the harmful effect of inducing oxidative stress by increasing the formation of lipid peroxidation and overall impairing enzymatic and non-enzymatic antioxidant defenses in the STI diet-fed mice, which cause structural damage and secretory dysfunction of the pancreas. Moreover, the RT-PCR results for the expression of SOD, GSH-Px, TPS, SST, and SSTR5 genes further demonstrated the above results. In addition, these harmful effects are periodic. Meanwhile, the inference that free radicals generated by STI intake where the main contributor to pancreatic injury was confirmed by the improvement in pancreatic injury after VC intake. This suggested that adding VC, especially soy protein products, to ingredients containing STIs, whether food or feed, is a good way to mitigate the damage caused by STIs to the pancreas or that there are practical implications of consuming soy protein (containing STI) along with Vc.

Author Contributions: Conceptualization, C.G.; methodology, Q.Y. and L.Z.; software, C.G.; data curation, Q.Y. and S.L. and B.L.; writing—original draft preparation, C.G. and Q.Y.; supervision, Y.W. and H.Y.; project administration, H.Y. All authors have read and agreed to the published version of the manuscript.

Funding: This research is in part financially supported by the Modern Agro-industry Technology Research System (CARS-04), the National Natural Science Foundation of China (NSFC, No.31000769), and the Postdoctoral Library of Jilin Agricultural University and the China Postdoctoral Science Foundation (No.2012M520690).

Institutional Review Board Statement: The study was approved by the Ethics Committee of Laboratory Animal Welfare and the Ethics Committee of Jilin Agricultural University. (Protocol code No.20130530001, May 2013).

Data Availability Statement: The data presented in this study are available on request from the corresponding author.

Conflicts of Interest: The authors declare no conflict of interest.

References

1. Haidar, C.N.; Coscueta, E.; Cordiso, E.; Nerli, B.B.; Malpiedi, L.P. Aqueous micellar two-phase system as an alternative method to selectively remove soy antinutritional factors. *LWT* **2018**, *93*, 665–672. [CrossRef]
2. Vagadia, B.H.; Vanga, S.K.; Raghavan, V. Inactivation methods of soybean trypsin inhibitor—A review. *Trends Food Sci. Technol.* **2017**, *64*, 115–125. [CrossRef]
3. Li, J.; Xiang, Q.; Liu, X.; Ding, T.; Zhang, X.; Zhai, Y.; Bai, Y. Inactivation of soybean trypsin inhibitor by dielectric-barrier discharge (DBD) plasma. *Food Chem.* **2017**, *232*, 515–522. [CrossRef] [PubMed]
4. Flavin, D.F. The effects of soybean trypsin inhibitors on the pancreas of animals and man: A review. *Vet. Hum. Toxicol.* **1982**, *24*, 25–28.

5. Kunitz, M. Crystalline soybean trypsin inhibitor: Ii. *General properties*. *J. Gen. Physiol.* **1947**, *30*, 291–310. [CrossRef]
6. Zhao, W.-P.; Wang, H.-W.; Liu, J.; Zhang, Z.-H.; Zhu, S.-Q.; Zhou, B.-H. Mitochondrial respiratory chain complex abnormal expressions and fusion disorder are involved in fluoride-induced mitochondrial dysfunction in ovarian granulosa cells. *Chemosphere* **2019**, *215*, 619–625. [CrossRef]
7. Svegliati, S.T.; Spadoni, G. Moroncini and A. Gabrielli. "Nadph oxidase, oxidative stress and fibrosis in systemic sclerosis. *Free Radic. Biol. Med.* **2018**, *125*, 90–97. [CrossRef]
8. Ramírez-Camacho, I.; Correa, F.; El Hafidi, M.; Silva-Palacios, A.; Ostolga-Chavarría, M.; Esparza-Perusquía, M.; Olvera-Sánchez, S.; Flores-Herrera, O.; Zazueta, C. Cardioprotective strategies preserve the stability of respiratory chain supercomplexes and reduce oxidative stress in reperfused ischemic hearts. *Free Radic. Biol. Med.* **2018**, *129*, 407–417. [CrossRef]
9. Homma, T.; Kobayashi, S.; Sato, H.; Fujii, J. Edaravone, a free radical scavenger, protects against ferroptotic cell death in vitro. *Exp. Cell Res.* **2019**, *384*, 111592. [CrossRef]
10. Premaratne, S.; Amaratunga, D.T.; Mensah, F.E.; McNamara, J.J. Significance of oxygen free radicals in the pathophysiology of hemorrhagic shock—A protocol. *Int. J. Surg. Protoc.* **2018**, *9*, 15–19. [CrossRef]
11. Losada-Barreiro, S.; Bravo-Díaz, C. Free radicals and polyphenols: The redox chemistry of neurodegenerative diseases. *Eur. J. Med. Chem.* **2017**, *133*, 379–402. [CrossRef]
12. Ahn, B.; Smith, N.; Saunders, D.; Ranjit, R.; Kneis, P.; Towner, R.A.; Van Remmen, H. Using MRI to measure in vivo free radical production and perfusion dynamics in a mouse model of elevated oxidative stress and neurogenic atrophy. *Redox Biol.* **2019**, *26*, 101308. [CrossRef]
13. Taleb, A.; Ahmad, K.A.; Ihsan, A.U.; Qu, J.; Lin, N.; Hezam, K.; Koju, N.; Hui, L.; Qilong, D. Antioxidant effects and mechanism of silymarin in oxidative stress induced cardiovascular diseases. *Biomed. Pharmacother.* **2018**, *102*, 689–698. [CrossRef]
14. Fonin, A.V.; Stepanenko, O.; Povarova, O.I.; Volova, C.A.; Philippova, E.M.; Bublikov, G.S.; Kuznetsova, I.M.; Demchenko, A.P.; Turoverov, K.K. Spectral characteristics of the mutant form GGBP/H152C of D-glucose/D-galactose-binding protein labeled with fluorescent dye BADAN: Influence of external factors. *PeerJ* **2014**, *2*, e275. [CrossRef]
15. Zhong, G.S.; Qin, D.; Townsend, B.A.; Schulte, K.D.T.; Wang, G.Y. Oxidative stress induces senescence in breast cancer stem cells. *Biochem. Biophys. Res. Commun.* **2019**, *514*, 1204–1209. [CrossRef]
16. Poprac, P.; Jomova, K.; Simunkova, M.; Kollar, V.; Rhodes, C.J.; Valko, M. Targeting Free Radicals in Oxidative Stress-Related Human Diseases. *Trends Pharmacol. Sci.* **2017**, *38*, 592–607. [CrossRef]
17. Abudawood, M.; Tabassum, H.; Almaarik, B.; Aljohi, A. Interrelationship between oxidative stress, DNA damage and cancer risk in diabetes (Type 2) in Riyadh, KSA. *Saudi J. Biol. Sci.* **2019**, *27*, 177–183. [CrossRef]
18. Koca, K.; Yurttas, Y.; Bilgic, S.; Cayci, T.; Topal, T.; Durusu, M.; Kaldirim, U.; Akgul, E.O.; Ozkan, H.; Yanmis, I.; et al. Effect of Preconditioned Hyperbaric Oxygen and Ozone on Ischemia-Reperfusion Induced Tourniquet in Skeletal Bone of Rats. *J. Surg. Res.* **2010**, *164*, e83–e89. [CrossRef]
19. Beauchamp, C.; Fridovich, I. Superoxide dismutase: Improved assays and an assay applicable to acrylamide gels. *Anal. Biochem.* **1971**, *44*, 276–287. [CrossRef]
20. Sabuncu, T.; Vural, H.; Harma, M.; Harma, M. Oxidative stress in polycystic ovary syndrome and its contribution to the risk of cardiovascular disease. *Clin. Biochem.* **2001**, *34*, 407–413. [CrossRef]
21. Mineo, H.; Ishida, K.; Morikawa, N.; Ohmi, S.; Machida, A.; Noda, T.; Fukushima, M.; Chiji, H. Ingestion of potato starch decreases chymotrypsin but does not affect trypsin, amylase, or lipase activity in the pancreas in rats. *Nutr. Res.* **2007**, *27*, 113–118. [CrossRef]
22. Li, W.; Shi, Y.H.; Yang, R.L.; Cui, J.; Xiao, Y.; Wang, B.; Le, G.W. Effect of somatostatin analog on high-fat diet-induced metabolic syndrome: Involvement of reactive oxygen species. *Peptides* **2010**, *31*, 625–629. [CrossRef] [PubMed]
23. Peña-Bautista, C.M.; Baquero, M.V.; Cháfer-Pericás, C. Free radicals in alzheimer's disease: Lipid peroxidation biomarkers. *Clin. Chim. Acta* **2019**, *491*, 85–90. [CrossRef]
24. Sahna, E.; Parlakpinar, H.; Turkoz, Y.; Acet, A. Protective effects of melatonin on myocardial ischemia-reperfusion induced infarct size and oxidative changes. *Physiol. Res.* **2005**, *5*, 491–495. [CrossRef]
25. Ni, H.; Li, J.; Jin, Y.; Zang, H.; Peng, L. The experimental animal model of hyperlipidemia and hyperlipidemic fatty liver in rats. *Chin. Pharmacol. Bull.* **1986**, *12*, wpr-555126.
26. Min, Y.; Niu, Z.; Sun, T.; Wang, Z.; Jiao, P.; Zi, B.; Chen, P.; Tian, D.; Liu, F. Vitamin E and vitamin C supplementation improves antioxidant status and immune function in oxidative-stressed breeder roosters by up-regulating expression of GSH-Px gene. *Poult. Sci.* **2018**, *97*, 1238–1244. [CrossRef]
27. Mazzawi, T.; Hausken, T.; Gundersen, D.; El-Salhy, M. Dietary guidance normalizes large intestinal endocrine cell densities in patients with irritable bowel syndrome. *Eur. J. Clin. Nutr.* **2015**, *70*, 175–181. [CrossRef]
28. Streuli, J.; Harris, A.G.; Cottiny, C.; Allagnat, F.; Daly, A.F.; Grouzmann, E.; Abid, K. Cellular effects of AP102, a somatostatin analog with balanced affinities for the hSSTR2 and hSSTR5 receptors. *Neuropeptides* **2018**, *68*, 84–89. [CrossRef]
29. Bustamante, J.; Lobo, M.V.T.; Alonso, F.J.; Mukala, N.-T.A.; Giné, E.; Solís, J.M.; Tamarit-Rodriguez, J.; Del Río, R.M. An osmotic-sensitive taurine pool is localized in rat pancreatic islet cells containing glucagon and somatostatin. *Am. J. Physiol. Metab.* **2001**, *281*, E1275–E1285. [CrossRef]
30. Virgolini, I.; Traub-Weidinger, T.; Decristoforo, C. Nuclear medicine in the detection and management of pancreatic islet-cell tumours. *Best Pr. Res. Clin. Endocrinol. Metab.* **2005**, *19*, 213–227. [CrossRef]

31. Wenger, F.A.; Kilian, M.; Mautsch, I.; Jacobi, C.A.; Steiert, A.; Peter, F.J.; Guski, H.; Schimke, I.; Müller, J.M. Influence of Octreotide on Liver Metastasis and Hepatic Lipid Peroxidation in BOP-Induced Pancreatic Cancer in Syrian Hamsters. *Pancreas* **2001**, *23*, 266–272. [CrossRef]
32. Schwetz, T.A.; Ustione, A.; Piston, D.W. Neuropeptide Y and somatostatin inhibit insulin secretion through different mechanisms. *Am. J. Physiol. Metab.* **2013**, *304*, E211–E221. [CrossRef]
33. Fang, Y.-Z.; Yang, S.; Wu, G. Free radicals, antioxidants, and nutrition. *Nutrition* **2002**, *18*, 872–879. [CrossRef]

Disclaimer/Publisher's Note: The statements, opinions and data contained in all publications are solely those of the individual author(s) and contributor(s) and not of MDPI and/or the editor(s). MDPI and/or the editor(s) disclaim responsibility for any injury to people or property resulting from any ideas, methods, instructions or products referred to in the content.

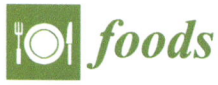

Article

Impact of Cavitation Jet on the Structural, Emulsifying Features and Interfacial Features of Soluble Soybean Protein Oxidized Aggregates

Yanan Guo, Caihua Liu, Yichang Wang, Shuanghe Ren, Xueting Zheng, Jiayu Zhang, Tianfu Cheng, Zengwang Guo * and Zhongjiang Wang

College of Food Science, Northeast Agricultural University, Harbin 150030, China
* Correspondence: gzwname@163.com

Abstract: A cavitation jet can enhance food proteins' functionalities by regulating solvable oxidized soybean protein accumulates (SOSPI). We investigated the impacts of cavitation jet treatment on the emulsifying, structural and interfacial features of soluble soybean protein oxidation accumulate. Findings have shown that radicals in an oxidative environment not only induce proteins to form insoluble oxidative aggregates with a large particle size and high molecular weight, but also attack the protein side chains to form soluble small molecular weight protein aggregates. Emulsion prepared by SOSPI shows worse interface properties than OSPI. A cavitation jet at a short treating time (<6 min) has been shown to break the core aggregation skeleton of soybean protein insoluble aggregates, and insoluble aggregates into soluble aggregates resulting in an increase of emulsion activity (EAI) and constancy (ESI), and a decrease of interfacial tension from 25.15 to 20.19 mN/m. However, a cavitation jet at a long treating time (>6 min) would cause soluble oxidized aggregates to reaggregate through an anti-parallel intermolecular β-sheet, which resulted in lower EAI and ESI, and a higher interfacial tension (22.44 mN/m). The results showed that suitable cavitation jet treatment could adjust the structural and functional features of SOSPI by targeted regulated transformation between the soluble and insoluble components.

Keywords: soybean protein; soluble oxidized aggregates; emulsifying properties; rheological properties; cavitating jet

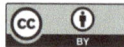

1. Introduction

Soybean is an important crop with seeds that contain abundant protein of approximately 40% [1]. The soybean protein has different physiological impacts including dropping blood lipids, blood pressure, and inhibiting cardiovascular and cerebrovascular disease indirectly [2]. Therefore, soybean proteins have been extensively exploited in food and feed plants due to their superior nutritious rate, high functional features, and low price [3]. Studies have revealed that in 2019, global soy production reached 366.67 million tons [4], which caused huge storage and transportation pressures. In addition, soy protein is vulnerable to oxidative attack during storage and transportation. The parties within the molecule re-syndicate to create oligomers following disclosure, owing to the oxidative denaturation of soy protein, which further forms macromolecular aggregates due to hydrophobicity and electrostatic attraction [5]. It is challenging to use oxidized soy protein in food manufacturing, because the formation of insoluble aggregates in protein aggregates is a significant factor in the loss of some biological and functional features of proteins, for instance, protein solubility, emulsifying effects, and emulsifying stability [6].

The physical control of oxidized protein aggregates is currently the subject of extensive research. The degree of whey protein isolate (WPI) aggregation's cross-linking could be controlled, and its gel and emulsifying characteristics could be improved, expanding the use of WPI in food processing, according to [7]. A decrease in the aggregate concentration of β-conglycinin and a rise in the size of the solvable accumulates for glycinin and soy protein insulate were found by Keerati-U-Rai et al. (2009) [8], who also established that dynamic extra-pressure homogenization triggered a transformation from insoluble aggregate to soluble aggregate. Additionally, Cao et al. (2021) [9] discovered that using ultrasound might modify the intermolecular interactions, alter the shape and accumulation of oxidized quinoa proteins, and increase the quantity of soluble aggregates, refining the functional attributes of the quinoa proteins. In a study by Zhang (2020) [10], it was demonstrated that ultrasonic treatment could prevent casein molecules from self-aggregating in a solution, as well as deteriorate the accumulation brought on by interfacial adsorption through foam fractional process, resulting in an improved protein aggregate function. Physical fields can therefore cause subunit dissociation and aggregation to directly regulate the protein structure, which eventually results in an improvement in the functional characteristics of protein aggregates. However, because of their high power requirements and limited effort capabilities in food processing procedures, high-pressure homogenization and ultrasonic processes were unable to be extensively utilized.

A cavitation jet is a water jet that can produce the cavitation effect; it can induce the rapid vaporization of the liquid to form many cavitation bubbles. After the liquid flows into the high-pressure zone, these cavitation bubbles will collapse and extinguish, resulting in the generation of an extra-velocity turbulent shear and a substantial pressure differential and molecular impact, which could cause big particles to break up into smaller ones and the structure of food to be refined, which will affect its functional characteristics [11]. The cavitation jet technique provides benefits over alternative mechanical treatments, including ease of use, speedy processing, low processing temperatures, and cheap processing costs [12]. Thus, in the realm of food processing, the cavitation jet treatment may be employed as an effective and energy-saving processing method. Cavitating jets could alter the structure and characteristics of proteins, as well as eliminate the hydrophobic and electrostatic connections between molecules. Based on this, researchers have shown that cavitation treatments may change the structures of the protein isolate and promote emulsifying characterizations [13]. The previous research results revealed that the appropriate time of cavitation jet treating could damage the structure of protein-oxidized accumulates and improve the emulsification and interface properties. In addition, this outcome might be associated with the regulation of the cavitation jet on the oxidized masses and the induction of conversion between the soluble and insoluble oxidized aggregates. Nevertheless, in the current work, the research on the transformation law between the soluble and insoluble components of protein oxidative aggregates was less. It is limited by the tender of the cavitation jet physical field in the governing of the protein accumulates and the analysis of its mechanism.

Thus, in this study, soybean protein was utilized as the investigation entity, and 2,2′-azobis(2-amidinopropane) dihydrochloride (AAPH) was employed to create an oxidation aggregation system of soy protein. By mimicking the definite creation of oxidized protein accumulates in the means of factory storing, the oxidized protein accumulates were treated with several cavitation jet times (0–15 min), and the soluble aggregates with the cavitation jet treatment were obtained during the centrifugation. We studied the change of the structure and the emulsifying and interfacial descriptions of the soluble component in protein accumulates after cavitation jet treatment. The mechanisms of the cavitation jet governing the oxidative accumulates of soybean protein and transformation law between soluble and insoluble components were explained at the molecular level. This might cause enhancements in the function of the cavitation jet in the soy protein plant, and deliver a theoretic base for the claim of the development, alterations, storing, and shipping of the soybean protein stuffs.

2. Materials and Methods

2.1. Materials

Shandong Yuwang ecological food industry Plant Limited provided the soy protein isolate (92.4% protein) (Shandong, China). From Beijing Dingguo Changsheng Biotechnology Co. Ltd., chemicals such as 2,2′-dithiobis(5-nitropyridine) (DTNP) and 8-Anilino-1-Naphthalene Sulfonate (ANS) were acquired (Beijing, China).

2.2. Formulation of Soluble Soybean Protein Oxidized Accumulates

According to a prior work, the soluble oxidized accumulates of soybean protein (SOSPI) were produced [14]. To generate a 10 mg mL^{-1} soybean protein mix, the soybean protein was liquified in a phosphate buffer solution (PBS) with a phosphate dose of 0.01 mol L^{-1}, a pH of 7.2, and 0.5 mg mL^{-1} of NaN$_3$. The final concentration of AAPH was increased to 0.5 mmol L^{-1} by adding AAPH. The soybean protein oxidized accumulate mix with a 12 h oxidation period was prepared after oxidating treatment for 12 h at 37 °C and became murky. Dialysis was performed at 4 °C for 72 h using a 14,000 kDa dialysis bag, and the deionized water (dH$_2$O) was replaced every 6 h. The samples were gathered and given the designation OSPI after spray drying. The soybean protein oxidized accumulate mix underwent a 12 h oxidation process before standing centrifugated at 4 °C for 20 min at a rapidity of 9000 rpm to discrete the soluble components from the insoluble components. The samples were gathered and given the name SOSPI after spray drying.

2.3. Formulation of Samples for Cavitation Jet Treatment

The 2 L OSPI (25 °C, 10 mg mL^{-1}) was poured into the SL-2 cavitation jet machine (Zhongsen Huijia Technology Development Co., Ltd., Beijing, China) to treat at 80 MPa for six diverse times: 2, 4, 6, 8, 10, and 15 min. The SOSPI was liquified in 0.01 mol/L PBS (pH 7.2, comprising 0.5 mg mL^{-1} NaN$_3$). After treatment, the protein was immediately chilled in an ice bath for 15 min, and trailed by 20 h of centrifugal treatment at 4 °C and 9000 rpm to remove the insoluble parts. Spray drying was used to create all sample solutions, which were given the names SCOSPI-2 min, SCOSPI-4 min, SCOSPI-6 min, SCOSPI-8 min, SCOSPI-10 min, and SCOSPI-15 min. Three groups of parallel samples were taken.

2.4. Measuring the Particle Size Dispersal

Based on the technique labeled by Ma et al. (2019), the particle size dispersal (PSD) was estimated via a laser scattering Mastersizer S (Malvern, UK) and a 300 inverse Fourier lens with the relief of a He–Ne laser λ = 633 [15]. The protein's refractive index was 1.33 when the amount was made at room temperature (RT, 25 ± 2 °C). Before measurement, the samples were diluted with dH$_2$O to 50 mg/mL, and the particle sizes ranged between 0–10,000 μm.

2.5. Measurement of the Molecular Weight Circulation

Following Ma et al. (2019) [15], examples of soybean protein were examined using an HPLC unit (Milford, MA, USA). Briefly, the molecular weight of the proteins at 280 nm was determined via a Waters 2175 UV finder (Milford, MA, USA).

2.6. Measurement of the Fourier Transform Infrared Spectroscopy (FTIR) Spectroscopy

A Bruker Vertex 70 was used to analyze the materials using Fourier transform infrared (FTIR) (Bruker Optics GmbH, Ettlingen, Germany). At 0.5 cm^{-1} tenacity and RT (25 ± 2 °C), a total of 64 scans were found between 4000 and 400 cm^{-1}. The secondary structure was determined using the FTIR spectra's secondary-derivation and deconvolution processes, and it was based on the amide I band (1600–1700 cm^{-1}). According to Tang et al. (2009), the method involved the secondary structure of the proteins being examined using Peakfit Ver., 4.12 software, and the algorithm utilized was Gaussian peak fitting [16].

2.7. Measuring of the Fluorescence Emission Spectra

According to the technique used by Jiang et al. (2014), the fluorescence emission spectra of the materials were found via a Hitachi F-7000 fluorescence spectrophotometer (Hitachi Inc., Tokyo, Japan) [17]. The soybean protein trials were thinned in 0.01 mol L^{-1} PBS to a protein dose of 0.2 mg mL^{-1} to produce emission spectra at an excitation wavelength of 295 nm and from 300 to 400 nm. By employing a fixed 5 nm for both the emission and excitation in triplicate, the bandwidths were attained.

2.8. Measurement of the Sulfhydryl Content

According to the Wu et al. (2019) approach, the amounts of disulfide bonds and free sulfhydryl (SH) assemblies were measured [18]. DTNP was used in a variation of Ellman's approach to ascertain the SH cluster insides in the trial. The molar extinction constant (13,600 M^{-1} cm^{-1}) was utilized to represent the SH contents as a nmol mg^{-1} protein.

2.9. Measuring of the Transmission Electron Microscopy (TEM)

TEM was dedicated by utilizing a previously described technique [19]. After being diluted 350 times in dH2O, the sample was dispensed in 30 μL droplets and applied on a carbon net (200 mesh). The surplus was wiped away using permeable paper after 120 s. The net was air-dehydrated on sieve paper after the samples were dyed for 3 min with a 2% uranyl acetate solution. Benefitting a TEM-JEM-1230 (JEOL, Tokyo, Japan) with a hastening voltage of 80 kV, the morphology of the sample was examined.

2.10. Measuring of the Emulsifying Activity Index (EAI) and Emulsion Solidity Index (ESI)

The Kevin et al. (1978) approach was used to evaluate the EAI and ESI [20]. A high-rapidity homogenizer (T-25 homogenizer, IKA, Staufen, Germany) was used to combine a 15 mL sample of a 0.1% (w/v) protein mix with 5 mL of maize oil at 7200× g for 10 min to create an emulsion. The emulsion was then detached from the lowest of the centrifuge tubes and normalized for 0 and 30 min before being diluted 100 times with 5 mL 0.1% sodium dodecyl sulfate. A spectrophotometer was used to test the absorbance at 500 nanometers (Beckman DU 500, Fullerton, CA, USA). The EAI and ESI were stated as:

$$\text{EAI}(m^2/g) = \frac{2 \times 2.303 \times \text{DF} \times A_0}{(1-\theta) \times C \times \phi \times 10000}$$
$$\text{ESI}(\%) = \frac{A_0}{A_0 - A_{30}} \times 10$$

where A_0 is the absorbance at 0 min of the thinned emulsion, DF is the dilution aspect (×100), c is the model dose (g mL^{-1}), φ is the pictorial path, θ is the portion of the oil (0.25), and A_{30} is the absorbance after 30 min.

2.11. Measurement of the Confocal Laser Scanning Microscope (CLSM)

The Leica TCS SP2 CLSM was used to study the microstructure of emulsions. To create an emulsion, 15 mL of a 0.1% (w/v) protein mix was normalized with 5 mL of maize oil at 7200× g for 30 min. A 1 mL of emulsion was added to the dye (40 μL), which included 0.02% Nile red dye and 0.1% Nile blue dye. After that, a coverslip was put on top of the colored emulsion in the middle of the slide. To prevent the water from evaporating, silicone oil was sprayed to the superiority of the coverslip. The emphasis plane was originally changed following an inspection with a 100× impartial lens, while the slide was mounted on a laser confocal microscope phase. Pre-examining was performed with Ar ion at 488 nm and a He/Ne ion laser at 633 nm. A fluorescence figure was composed with a visualizing intensity of 1024 × 1024.

2.12. Measuring of the Quantity of Adsorbed Proteins at Interface (AP%)

According to Liang and Tang, the amount of adsorbed proteins at the interface (AP%) of these emulsion samples was calculated [21]. A 10,000 g centrifuge was used to spin each new emulsion (1 mL) for 45 min at RT. A cream coat (or concerted oil droplets) at the upper of the tube and the aqueous stage of the emulsion at the bottom were visible after centrifugation. A 0.22 μm filter was utilized to sieve the supernatant after the cream layer was delicately detached using a syringe (Millipore Corp.). The Lowry technique was utilized to estimate the filtrate's protein content, with a BSA serving as the reference. To estimate the protein intensity (C_s) in the upper phase, the initial protein mix was likewise centrifuged under identical circumstances. The AP (%) was expressed as:

$$AP\ (\%) = \frac{C_S - C_f}{C_0} \times 100$$

where C_s is the content of preliminary protein solution in the supernatant (mg), C_f is the content of protein in filtrate after centrifugation (mg), and C_0 is the preliminary protein intensity of the protein mixes concerned for the emulsion formulation (mg).

2.13. Measurement of the Interfacial Tension

Various materials' surface tension was estimated via an automated surface tensiometer (DCAT21, Data Physics Instruments GmbH, Filderstadt, Germany). A total of 20 mL of the sample mix was then put into a 25 mL cylinder after the protein model had first been dissolved in dH$_2$O (1%, m/v). The apparatus's measuring variety was always between 1 and 100 mN m^{-1}, with a SD that never went beyond 0.03 mN m^{-1}.

2.14. Measurement of the Viscoelastic Properties

The Sun et al. (2012) approach is used to assess the viscoelastic characteristics of emulsions [22]. An RST-CPS rheometer was used to measure the sample emulsions' rheological characteristics (Brookfield, Middleboro, MA, USA). At a temperature of 40 °C, the samples were sandwiched between two parallel plates with 1 mm space among them. A strain examining the analysis performed at an incidence of 1 Hz was used to identify the linear viscoelastic area of each sample. Each protein sample's elastic and storage moduli were determined in the linear viscoelastic area.

2.15. Measurement of the Apparent Viscosity

Rendering to the technique delineated by Swa et al. (2020), rheological tests were carried out via an AR 1500 regulated stress rheometer (TA, West Sussex, UK) outfitted with cone and bowl geometries (40 mm, angle 1°, and gap 0.100 mm) [23]. The same technique was used to create the sample emulsions. The sample emulsions were divided into 2.0 mL aliquots and placed on the stage for measurement at 25 ± 0.1 °C. After 5 min, the viscosity ranged from 0 to 200 s^{-1}. Using the program, the measuring was performed in triplicate. We matched the investigational flow curves to Sisko's pattern that provided the finest fit and was signified by:

$$\eta = \eta_0 + K\gamma^{n-1}$$

where η is the ostensible viscosity (Pa·s), η_0 is the vintage ostensible viscosity (Pa·s), K is the consistency index (Pa·s^n), γ is the shear ratio (s^{-1}), and n is the performance index (dimensionless).

2.16. Statistical Analysis

Statistical assessment was accomplished via SPSS ver. 20.0. The outcomes were imperiled to Duncan's multiple series and ANOVA tests. All the rates gained are stated as the mean ± SD in triplicate. A p-value ≤ 0.05 was measured significantly.

3. Results

3.1. Particle Size Distribution and Molecular Weight Circulation

The SEC-HPLC and particle size dispersal can characterize the molecular weight, size, and aggregation degree of the soluble components in soybean protein oxidized aggregates treated by cavitation jet. It can be seen from Figures 1 and 2 and Table 1 that, equated with SPI, the particle size of OSPI showed a unimodal particle size and lifted to the right, meaning the average particle size increased significantly. Furthermore, the elution time of the first molecular weight peak of OSPI diminished and the peak quantity increased. However, as a soluble component in OSPI, the particle size of SOSPI displayed a bimodal particle size, the initial particle size peak transferred to the left, and the average particle size decreased. The elution time of the first molecular weight peak of SOSPI increased and the peak area decreased. The results revealed that after the oxidation treatment, the oxidized accumulates with a huge particle size and a high molecular weight were insoluble aggregates, and the soluble components were proteins with a small particle size and a low molecular weight. Radicals in the oxidative environment could induce proteins to form insoluble oxidative aggregates through covalent crosslinking, but they will also attack protein side chains to form small molecular weight soluble proteins [24].

With the increase of the cavitation jet treatment time, the retention time of the initial elution peak and the peak area of the protein components with a small molecular weight of SCOSPI decreased, and the particle size peak of SCOSPI lifted to the right. When the cavitation jet treatment time was 8 min, the first particle size peak of SCOSPI moved to the maximum right, and the average particle size achieved the highest. The outcomes displayed that the molecular weight and particle size of SCOSPI with the cavitation jet treatment increased, and the low molecular weight and small particle size protein components declined. The cavitation jet treatment could promote the depolymerization of insoluble aggregates in OSPI and transform them into soluble oxidized aggregates through high shear and cavitation effects, developing an increase of the particle size and molecular weight of the soluble oxidized accumulates [8]. Moreover, the cavitation jet would intensify the collision between the small molecule soluble aggregates, and then polymerize into a bigger particle size and molecular weight soluble protein molecule, resulting in the reduction of small molecular weight protein components [16,25]. When the cavitation jet treatment time exceeded 8 min, the first particle size peak of SCOSPI moved to the left and the retaining time of the initial elution peak and the peak area of protein substances with small molecular weight of SCOSPI amplified, indicating that when the treatment time was too long, the protein molecular weight of SCOSPI decreased and the small molecular weight protein component increased. The thermal effect and free radical effect of the cavitation jet, on the one hand, could promote the further aggregation among proteins to form insoluble aggregates, which were removed by centrifugation. On the other hand, it would split some peptide chains, resulting in soluble protein components dominated by small molecular weight and particle size protein molecules [16,26]. Combined with the research of the team in the early stage [27], cavitation jets can break losing the disulfide bonds and protein skeleton structures that declined the amassed sizes and molecular weights of oxidized aggregates. However, how these components of protein aggregates mutually transform is unclear. Through the particle size and molecular weight of this research, we can obtain that a cavitation jet can also induce the insoluble aggregates to break down under high shear stress and transform into soluble aggregates, ensuing in the rise of the particle size and molecular weight of the solvable accumulates. Consequently, a suitable cavitation jet treatment could adjust the structural and functional attributes of OSPI by inducing the cleavage of insoluble oxidized aggregates and transforming them into soluble aggregate components.

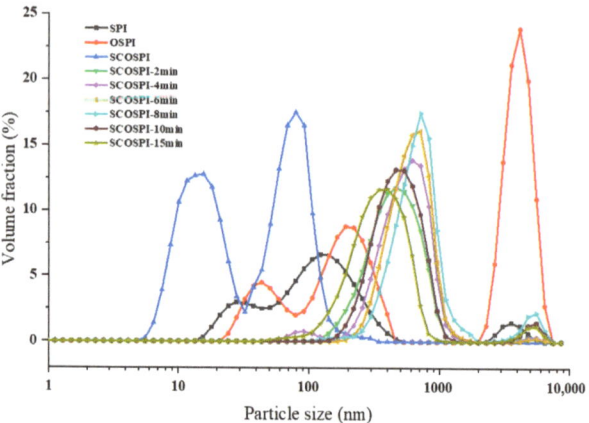

Figure 1. Particle size distribution (PSD) of natural, oxidized soybean protein, and the cavitation jet treated on soluble soybean protein oxidized accumulates at several times (2, 4, 6, 8, 10, and 15 min).

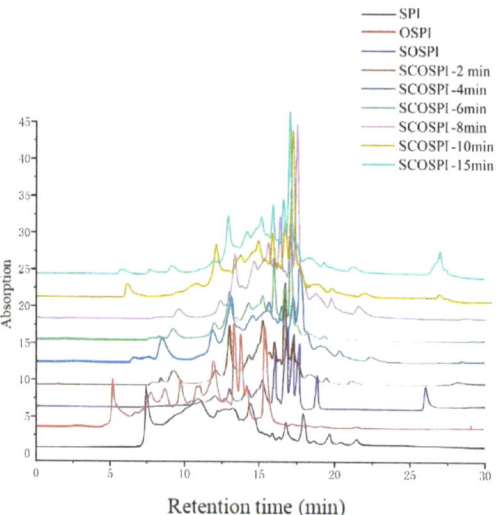

Figure 2. SEC profiles of natural, oxidized soybean protein, and cavitation jet treated on soluble soybean protein oxidized accumulates at several times (2, 4, 6, 8, 10, and 15 min).

Table 1. Particle size and protein dispersibility index (PDI) of natural, oxidized soybean protein, and cavitation jet treated on soluble soybean protein oxidized accumulates at several times (2, 4, 6, 8, 10, and 15 min).

Samples	Particle Size (nm)	PDI
SPI	181.59 ± 2.77 [h]	0.76 ± 0.11 [a]
OSPI	3836.18 ± 66.82 [a]	0.19 ± 0.03 [d]
SOSPI	97.38 ± 1.63 [i]	0.17 ± 0.01 [d]
SCOSPI-2 min	551.03 ± 5.07 [e]	0.14 ± 0.02 [ef]
SCOSPI-4 min	639.27 ± 18.31 [d]	0.11 ± 0.04 [f]
SCOSPI-6 min	705.81 ± 15.33 [c]	0.29 ± 0.04 [c]
SCOSPI-8 min	776.14 ± 11.91 [b]	0.15 ± 0.01 [e]
SCOSPI-10 min	538.15 ± 9.52 [f]	0.28 ± 0.03 [c]
SCOSPI-15 min	443.96 ± 22.28 [g]	0.33 ± 0.01 [b]

Note: Comparisons were carried out between values of the same column; values with a different letter(s) indicate a significant difference at $p \leq 0.05$.

3.2. FTIR Spectroscopy

Fourier transform infrared spectroscopy can be utilized to elucidate the secondary structure change of proteins during aggregation and disaggregation [28]. Figure 3 is the FTIR spectra, and Table 2 is the secondary structure of oxidized accumulates and soluble oxidized aggregates after the cavitation jet treatment. Oxidized treatment raised the compounds of β1, β-turn, and γ-random coil in the OSPI and declined the compounds of α-helix. Compared with OSPI, the components of β1 and γ-random coil in SOSPI declined, and the compounds of α-helix increased. α-helix has structured secondary structures featured by high inflexibility and recurrence structure, while γ-random coil has unordered secondary structures featured by plasticity and the deficiency of a recurrence structure [29]. The marker structure of aggregation (β1) is created by molecular interactions during protein oxidation [30]. Changes in the constancy of the H-bond between the amino parties and the polypeptide chain's carbonyl parties are primarily responsible for the changes in the amount of α-helices [31]. Since the hydrogen connection among the amino and carbonyl groups in the polypeptide chain is unstable, oxidation may attack the amino acid residues in the primary peptide chain, reducing the amount of α-helix present. The spatial structure of a protein heavily influences its functional activities, and proteins with a suitably organized and compact structure exhibit beneficial functional behaviors [32]. Compared with other samples, the lowest α-helix content of OSPI referred that excessive oxidation would seriously demolish the ordered structure of protein. This might be one of the important reasons for the decline of OSPI functional activity [33]. Comparing the results of OSPI and SOSPI, we can find that oxidized protein with several β1 existed in OSPI, while SOSPI has more rigid and ordered structures.

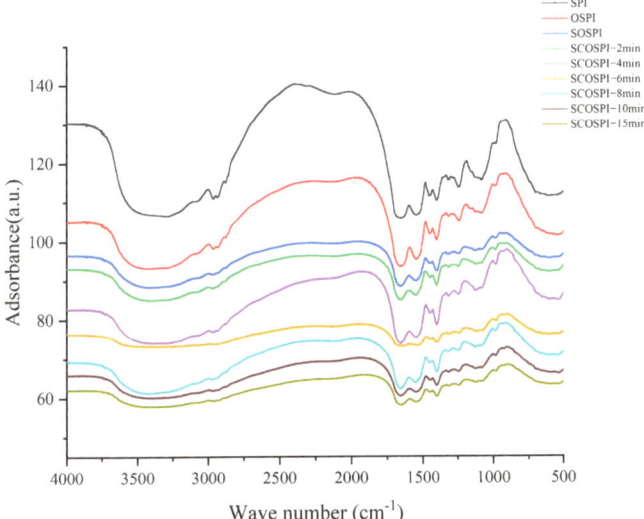

Figure 3. FTIR spectra of natural, oxidized soybean protein, and cavitation jet treated on soluble soybean protein oxidized accumulates at several times (2, 4, 6, 8, 10, and 15 min).

With the increase of the cavitation jet treatment time, β1 of SCOSPI increased first, then decreased and then increased, and other structures showed no obvious regular change trend. Combined with the outcomes of particle size and molecular weight, the superior pressure and superior shear strengths of the cavitation jet at a fleeting treatment time could lead to the cleavage of protein accumulates by weakening the protein–protein interactions and induce insoluble aggregates with high contents of β1 to transform into soluble aggregates resulting in the increase of the β1 contents [34]. Nevertheless, after the treatment time of the cavitation jet exceeded 6 min, the components of β1 of SCOSPI decreased first and then increased. The cavitation jet with long treatment time could induce the soluble aggregate in OSPI to aggregate further, due to the thermal impact and extra-speed instability and formed the insoluble aggregates with high β1 components which were centrifuged and removed, resulting in the decrease of the β1 content. When the cavitation jet treatment time was 8–15 min, the β1 content of SCOSPI increased. Combined with the previous research results of the team [27] during this timeframe, the β1 of the protein oxidized accumulates and soluble aggregates both increased, which showed that continuously extreme cavitation jet treatment can cause the formation of more β1 structures with the aggregation characteristics of soluble and insoluble components. Integrated with the particle size and molecular weight findings, we could find that the particle size and molecular weight of SCOSPI decreased with a long cavitation jet treatment time. This showed that the cavitation jet could depolymerize the soluble components and at the same time could induce the aggregation reaction between protein molecules, resulting in more β1 structures. The above results showed that the control of cavitating jet is an extremely complex process. The cavitation jet might dynamically govern the depolymerization and reaggregation of soluble soybean protein oxidized accumulates through the transformation of the protein spatial structure.

Table 2. Secondary structure content of natural, oxidized soybean protein, and cavitation jet treated on soluble soybean protein oxidized accumulates at several times (2, 4, 6, 8, 10, and 15 min).

Content (%)	Anti-Parallel Intermolecular β-Sheet (β1)	Parallel Intermolecular β-Sheet (β2)	Intramolecular β-Sheet	α-Helix	β-Turn	γ-Random Coil
Wavenumber (cm^{-1})	1608–1622	1682–1700	1622–1637	1646–1662	1662–1681	1637–1645
SPI	9.27 ± 0.28 [d]	15.95 ± 0.23 [a]	18.41 ± 0.18 [a]	26.35 ± 0.18 [c]	21.33 ± 0.17 [f]	8.69 ± 0.15 [e]
OSPI	13.58 ± 0.19 [a]	7.16 ± 0.18 [f]	17.18 ± 0.13 [b]	17.82 ± 0.19 [d]	26.66 ± 0.20 [e]	17.41 ± 0.20 [a]
SOSPI	9.05 ± 0.26 [d]	9.74 ± 0.22 [b]	13.58 ± 0.25 [f]	27.84 ± 0.19 [a]	28.28 ± 0.18 [d]	10.51 ± 0.22 [b]
SCOSPI-2 min	11.28 ± 0.08 [c]	8.54 ± 0.26 [d]	13.38 ± 0.07 [g]	26.27 ± 0.08 [c]	30.61 ± 0.13 [b]	9.92 ± 0.17 [c]
SCOSPI-4 min	12.70 ± 0.10 [b]	7.84 ± 0.19 [e]	13.80 ± 0.26 [e]	24.52 ± 0.19 [e]	31.82 ± 0.02 [a]	9.32 ± 0.18 [d]
SCOSPI-6 min	12.77 ± 0.01 [b]	9.02 ± 0.25 [c]	13.58 ± 0.05 [f]	23.36 ± 0.04 [f]	31.92 ± 0.22 [a]	9.35 ± 0.06 [d]
SCOSPI-8 min	11.42 ± 0.19 [c]	9.83 ± 0.01 [b]	15.80 ± 0.19 [c]	22.72 ± 0.14 [g]	29.66 ± 0.22 [c]	10.57 ± 0.16 [b]
SCOSPI-10 min	12.78 ± 0.06 [b]	6.78 ± 0.22 [g]	13.70 ± 0.03 [ef]	26.68 ± 0.20 [b]	30.73 ± 0.24 [b]	9.33 ± 0.30 [d]
SCOSPI-15 min	13.51 ± 0.13 [a]	6.76 ± 0.05 [g]	15.36 ± 0.15 [d]	25.09 ± 0.06 [d]	29.79 ± 0.15 [c]	9.49 ± 0.18 [d]

Note: Comparisons were carried out between values of the same column; values with a different letter(s) indicate a significant difference at $p \leq 0.05$.

3.3. Fluorescence Emission Spectra

Fluorescence spectra can characterize the polarity changes of aromatic amino acids in the microenvironment, so as to predict alterations in the tertiary structure of soluble protein aggregates [35]. Figure 4 is the intrinsic fluorescence spectra of the soluble soybean protein oxidized aggregates. Compared with SPI, the fluorescence intensity of OSPI declined significantly and λmax was blue shifted. Compared with OSPI, the fluorescence intensity of SOSPI raised and λmax was red shifted. Free radicals in the oxidizing situation could induce the crosslinking, condensation, and nucleation of SPI, and then form the protein aggregation with a tighter structure [36]. Comparing the fluorescence spectrum of OSPI and SOSPI, we could find that the components with tighter structures in the OSPI components exist in insoluble oxidized aggregates. On the other hand, this showed that the change of the structural tightness degree could reflect the conformational change law of the transformation from a soluble protein to an insoluble protein. With the prolongation of the cavitation jet treatment time, SCOSPI λmax initially raised and then declined, and achieved the supreme when the treatment time was 6 min. This showed that the cavitation jet could alter the spatial structure of SCOSPI to regulate the functional activity. The cavitation jet could cleave and break some insoluble soybean protein oxidation aggregates and induce the creation of soluble oxidation accumulates with a loose structure and a larger particle size. This could cause the increase of the number and exposed degree of aromatic amino acid elements of SCOSPI; to show polar solute circumstances, a red move of λmax of SCOSPI was noted. However, with the further extension of the treatment time, some soluble oxidized aggregates of the soybean protein regrouped and transformed into insoluble aggregates, which were centrifuged, resulting in the reduction of the number of aromatic amino acid elements of SCOSPI [37]. In addition, the other soluble aggregates could form β1 structures and aggregate through covalent cross-linking and hydrophobic interaction in the collision, so that the aromatic amino acids of SCOSPI were buried in the structure [38]. Consequently, excessive cavitation jet treatment will, through this dual effect of aggregation and depolymerization together, cause the λmax of SCOSPI blue shift.

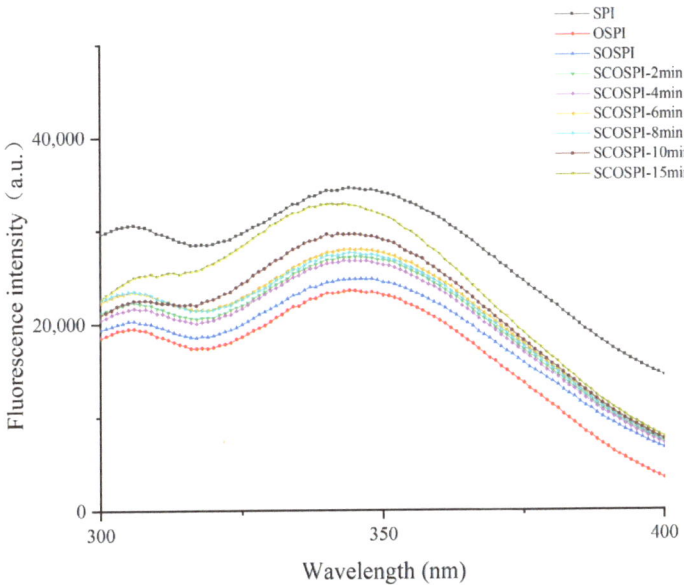

Figure 4. Fluorescence emission spectra of natural, oxidized soybean protein, and cavitation jet treated on soluble soybean protein oxidized accumulates at several times (2, 4, 6, 8, 10, and 15 min).

3.4. Sulfhydryl Content

SH/SS replacement reactions play a key role in protein accumulation, which can reproduce the impact of physical fields on the depolymerization mechanisms of protein. As shown in Table 3, the free sulfhydryl and total sulfhydryl quantity of OSPI decreased, and the disulfide bond quantity increased compared with SPI. However, compared with OSPI, the free sulfhydryl content of SOSPI rose, and the disulfide bond content decreased. The oxidation treatment could promote the creation of disulfide bonds via the disulfide/sulfhydryl switch reaction. More disulfide bonds reflect the tighter spatial structure of soybean protein, so that the oxidation increased the tightness of the soybean protein molecular space structure [39]. This showed that oxidation could adjust the compactness of the protein structure by changing the disulfide bond, thus affecting its functional activity [40]. In addition, the total sulfhydryl content was also decreasing, and the decay of free sulfhydryl quantity was higher than the raise of disulfide bond content, signifying that oxidation also had a non-reversible oxidation reaction on the soybean protein, inducing the transformation of free sulfhydryl into sulfur compounds without a disulfide bond [41]. For soluble components in OSPI, namely SOSPI, the disulfide bond quantity decreased. Combined with the results of the particle size and fluorescence emission spectra, the oxidized treatment diminished the particle size and amplified the fluorescence intensity of SOSPI, indicating that the oxidized masses of soybean protein after the oxidation treatment were mainly insoluble aggregates, and most of the soluble components show a small particle size and a loose and unfolded structure [40]. With the addition of the cavitation jet treatment time, the contents of free sulfhydryl, total sulfhydryl, and disulfide bonds of SCOSPI amplified first and then declined, but the processing time, corresponding to a maximum value of the three, is inconsistent. This is because there was more than one conversion reaction between free sulfhydryl and disulfide bonds in the system. The cavitation jet treatment could break the core aggregation skeleton of SCOSPI, destroy the intermolecular force and spatial structure, and induce the conversion of disulfide bonds into free sulfhydryl groups, resulting in the increase of the free sulfhydryl content of the soluble oxidized aggregates. At the identical time, combining with the increase particle size findings of SOSPI after the cavitation jet, cavitation could also promote the transformation from insoluble aggregates with high disulfide bonds content into soluble aggregates, so the number of soluble aggregates increased [42], which instigated the expansion of disulfide bond content and free sulfhydryl content of soluble oxidized aggregates. Nevertheless, when the cavitation jet treatment time was too long, high intensity, long-time cavitation, turbulence, and thermal effects would cause the re-aggregation of soluble aggregates and also cause the cracking of all accumulates, which was an irreversible denaturation for protein [43]. To be more specific, when the treatment time was maximized, the cavitation jet would destroy the spatial structure and intermolecular force of the oxidized aggregates, resulting in the reduction of the disulfide bond content, which is well matched with the finding of a decreased particle size. However, the free sulfhydryl groups, formed by the disulfide bond breaking in OSPI, would aggregate with each other to form SCOSPI with a tighter spatial structure, ending in a reduction in the quantity of free sulfhydryl groups. This is matched with the findings of FTIR spectroscopy and fluorescence emission spectra. At the same time, cavitation jet also induced the irreversible reaction of protein sulfhydryl groupings to generate the sulfur-comprising components with non-disulfide bonds. Moreover, the conversion of soluble oxidized aggregates to insoluble oxidized aggregates will also lead to the fluctuation of the disulfide bond and free sulfhydryl quantity. These factors together caused the reduction of free sulfhydryl and disulfide bond quantity. The inconsistent processing time, corresponding to the maximum value of the free sulfhydryl, total sulfhydryl, and disulfide bond, showed that the process of aggregation and depolymerization and the conversion between soluble and non-soluble was a very complex process and needs further research.

Table 3. Sulfhydryl content of natural, oxidized soybean protein, and cavitation jet treated on soluble soybean protein oxidized accumulates at several times (2, 4, 6, 8, 10, and 15 min).

Samples	Free Sulfhydryl (nmol/mg)	Total Sulfhydryl (nmol/mg)	Disulfide Bond (nmol mg^{-1})
SPI	11.72 ± 0.15 [a]	15.64 ± 0.32 [a]	1.96 ± 0.11 [c]
OSPI	4.05 ± 0.23 [h]	10.78 ± 0.14 [g]	3.37 ± 0.13 [a]
SOSPI	8.06 ± 0.22 [e]	10.99 ± 0.12 [f]	1.47 ± 0.16 [d]
SCOSPI-2 min	8.65 ± 0.17 [c]	11.95 ± 0.16 [e]	1.65 ± 0.17 [cd]
SCOSPI-4 min	8.92 ± 0.21 [b]	12.56 ± 0.18 [c]	1.82 ± 0.13 [c]
SCOSPI-6 min	8.87 ± 0.19 [bc]	13.29 ± 0.22 [b]	2.21 ± 0.15 [b]
SCOSPI-8 min	8.21 ± 0.14 [d]	12.15 ± 0.19 [d]	1.97 ± 0.16 [c]
SCOSPI-10 min	7.65 ± 0.16 [f]	10.69 ± 0.15 [g]	1.52 ± 0.16 [d]
SCOSPI-15 min	7.15 ± 0.18 [g]	10.07 ± 0.16 [h]	1.46 ± 0.19 [d]

Note: Comparisons were carried out between values of the same column; values with a different letter(s) indicate a significant difference at $p \leq 0.05$.

3.5. Transmission Electron Microscopy (TEM)

To better understand SPI and compare the differences among SPI, OSPI, SOSPI, and SCOSPI, the apparent morphology was visualized by TEM, as shown in Figure 5. Compared with SPI, the aggregation degree of OSPI was increased, and OSPI formed a dense network structure with intense central part. The skeleton structure of SOSPI mainly presented short and small wormlike structures. Oxidation led to the conformational changes of SPI and exposed the side chain groups of hydrophobic aliphatic and aromatic amino acids entrenched within, inducing cross-linking aggregation through hydrophobic interaction. Furthermore, they can also attack the sulfhydryl groups of proteins and convert them into disulfide bonds, showing insoluble protein accumulates with a large particle size and highly cross-linked clusters in OSPI [44]. However, SOSPI showed short rod protein molecules with a small particle size; this is because the proteins with a high degree of cross-linking were transformed into insoluble aggregates and removed by centrifugation [25], as the soluble components of the protein are mainly in the shape of short and small rods. With the increase of the cavitation jet treatment time from 2 min to 8 min, the aggregation degree of SCOSPI increased. Most of the protein aggregates heavily bonded, which consisted of agglomerated smaller worm-like particles, and the skeleton structure became larger and more branches appeared. This is well matched with the outcomes of the particle size and molecular weight. On the one hand, it might be because the cavitation jet broke the disulfide bond of the aggregates, and the insoluble aggregation with large, clustered morphology, resembling those of compact reticulation, was cracked. Then, the insoluble aggregation transformed into soluble aggregates, which led to the amplification of the number of soluble aggregates in the supernatant and presented a cluster structure. On the other hand, it might be that under the cavitation treatment, the fragmentation of the skeleton structure increased. This result promoted the mutual collision between soluble protein molecules and the binding probability of free sulfhydryl clusters, resulting in the enlargement and additional branches of the originally short rod-shaped skeleton structure [26]. However, with the further conservation of the cavitating jet treatment time, the mesh skeleton structure was seriously broken and gradually transformed into a short bar structure. When the treatment time reached 15 min, the mesh structure disappeared, and the skeleton structure presented a slender bar. Combined with the above results, the cavitation jet has the dual effects of breaking and reassembling the protein skeleton structure. In addition, it also induces a mutual transformation between the soluble and insoluble aggregates. Therefore, the long-time cavitation jet can induce the soluble aggregates to transform into insoluble aggregates and be removed by centrifugation, and decrease the content of the soluble aggregates. In addition, under high temperatures, great pressure, and the shear force conditions of the long-time cavitation jet, the skeleton structure of the protein was broken. These two works together resulted in the decrease of the cementation and intercross network structure of the soluble aggregates, and the formation of a small and slender skeleton structure.

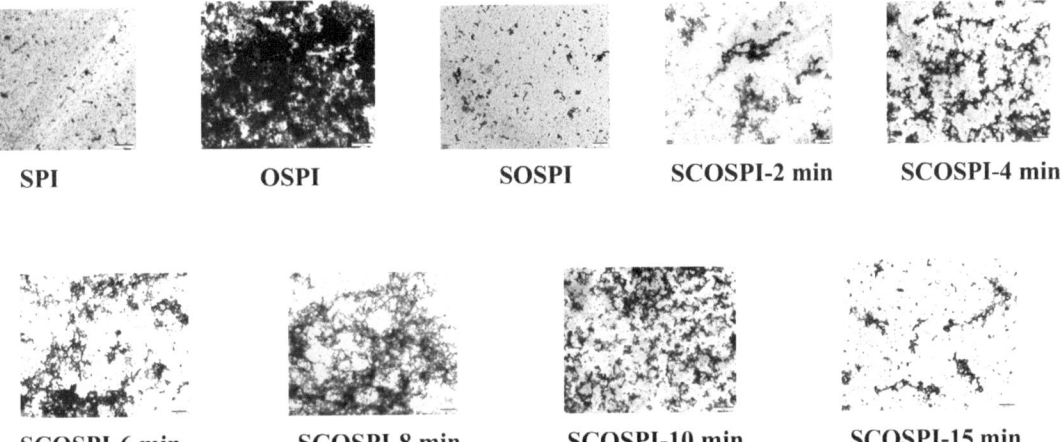

Figure 5. Backbone structure of natural, oxidized soybean protein, and cavitation jet treated on soluble soybean protein oxidized accumulates at several times (2, 4, 6, 8, 10, and 15 min).

3.6. Emulsion Capacity and Stability

Due to its good emulsifying activity, proteins are usually used in food emulsions and artificial fats. However, emulsifying features differ both on the capability of the protein adsorbed on the oil droplet superficially and the protein intermolecular binding, and it is related to the shape, size, and superficial hydrophobicity of the protein molecules [45]. The EAI and ESI of the emulsions stabilized by the soluble soybean protein oxidized accumulates are shown in Table 4. The oxidization treatment decreased the EAI and ESI of emulsions steadied by OSPI and SOSPI. In addition, the EAI of SOSPI was superior to that of SPI, but the ESI was relatively inferior. The oxidation treatment could form a highly ordered intermolecular β-sheet between proteins, which were poor supports to the flexible body. The molecular flexibility of OSPI decreased and formed insoluble oxidized aggregates whose structure is difficult to relax, resulting in the reduction of protein interface activity and the decline of the binding ability between the protein and oil, which induced the EAI and ESI of OSPI, inferior than that of SPI [46]. However, compared with the OSPI, the SOSPI contained abundant free sulfhydryl groups and short worm-like skeleton structures. In the process of forming the emulsions, the SOSPI moved to the interface in smaller particle size aggregates, which increased the exchange area between the protein and the oil–water interface and made SOSPI easier to absorb and relax at the interface, so that the EAI of SOSPI were higher than that of OSPI. Nevertheless, it is difficult for proteins with a miniature particle size to adsorb stably on the interface for a long time, resulting in a decrease of the ESI of SOSPI.

Table 4. Emulsion capacity and solidity of natural, oxidized soybean protein, and cavitation jet treated on soluble soybean protein oxidized accumulates at several times (2, 4, 6, 8, 10, and 15 min).

Samples	EAI/(m^2·g^{-1})	ESI/min
SPI	91.61 ± 1.17 [a]	186.19 ± 3.89 [a]
OSPI	46.97 ± 2.24 [g]	137.20 ± 3.51 [e]
SOSPI	89.92 ± 2.37 [a]	126.75 ± 3.18 [f]
SCOSPI-f-2 min	57.17 ± 1.89 [f]	149.08 ± 3.15 [d]
SCOSPI-f-4 min	71.92 ± 1.91 [e]	156.24 ± 2.89 [c]
SCOSPI-f-6 min	86.24 ± 2.39 [b]	163.17 ± 2.68 [b]
SCOSPI-f-8 min	81.64 ± 2.64 [c]	152.56 ± 3.37 [cd]
SCOSPI-f-10 min	76.95 ± 2.19 [d]	147.89 ± 2.90 [d]
SCOSPI-f-15 min	72.68 ± 2.64 [e]	140.27 ± 3.64 [e]

Note: Comparisons were carried out between values of the same column; values with a different letter(s) indicate a significant difference at $p \leq 0.05$.

With the extension of the cavitation jet treatment time, the EAI and ESI of SOSPI initially amplified and then declined, and achieved the highest when the cavitation jet treatment time was 6 min. The high pressure, shear, and cavitation effects shaped by the cavitating jet could cleave oxidized aggregates and induce some insoluble aggregates to change into soluble aggregates, so that the content of the soluble protein accumulates increased. The cavitation jet could also abolish the intermolecular binding of SCOSPI, and the structure of SCOSPI is altered. These two results result in the amplification of the number of exterior hydrophobic parties and polar groups, particle size, and molecular flexibility of SCOSPI to improve the emulsifying activity and emulsifying constancy [47]. Additionally, the intercross networks structure, cross-connected by the protein, were useful in the creation of the emulsion [48]. Combined with the TEM results, it can be found that after the cavitation jet treatment, the mesh skeleton structure of SCOSPI became larger than was beneficial to the formation and stability of the emulsion. However, when the cavitation jet treating time exceeded 6 min, the long-time high temperature, pressure, and shear force produced by cavitation jet impacted the hydrophilic and hydrophobic clusters and interior binding of the protein molecules, which unfavored the aptitude of SCOSPI to adsorb at the oil–water interface. In addition, during the long time cavitation jet, the SCOSPI gradually formed a small molecular protein with a more highly ordered β-sheet structure, difficult relaxation, and low molecular flexibility, resulting in the reduction of the emulsifying activity and emulsifying stability of SCOSPI [49].

3.7. Confocal Laser Scanning Microscope (CLSM)

The CLSM was utilized to explore the fluctuations in the microstructure of the soybean protein emulsion after pretreating it with the cavitation jet, as displayed in Figure 6. The green fluorescence in CLSM micrographs signified the protein piece, the red fluorescence represented the soybean oil, and the vivid yellow fluorescence signified the proteins adsorbed on the oil droplets. The small spherical droplets were evenly distributed throughout the emulsion system, which was prepared from SPI. After the oxidation treating, the flocculation of the emulsion dewdrops prepared from OSPI and SOSPI were serious, and the red areas in the unceasing phase increased significantly and gathered on the surface of emulsion droplets, showing the phenomenon of oil–water separation. The oil–water separation of OSPI was more serious than SOSPI. The oxidative treatment caused the accumulation and solubility of the protein molecules to decrease, causing difficulty for the formation of steady interfacial film in the emulsification procedure, thus showing a red oil droplet accretion area in a large aggregation area [50]. Nevertheless, compared with OSPI, the particle size and skeleton structure of SOSPI were smaller, and it had better adsorption ability at the oil–water interface. Most of the oil droplets are encapsulated in the emulsion droplets prepared by SCOSPI, and there was only a small-scale accumulation of red oil droplets. This shows that macromolecules and insoluble protein oxidation aggregates formed during the oxidation were the key to causing significant decline in emulsifying activity. Therefore, regulating the macromolecules and insoluble proteins aggregates could improve the function activity of OSPI.

During the treatment of the cavitation jet, the green area of the emulsion prepared with SCOSPI in the CLSM image increased gradually, and the red area gradually decreased and showed the wrapped state in the green area, and a steady protein interfacial film was shaped at the oil–water interface. The cavitation jet treatment could induce the insoluble oxidation aggregates, which are difficult to relax at the interface, to transform into soluble aggregates with smaller steric hindrance and a more flexible structure, as well as to expand the adsorption, relaxation, and reordering effects of SCOSPI at the interface, so as to improve the steadiness of the oil–water interface [51]. In addition, the number of surface hydrophobic groups and polar groups in SCOSPI were increased, which promoted additional protein molecules to be adsorbed at the oil–water interface to produce a steadier interfacial film, and could improve the interfacial activity and emulsifying features [52,53]. Therefore, the proteins discolored green were consistently and firmly spread across the oil droplets that efficiently avoided coalescence. However, with the further delay of the cavitation jet treatment time, in the CLSM images of the emulsion prepared by SCOSPI, the red area of oil increased gradually, and the green area of the protein was mainly concentrated. Excessive cavitation jet treatment would increase the content of the anti-parallel intermolecular β-sheet, surface hydrophobicity, and ζ-potential reduction of SCOSPI, and the specific surface area declined, which was not encouraging for distribution to crossing and extension on the oil–water interface [54]. Finally, the binding capacities of SCOSPI to oil were weakened, resulting in the increase of free oil droplets and serious oil–water separation. A cavitation jet can affect the flocculation and stability of the emulsion by regulating the transformation between insoluble and soluble aggregates.

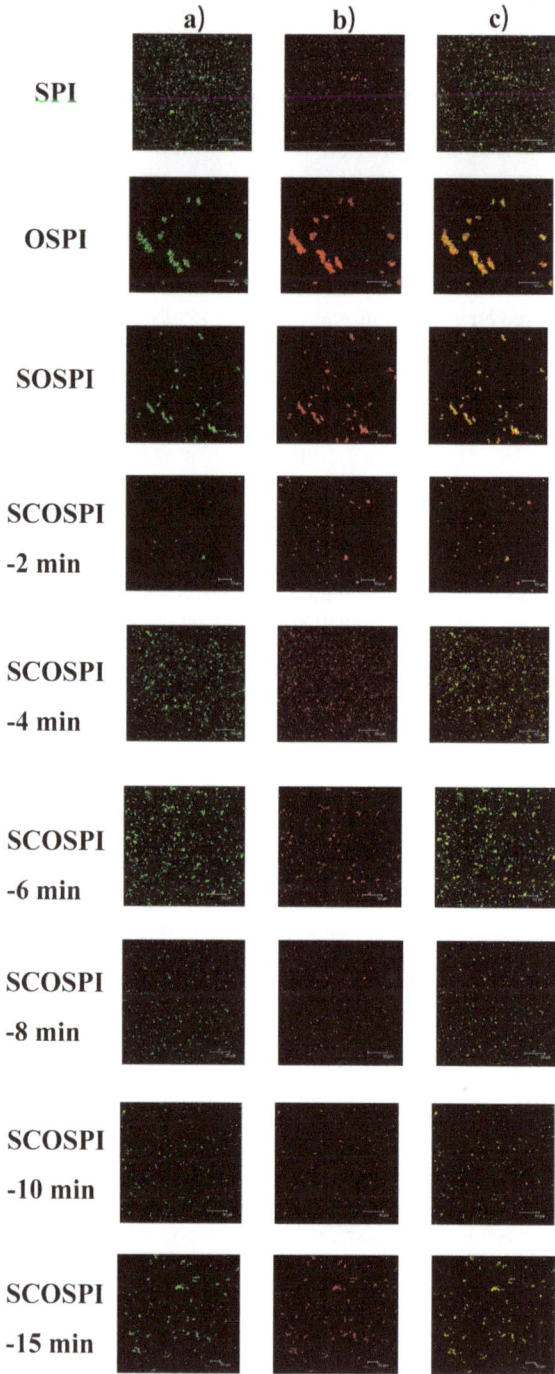

Figure 6. CLSM micrographs of natural, oxidized soybean protein, and cavitation jet treated on soluble soybean protein oxidized accumulates at several times (2, 4, 6, 8, 10, and 15 min). Note: (**a**) represents the proteins, (**b**) represents the oil droplets, and (**c**) represents the proteins adsorbed on the oil droplet.

3.8. Quantity of Adsorbed Proteins at Interface (AP%)

The quantity of the adsorbed proteins at the interface has a key impact on the constancy of the emulsion. The higher interfacial protein amount, the stronger capability of protein adsorption to the oil–water interface [55]. As shown in Figure 7, the AP% of the emulsion made by OSPI and SOSPI decreased compared with SPI, and the AP% of the emulsion made by SOSPI was lower than OSPI. It is generally considered that proteins undergo a certain amount of structural extension and relaxation when dissolved in an aqueous solution [56]. The more flexible the structure of the proteins, the better it is for structural expansion and the more prone they are to bulk diffusion, adsorption at the interface, unfolding, and rearrangement, inducing the increase of AP% [57]. During oxidation, the level of protein accumulation creased, and the structural flexibility of highly clustered OSPI was reduced and its rigidity was enhanced, which was not favorable to the expansion and adsorption at the interface, resulting in the decrease of AP% [58]. In addition, the decrease of AP% might be largely ascribed to the fabrication of the bridged emulsions, e.g., two particular oil droplets allocated an identical protein particle layer, facilitated by the oxidization-induced aggregation of SPI [59]. At the time of the formulation of the emulsion, large molecules can be transported to the oil–water interface in preference to small molecules because of the convective mass transport effect of high-pressure homogenization, i.e., large molecules can adsorb more quickly than small molecules [60]. Compared with OSPI, SOSPI had a small particle size and low molecular weight, which affected the protein adsorption ratio to the oil–water interface, subsequent in lower AP% [61]. However, the protein with a small particle size, low molecular weight, and a high solubility contributes to improving the connection region with the oil–water interface and the affinity of protein to the interface; foremost there was only a small-scale accumulation of red oil droplets in the emulsion prepared by SOSPI. Therefore, the AP% is not the only consideration in deciding the characteristics of emulsion.

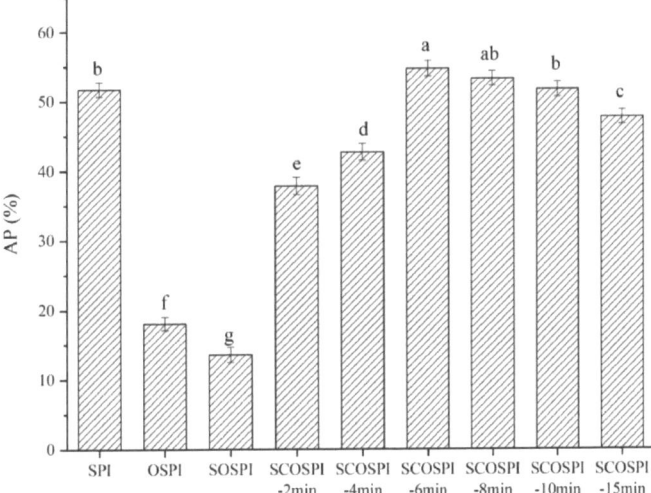

Figure 7. AP% of emulsions of natural, oxidized soybean protein, and cavitation jet treated on soluble soybean protein oxidized accumulates at several times (2, 4, 6, 8, 10, and 15 min). Note: Values with a different letter(s) indicate a significant difference at $p \leq 0.05$.

With the expansion of the cavitation jet treatment time, the AP% of SCOSPI boosted first and then diminished, and touched the highest when the treatment time was 6 min. The high-velocity turbulent flow, high-speed shearing, and large pressure produced by the cavitation jet acted on cross-linked aggregates to realize the transformation from insoluble aggregates to soluble aggregates and directional regulation for amorphous soluble aggregation, which improved the soluble protein content and molecular flexibility of the soluble proteins. It promoted more proteins with structural relaxation and overall flexibility to be adsorbed, unfolded, and rearranged at the interface. Then, it enhanced the AP% of the emulsion prepared by SCOSPI, and increased to interfacially prepare and bulk stabilize the oil–water systems [62]. Nevertheless, when the cavitation jet treating time was too long, the majority of the soluble protein components were dominated by a small molecular weight and particle size protein molecules, and the content of β1 in SCOSPI was increased, designating that the content of the methodical structure augmented and that the structure was relatively tight and complex, which was not favorable for the adsorption and unfolding of protein at the oil–water interface and the formation of a dense interface interfacial film. These results together led to the decrease of AP% of emulsion prepared by SCOSPI [63].

3.9. Interfacial Tension

A key element in the investigation and analysis of emulsion stability is the interfacial tension at the liquid–liquid interface, which can also describe the exterior activity of proteins at the oil–water interface [64]. As shown in Figure 8, the interfacial tension of the emulsion prepared with natural soy protein was 21.29 mN/m. After the oxidation treatment, the interfacial tension of the emulsions made by OSPI and SOSPI were raised, and SOSPI was higher than OSPI. The oxidation treatment would promote a protein aggregate to form insoluble oxidation aggregates with a larger particle size, low molecular flexibility, and poor solubility [39]. In addition, the exact surface region of the protein molecules was reduced, and the steric hindrance was increased, which were not beneficial to the adsorption and reordering of protein at the oil–water interface, resulting in an increase in the protein interfacial tension [65]. The soluble components in SOSPI were more easily dissolved in the water phase, the particle size was lesser, and the ordered structure was greater. The ability to form stable interfacial film was significantly reduced, resulting in a higher interfacial tension and lower emulsion stability.

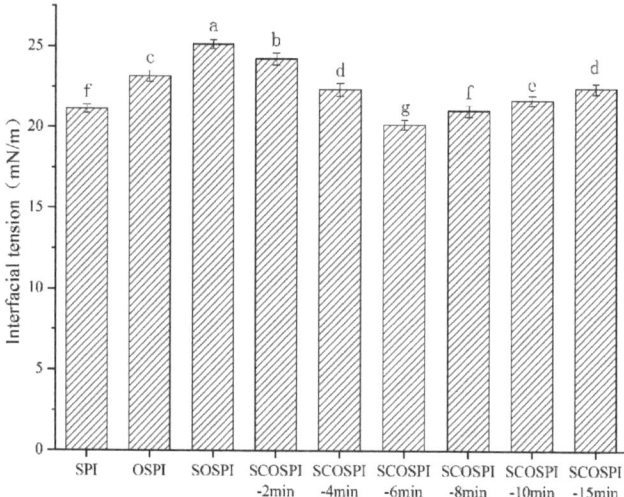

Figure 8. Interfacial tension of emulsions of natural, oxidized soybean protein, and cavitation jet treated on soluble soybean protein oxidized accumulates at several times (2, 4, 6, 8, 10, and 15 min). Note: Values with a different letter(s) indicate a significant difference at $p \leq 0.05$.

After the cavitation jet treatment, the interfacial tension of SCOSPI decreased first and was then amplified, achieving the bottom when the treatment time was 6 min. Combined with the results of the particle distribution and TEM, it could be seen that the particle size of SCOSPI increased and the protein skeleton widened, indicating that the cavitation jet could break the insoluble soybean protein oxidation aggregate and transform it into soluble oxidation aggregate, resulting in the increase of hydrophobic clusters of soluble protein components and a more complex conformational space [53]. Protein molecules were not easily soluble in the aqueous phase, which improved the expansion and reordering of the protein molecules at the interface and declined the interfacial tension [66]. However, when the cavitation jet treatment time was too long, the quantity of β1 increased and the γ-random coil (Table 2) decreased. Additionally, particle size (Table 1) was reduced and soluble oxidized aggregates with a more orderly structure and lower molecular flexibility were formed, with the result that adsorption energy barricaded at the boundary was higher, and the adsorption efficacy was decreased. This affected the adsorption and evolving of the protein at the oil–water interface and caused an increase of interfacial tension [67]. Combined with the results of EAI, ESI, CLSM, and AP%, we can find that when the cavitation jet treatment was 6 min, the soluble soybean protein oxidized aggregates showed the best emulsification interface characteristics. This provided a simple and effective technology for the application of soybean protein in the food industry.

3.10. Viscoelastic Properties

Rheological quantities deliver evidence on the physical performance and steadiness of lotion [68]. Elastic modulus G' is a measurement of elasticity and signifies the storing modulus of the energy of stress that could be reinstated when the stress is liberated, while the viscous modulus G'' signifies the viscous substances, which assumes the flow defiance of the sample [69,70]. G' and G'' of emulsion are shown in Figure 9. Both the elastic modulus (G') and viscous modulus (G'') gradually amplified within the oscillation frequency range. In all samples, the G' was superior to the G'' and exhibited an elastic character. It showed that the protein on the interface formed a viscoelastic adsorbed film and suggested an elastic network structure of emulsion. The G' and G'' of the emulsion formulated by OSPI were both higher than SPI, while the SOSPI showed the opposite results. The rheological features of the interface layer were mainly impacted by the hydrophobic interaction and disulfide bonds among proteins adsorbed at the oil–water interface [71]. After the oxidation treatment, the quantity of the disulfide bonds in the protein aggregates increased significantly. In addition, under the hydrophobic interaction, they were bound to the proteins that have been adsorbed on the interface layer. Therefore, the formation of the oxidative aggregates enhanced the binding between protein molecules at the interface, thus amending the interfacial elastic modulus of the emulsion prepared by OSPI. However, the soluble soybean protein aggregates were transformed into insoluble oxidized aggregates after the oxidation treatment. The soluble components with smaller molecular proteins were more likely to dissolve in the water phase and were unable to shape a protein-bound film, resulting in a decline in G' and G'' of emulsion equipped by SOSPI [72].

With the cavitation jet treatment, the G' of the emulsion fabricated by SCOSPI increased first and then declined, and the G'' presented no obvious change. With the delay of cavitation jet treatment time, the skeleton of soluble oxidized aggregates became wider, the particle size was larger, the exposure of hydrophilic and lipophilic groups in components raised, the electrostatic revulsion among emulsion droplets was also amplified, the protein content adsorbed on the oil–water interface layer was more and more, and the thickness of the interfacial film slowly augmented, subsequent to the increase of interfacial elastic modulus. When the cavitation jet treating time was maximized, the SCOSPI through β1 would form protein aggregates with a high aggregation degree, small particle size, and weak reticular structure, which had negative impacts on the interface activity and resulted in the decrease of G' [73,74].

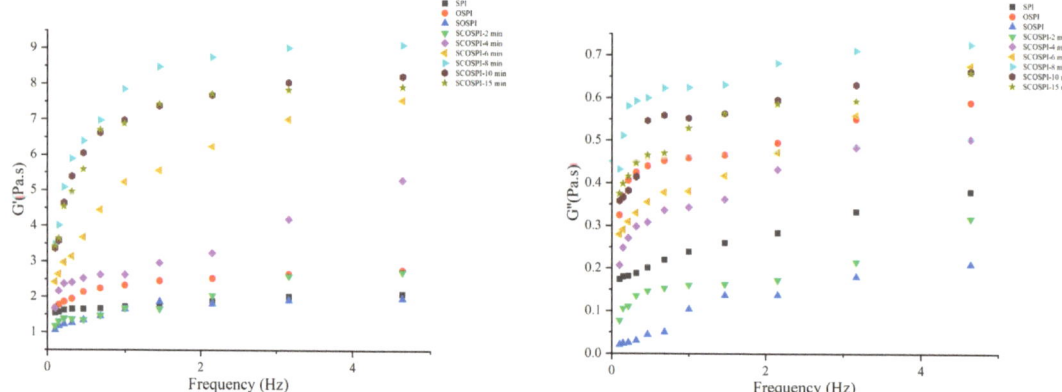

Figure 9. Viscoelastic properties of natural, oxidized soybean protein, and cavitation jet treated on soluble soybean protein oxidized accumulates at several times (2, 4, 6, 8, 10, and 15 min).

3.11. Apparent Viscosity

Figure 10 and Table 5 depict the emulsions' rheological behavior. All the emulsions' flow curves could be matched with Sisko's model. With flow performance indices fluctuating from 0.059 to 0.271, all the emulsions displayed shear-thinning behavior. Intermolecular bindings among aggregated molecules, which result in the creation of weak transient networks, may be the motive of shear-thinning actions for the stabilized emulsions [65]. Emulsions steadied by OSPI exhibited a higher ostensible viscosity and K than those stabilized by SPI, but those steadied by SOSPI had an inverse relationship between their apparent viscosity and K. The volume proportion of the dispersed phase and the size of the combinations created from the proteins determined the rheological parameters of the emulsion. The higher the number and size of these masses, the higher the viscosity [75,76]. This led to a higher initial apparent viscosity in the emulsion made from oxidized soy protein aggregates. After the oxidation process, the initially soluble oxidized aggregates eventually changed into insoluble oxidized aggregates. A reduction in the K and apparent viscosity resulted from the remaining soluble components, which were primarily made up of tiny protein molecules that tended to dissolve in the aqueous phase and enclose oil droplets [42,77,78]. The ostensible viscosity and K of the emulsion produced by SCOSPI grew initially and subsequently dropped with the length of the cavitation jet treatment time. Particle size and TEM results show that an effective cavitation jet treatment could encourage the conversion of insoluble aggregates into soluble aggregates, increase the particle size and skeleton structure of soluble soybean protein oxidation masses, and ultimately, increase the ostensible viscosity and K of the emulsion created by SCOSPI. However, the prolonged cavitation jet treating period might lead to an increase in insoluble aggregates that were unfavorable to the steadiness of the emulsion, lowering K and its apparent viscosity. By modifying the structure and content of the soy protein soluble oxidized accumulates and controlling the reciprocal transformation of protein constituents, the cavitation jet treatment can alter the rheological characteristics of the emulsion.

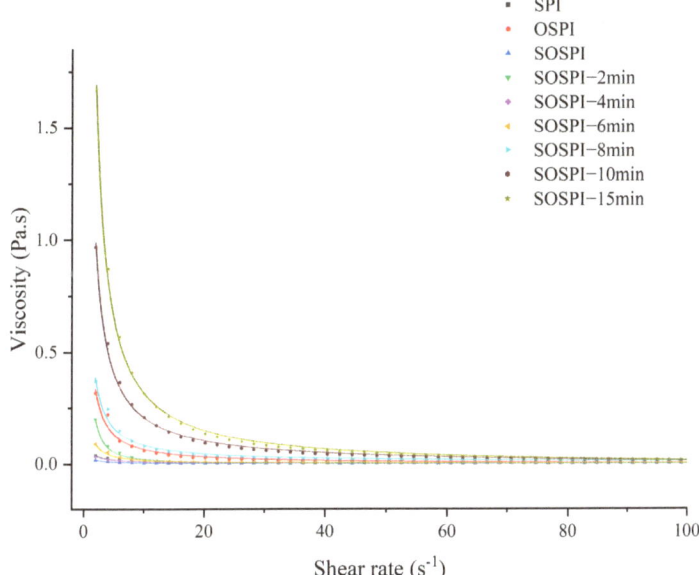

Figure 10. Apparent viscosity and shear rate relationship of emulsions of natural, oxidized soybean protein, and cavitation jet treated on soluble soybean protein oxidized accumulates at several times (2, 4, 6, 8, 10, and 15 min).

Table 5. Fitting result of Sisko's model of emulsion of natural, oxidized soybean protein, and cavitation jet treated on soluble soybean protein oxidized accumulates at several times (2, 4, 6, 8, 10, and 15 min).

Samples	K (Pa·s^n)	n	R^2
SPI	0.066	0.271	0.99
OSPI	0.626	0.059	0.99
SOSPI	0.021	0.169	0.99
SCOSPI-2 min	0.539	0.183	0.99
SCOSPI-4 min	1.380	0.216	0.99
SCOSPI-6 min	2.673	0.219	0.99
SCOSPI-8 min	3.343	0.173	0.99
SCOSPI-10 min	3.123	0.154	0.99
SCOSPI-15 min	2.676	0.152	0.99

Note: The K signifies the consistency index. The n signifies the behavior index.

4. Conclusions

Oxidized treatment influenced the structure of the SOSPI, causing a decline in their emulsifying properties and interfacial features. A cavitation jet at a short treating time can break the insoluble soybean protein oxidation aggregate and transform it into a soluble oxidation aggregate, causing the expansion of particle size, protein skeleton, and disulfide bond content. This also improved the emulsion activity and state of SOSPI and raised the quantity of adsorbed proteins at the interface while decreasing the interfacial tension of the emulsion. A long cavitation jet treatment time could induce the soluble oxidized aggregate to gradually form a small molecular weight protein with difficult relaxation and low molecular flexibility, which were not favorable to the solidity of emulsion, resulting in the decrease of EAI, ESI, apparent viscosity, K, and an increase of interfacial tension.

Author Contributions: Y.G.: Conceptualization, Software, Writing-original draft. C.L.: Data curation. Y.W.: Investigation, Writing. S.R.: Visualization. X.Z.: Methodology. J.Z.: Investigation. T.C.: Investigation. Z.G.: Supervision. Z.W.: Funding acquisition, Project administration. All authors have read and agreed to the published version of the manuscript.

Funding: This research was funded by The National Natural Science Foundation, grant number "32202228"; National key R&D plan, grant number "2021YFD2100401"; National key R&D plan, grant number "2022YFF1100603"; Heilongjiang Province key R&D plan, grant number "GA21D001"; Heilongjiang Province Major Achievements Transformation Project, grant number "CG19A002"; China Fund on the surface of a postdoctoral project, grant number "2022M721995" and Heilongjiang Province million project, grant number "2021ZX12B02".

Data Availability Statement: The data presented in this study are available on request from the corresponding author.

Acknowledgments: The authors would like to thank the National Natural Science Foundation [32202228], the National key R&D plan [2021YFD2100401], the National key R&D plan [2022YFF1100603], the Heilongjiang Province key R&D plan [GA21B001] the Heilongjiang Province Major Achievements Transformation Project [CG19A002], the China Fund on the surface of a postdoctoral project [2022M721995], and the Heilongjiang Province million project [2021ZX12B02] for the support.

Conflicts of Interest: The authors declare no conflict of interest.

References

1. Boerma, H.R. *Managing Inputs for Peak Production*; American Society of Agronomy, Crop Science Society of America, and Soil Science Society of America: Madison, WI, USA, 2004; pp. 15–20.
2. Caponio, G.R.; Wang, H.; Ciaula, A.D.; Angelis, M.; Portincasa, P. Molecular Sciences Regulation of Cholesterol Metabolism by Bioactive Components of Soy Proteins: Novel Translational Evidence. *Int. J. Mol. Sci.* **2020**, *22*, 227. [CrossRef] [PubMed]
3. He, L.; Han, M.; Qiao, S.; He, P.; Li, D.; Li, N.; Ma, X. Soybean Antigen Proteins and their Intestinal Sensitization Activities. *Curr. Protein Pept. Sci.* **2015**, *16*, 613–621. [CrossRef] [PubMed]
4. Botta, G.F.; Antille, D.L.; Nardon, G.F.; Rivero, D.; Bienvenido, F.; Contessotto, E.E.; Ezquerra-Canalejo, A.; Ressia, J.M. Zero and controlled traffic improved soil physical conditions and soybean yield under no-tillage. *Soil Tillage Res.* **2022**, *215*, 105235. [CrossRef]
5. Yuan, C.A.; Yuan, C.B.; Xg, A.; Yc, A. Effect of 2,2′-azobis(2-amidinopropane) dihydrochloride (AAPH) induced oxidation on the physicochemical properties, in vitro digestibility, and nutritional value of egg white protein. *LWT Food Sci. Technol.* **2021**, *143*, 111103.
6. Hinderink, E.; Schrder, A.; Sagis, L.; Schron, K.; Berton-Carabin, C.C. Physical and oxidative stability of food emulsions prepared with pea protein fractions. *LWT Food Sci. Technol.* **2021**, *146*, 111424. [CrossRef]
7. Shi, R.; Li, T.; Li, M.; Munkh-Amgalan, G.; Jiang, Z. Consequences of dynamic high-pressure homogenization pretreatment on the physicochemical and functional characteristics of citric acid-treated whey protein isolate. *LWT Food Sci. Technol.* **2021**, *136*, 110303. [CrossRef]
8. Keerati-U-Rai, M.; Corredig, M. Effect of Dynamic High Pressure Homogenization on the Aggregation State of Soy Protein. *J. Agric. Food Chem.* **2009**, *57*, 3556–3562. [CrossRef]
9. Cao, H.; Sun, R.; Shi, J.; Li, M.; Guan, X.; Liu, J.; Huang, K.; Zhang, Y. Effect of ultrasonic on the structure and quality characteristics of quinoa protein oxidation aggregates. *Ultrason. Sonochemistry* **2021**, *77*, 105685. [CrossRef]
10. Zhang, Y.; Di, R.; Zhang, H.; Zhang, W.; Yang, C. Effective recovery of casein from its aqueous solution by ultrasonic treatment assisted foam fractionation: Inhibiting molecular aggregation. *J. Food Eng.* **2020**, *284*, 110042. [CrossRef]
11. Chi, H.; Li, G.; Liao, H.; Tian, S.; Song, X. Effects of parameters of self-propelled multi-orifice nozzle on drilling capability of water jet drilling technology. *Int. J. Rock Mech. Min. Sci.* **2016**, *86*, 23–28. [CrossRef]
12. Mitroglou, N.; Stamboliyski, V.; Karathanassis, I.K.; Nikas, K.S.; Gavaises, M. Cloud cavitation vortex shedding inside an injector nozzle. *Exp. Therm. Fluid Sci.* **2017**, *84*, 179–189. [CrossRef]
13. He, M.; Wu, C.; Li, L.; Zheng, L.; Teng, F. Effects of Cavitation Jet Treatment on the Structure and Emulsification Properties of Oxidized Soy Protein Isolate. *Foods* **2020**, *10*, 2. [CrossRef] [PubMed]
14. Wu, W.; Wu, X.; Hua, Y. Structural modification of soy protein by the lipid peroxidation product acrolein. *LWT Food Sci. Technol.* **2010**, *43*, 133–140. [CrossRef]
15. Ma, W.; Wang, J.; Xu, X.; Qin, L.; Wu, C.; Du, M. Ultrasound treatment improved the physicochemical characteristics of cod protein and enhanced the stability of oil-in-water emulsion. *Food Res. Int.* **2019**, *121*, 247–256. [CrossRef]
16. Tang, C.H.; Ma, C.Y. Effect of high pressure treatment on aggregation and structural properties of soy protein isolate. *LWT Food Sci. Technol.* **2009**, *42*, 606–611. [CrossRef]
17. Jiang, L.; Wang, J.; Li, Y.; Wang, Z.; Liang, J.; Wang, R.; Chen, Y.; Ma, W.; Qi, B.; Zhang, M. Effects of ultrasound on the structure and physical properties of black bean protein isolates. *Food Res. Int.* **2014**, *62*, 595–601. [CrossRef]
18. Wu, D.; Wu, C.; Wang, Z.; Fan, F.; Chen, H.; Ma, W.; Du, M. Effects of high pressure homogenize treatment on the physicochemical and emulsifying properties of proteins from scallop (Chlamys farreri). *Food Hydrocoll.* **2019**, *94*, 537–545. [CrossRef]

19. Keppler, J.K.; Heyn, T.R.; Meissner, P.M.; Schrader, K.; Schwarz, K. Protein oxidation during temperature-induced amyloid aggregation of beta-lactoglobulin. *Food Chem.* **2019**, *289*, 223–231. [CrossRef] [PubMed]
20. Pearc, K.N.; Kinsella, J.E. Emulsifying properties of proteins: Evaluation of a turbidimetric technique. *J. Agric. Food Chem.* **1978**, *26*, 716–723. [CrossRef]
21. Liang, H.N.; Tang, C.H. pH-dependent emulsifying properties of pea [Pisum sativum (L.)] proteins. *Food Hydrocoll.* **2013**, *33*, 309–319. [CrossRef]
22. Sun, X.D.; Arntfield, S.D. Gelation properties of myofibrillar/pea protein mixtures induced by transglutaminase crosslinking. *Food Hydrocoll.* **2012**, *27*, 394–400. [CrossRef]
23. Wang, S.; Yang, J.; Shao, G.; Qu, D.; Zhao, H.; Yang, L.; Zhu, L.; He, Y.; Liu, H.; Zhu, D. Soy protein isolated-soy hull polysaccharides stabilized O/W emulsion: Effect of polysaccharides concentration on the storage stability and interfacial rheological properties. *Food Hydrocoll.* **2020**, *101*, 105490. [CrossRef]
24. Ye, L.; Liao, Y.; Zhao, M.; Sun, W. Effect of Protein Oxidation on the Conformational Properties of Peanut Protein Isolate. *J. Chem.* **2013**, *2013*, 423254. [CrossRef]
25. Shen, L.; Tang, C.H. Microfluidization as a potential technique to modify surface properties of soy protein isolate. *Food Res. Int.* **2012**, *48*, 108–118. [CrossRef]
26. Oliete, B.; Potin, F.; Cases, E.; Saurel, R. Modulation of the emulsifying properties of pea globulin soluble aggregates by dynamic high-pressure fluidization. *Innov. Food Sci. Emerg. Technol.* **2018**, *47*, 292–300. [CrossRef]
27. Guo, Y.; Li, B.; Cheng, T.; Hu, Z.; Liu, S.; Liu, J.; Sun, F.; Guo, Z.; Wang, Z. Effect of cavitation jet on the structural, emulsifying properties and rheological properties of soybean protein-oxidised aggregates. *Int. J. Food Sci. Technol.* **2022**, *58*, 343–354. [CrossRef]
28. Sarroukh, R.; Goormaghtigh, E.; Ruysschaert, J.M.; Raussens, V. ATR-FTIR: A "rejuvenated" tool to investigate amyloid proteins. *BBA Biomembr.* **2013**, *1828*, 2328–2338. [CrossRef] [PubMed]
29. Xia, W.; Zhang, H.; Chen, J.; Hu, H.; Rasulov, F.; Bi, D.; Huang, X.; Pan, S. Formation of amyloid fibrils from soy protein hydrolysate: Effects of selective proteolysis on β-conglycinin. *Food Res. Int.* **2017**, *100*, 268–276. [CrossRef]
30. Fan, S.; Guo, J.; Wang, X.; Liu, X.; Chen, Z.; Zhou, P. Effects of lipoxygenase/linoleic acid on the structural characteristics and aggregation behavior of pork myofibrillar protein under low salt concentration. *LWT Food Sci. Technol.* **2022**, *161*, 113359. [CrossRef]
31. Li, F.; Wang, B.; Kong, B.; Shi, S.; Xia, X. Decreased gelling properties of protein in mirror carp (Cyprinus carpio) are due to protein aggregation and structure deterioration when subjected to freeze-thaw cycles. *Food Hydrocoll.* **2019**, *97*, 105223. [CrossRef]
32. Xu, Y.; Silva, W.; Qian, Y.; Gray, S.M. An aromatic amino acid and associated helix in the C-terminus of the potato leafroll virus minor capsid protein regulate systemic infection and symptom expression. *PLoS Pathog.* **2018**, *14*, e1007451. [CrossRef] [PubMed]
33. Phillips, L.G. Introduction to Functional Properties of Proteins. In *Structure–Function Properties of Food Proteins*; Academic Press: Cambridge, MA, USA, 1994; pp. 107–109.
34. Boora, K.A.; Amarjeet, K.; Kumar, K.S.; Nitin, M. Characterization of heat-stable whey protein: Impact of ultrasound on rheological, thermal, structural and morphological properties. *Ultrason. Sonochemistry* **2018**, *49*, 333–342.
35. Viseu, M.I.; Carvalho, T.I.; Costa, S. Conformational Transitions in β-Lactoglobulin Induced by Cationic Amphiphiles: Equilibrium Studies. *Biophys. J.* **2004**, *86*, 2392–2402. [CrossRef] [PubMed]
36. Zhang, Y.; Yang, R.; Zhang, W.; Hu, Z.; Zhao, W. Structural characterization and physicochemical properties of protein extracted from soybean meal assisted by steam flash-explosion with dilute acid soaking. *Food Chem.* **2017**, *219*, 48–53. [CrossRef] [PubMed]
37. Siddique, M.A.B.; Maresca, P.; Pataro, G.; Ferrari, G. Influence of pulsed light treatment on the aggregation of whey protein isolate. *Food Res. Int.* **2017**, *99*, 419–425. [CrossRef] [PubMed]
38. Evangelho, J.A.; Vanier, N.L.; Pinto, V.Z.; Berrios, J.J.; Dias, A.R.; Zavareze, E.R. Black bean (Phaseolus vulgaris L.) protein hydrolysates: Physicochemical and functional properties. *Food Chem.* **2017**, *214*, 460–467. [CrossRef] [PubMed]
39. Li, F.; Wu, X.; Wu, W. Effects of protein oxidation induced by rice bran rancidity on the structure and functionality of rice bran glutelin. *LWT Food Sci. Technol.* **2021**, *149*, 111874. [CrossRef]
40. Platt, A.A.; Gieseg, S.P. Inhibition of protein hydroperoxide formation by protein thiols. *Redox Rep.* **2003**, *8*, 81–86. [CrossRef]
41. Morzel, M.; Gatellier, P.; Sayd, T.; Renerre, M.; Laville, E. Chemical oxidation decreases proteolytic susceptibility of skeletal muscle myofibrillar proteins. *Meat Sci.* **2006**, *73*, 536–543. [CrossRef]
42. Guo, Z.; Huang, Z.; Guo, Y.; Li, B.; Yu, W.; Zhou, L.; Jiang, L.; Teng, F.; Wang, Z. Effects of high-pressure homogenization on structural and emulsifying properties of thermally soluble aggregated kidney bean (Phaseolus vulgaris L.) proteins. *Food Hydrocoll.* **2021**, *119*, 106835. [CrossRef]
43. Liu, C.M.; Zhong, J.Z.; Liu, W.; Tu, Z.C.; Wan, J.; Cai, X.F.; Song, X.Y. Relationship between Functional Properties and Aggregation Changes of Whey Protein Induced by High Pressure Microfluidization. *J. Food Sci.* **2011**, *76*, 341–347. [CrossRef]
44. Chen, N.; Zhao, M.; Sun, W.; Ren, J.; Cui, C. Effect of oxidation on the emulsifying properties of soy protein isolate. *Food Res. Int.* **2013**, *52*, 26–32. [CrossRef]
45. Jing, X.; Zijing, C.; Dong, H.; Yangyang, L.; Xiaotong, S.; Zhongjiang, W.; Hua, J. Structural and Functional Properties Changes of β-Conglycinin Exposed to Hydroxyl Radical-Generating Systems. *Molecules* **2017**, *22*, 1893.
46. Zhang, H.J.; Zhang, H.; Wang, L.; Guo, X.N. Preparation and functional properties of rice bran proteins from heat-stabilized defatted rice bran. *Food Res. Int.* **2012**, *47*, 359–363. [CrossRef]

47. Wu, C.; He, M.; Zheng, L.; Tian, T.; Teng, F.; Li, Y. Effect of cavitation jets on the physicochemical properties and structural characteristics of the okara protein. *J. Food Sci.* **2021**, *86*, 4566–4576. [CrossRef]
48. Li, T.; Wang, L.; Chen, Z.; Sun, D.; Li, Y. Electron beam irradiation induced aggregation behaviour, structural and functional properties changes of rice proteins and hydrolysates. *Food Hydrocoll.* **2019**, *97*, 105192. [CrossRef]
49. Fu, Z.; Popov, V. The ACA–BEM approach with a binary-key mosaic partitioning for modelling multiple bubble dynamics. *Eng. Anal. Bound. Elem.* **2015**, *50*, 169–179. [CrossRef]
50. Li, X.; Cheng, Y.; Yi, C.; Hua, Y.; Yang, C.; Cui, S. Effect of ionic strength on the heat-induced soy protein aggregation and the phase separation of soy protein aggregate/dextran mixtures. *Food Hydrocoll.* **2009**, *23*, 1015–1023. [CrossRef]
51. Sha, L.; Koosis, A.O.; Wang, Q.; True, A.D.; Xiong, Y.L. Interfacial dilatational and emulsifying properties of ultrasound-treated pea protein. *Food Chem.* **2021**, *350*, 129271. [CrossRef]
52. Cheng, Y.; Donkor, P.O.; Ren, X.; Wu, J.; Agyemang, K.; Ayim, I.; Ma, H. Effect of ultrasound pretreatment with mono-frequency and simultaneous dual frequency on the mechanical properties and microstructure of whey protein emulsion gels. *Food Hydrocoll.* **2019**, *89*, 434–442. [CrossRef]
53. Hu, H.; Wu, J.; Li-Chan, E.C.Y.; Zhu, L.; Zhang, F.; Xu, X.; Fan, G.; Wang, L.; Huang, X.; Pan, S. Effects of ultrasound on structural and physical properties of soy protein isolate (SPI) dispersions. *Food Hydrocoll.* **2013**, *30*, 647–655. [CrossRef]
54. Stathopulos, P.B.; Scholz, G.A.; Hwang, Y.M.; Rumfeldt, J.A.O.; Lepock, J.R.; Meiering, E.M. Sonication of proteins causes formation of aggregates that resemble amyloid. *Protein Sci.* **2010**, *13*, 3017–3027. [CrossRef] [PubMed]
55. Izmailova, V.N.; Yampolskaya, G.P.; Tulovskaya, Z.D. Development of the Rehbinder's concept on structure-mechanical barrier in stability of dispersions stabilized with proteins. *Colloids Surf. A Physicochem. Eng. Asp.* **1999**, *160*, 89–106. [CrossRef]
56. Graham, D.E.; Phillips, M.C. Proteins at liquid interfaces: III. Molecular structures of adsorbed films. *J. Colloid Interface Sci.* **1979**, *70*, 427–439. [CrossRef]
57. Damodaran, S.; Razumovsky, L. Role of surface area-to-volume ratio in protein adsorption at the air–water interface. *Surf. Sci.* **2008**, *602*, 307–315. [CrossRef]
58. Delahaije, R.; Wierenga, P.A.; Nieuwenhuijzen, N.V.; Giuseppin, M.; Gruppen, H. Protein concentration and protein-exposed hydrophobicity as dominant parameters determining the flocculation of protein-stabilized oil-in-water emulsions. *Langmuir ACS J. Surf. Colloids* **2013**, *29*, 11567–11574. [CrossRef]
59. Peng, L.P.; Xu, Y.T.; Li, X.T.; Tang, C.H. Improving the emulsification of soy β-conglycinin by alcohol-induced aggregation. *Food Hydrocoll.* **2019**, *98*, 105307. [CrossRef]
60. Nilsson, L.; Leeman, M.; Wahlund, K.G.; Bergenståhl, B. Competitive adsorption of a polydisperse polymer during emulsification: Experiments and modeling. *Langmuir ACS J. Surf. Colloids* **2007**, *23*, 2346–2351. [CrossRef] [PubMed]
61. Wang, J.M.; Xia, N.; Yang, X.Q.; Yin, S.W.; Qi, J.R.; He, X.T.; Yuan, D.B.; Wang, L.J. Adsorption and dilatational rheology of heat-treated soy protein at the oil-water interface: Relationship to structural properties. *J. Agric. Food Chem.* **2012**, *60*, 3302–3310. [CrossRef]
62. Alizadeh, V.; Amirkhizi, A. Modeling of Cavitation Erosion Resistance in Polymeric Materials Based on Strain Accumulation. 2019, Volume 2. Available online: https://www.researchgate.net/publication/326959965_Modeling_of_Cavitation_Erosion_Resistance_in_Polymeric_Materials_Based_on_Strain_Accumulation (accessed on 5 February 2023).
63. Yang, J.; Liu, G.; Zeng, H.; Chen, L. Effects of high pressure homogenization on faba bean protein aggregation in relation to solubility and interfacial properties. *Food Hydrocoll.* **2018**, *83*, 275–286. [CrossRef]
64. Qiu, H.; Chen, X.; Wei, X.; Liang, J.; Zhou, D.; Wang, L. The Emulsifying Properties of Hydrogenated Rosin Xylitol Ester as a Biomass Surfactant for Food: Effect of pH and Salts. *Molecules* **2020**, *25*, 302. [CrossRef]
65. Dapueto, N.; Troncoso, E.; Mella, C.; Zúñiga, R. The effect of denaturation degree of protein on the microstructure, rheology and physical stability of oil-in-water (O/W) emulsions stabilized by whey protein isolate. *J. Food Eng.* **2019**, *263*, 253–261. [CrossRef]
66. Fu, L.; Tang, C.H. Soy glycinin as food-grade Pickering stabilizers: Part. I. Structural characteristics, emulsifying properties and adsorption/arrangement at interface. *Food Hydrocoll.* **2016**, *60*, 606–619.
67. Sakuno, M.M.; Matsumoto, S.; Kawai, S.; Taihei, K.; Matsumura, Y. Adsorption and structural change of beta-lactoglobulin at the diacylglycerol-water interface. *Langmuir* **2008**, *24*, 11483–11488. [CrossRef] [PubMed]
68. Nurazwa, I.; Ahmad, L.; Rosfarizan, M.; Arbakariya, A.; Mohd, M.; Murni, H.; Helmi, W. Kinetics and Optimization of Lipophilic Kojic Acid Derivative Synthesis in Polar Aprotic Solvent Using Lipozyme RMIM and Its Rheological Study. *Molecules* **2018**, *23*, 501.
69. Antonio, L.; Annalisa, C.; Nunzio, D.; Mara, P.; Rosa, I.; Elisabetta, F.; Angela, L.; Nicoletta, D.; Modesto, D.C.; Massimo, F. Delivery of Proapoptotic Agents in Glioma Cell Lines by TSPO Ligand–Dextran Nanogels. *Int. J. Mol. Sci.* **2018**, *19*, 1155.
70. Toledo, L.; Ramos, M.; Silva, P.; Rodero, C.F.; Bauab, T.M. Improved in vitro and in vivo Anti-Candida albicans Activity of Cymbopogon nardus Essential Oil by Its Incorporation into a Microemulsion System. *Int. J. Nanomed.* **2020**, *15*, 10481–10497. [CrossRef] [PubMed]
71. Li, Y. *A Study on the Rheology and Fiber Extrusion of Polyacrylonitrile Gel*; Auburn University: Auburn, AL, USA, 2003.
72. Bos, M.A.; Vliet, T.V. Interfacial rheological properties of adsorbed protein layers and surfactants: A review. *Adv. Colloid Interface Sci.* **2001**, *91*, 437–471. [CrossRef] [PubMed]
73. Zhang, Z.; Regenstein, J.M.; Zhou, P.; Yang, Y. Effects of high intensity ultrasound modification on physicochemical property and water in myofibrillar protein gel. *Ultrason. Sonochemistry* **2017**, *34*, 960–967. [CrossRef] [PubMed]

74. Qin, X.S.; Chen, S.S.; Li, X.J.; Luo, S.Z.; Zhong, X.Y.; Jiang, S.T.; Zhao, Y.Y.; Zheng, Z. Gelation Properties of Transglutaminase-Induced Soy Protein Isolate and Wheat Gluten Mixture with Ultrahigh Pressure Pretreatment. *Food Bioprocess Technol.* **2017**, *10*, 866–874. [CrossRef]
75. Pal, R.; Yan, Y.; Masliyah, J. Advances in Food Rheology and Its Applications. *Rheol. Emuls.* **1992**, *12*, 437–457.
76. Walstra, P. Food emulsions: Principles, practice, and techniques. *Trends Food Sci. Technol.* **2001**, *36*, 223–224. [CrossRef]
77. Guo, Z.; Teng, F.; Huang, Z.; Lv, B.; Lv, X.; Babich, O.; Yu, W.; Li, Y.; Wang, Z.; Jiang, L. Effects of material characteristics on the structural characteristics and flavor substances retention of meat analogs. *Food Hydrocoll.* **2020**, *105*, 105752. [CrossRef]
78. Guo, Y.; Wang, Z.; Hu, Z.; Yang, Z.; Liu, J.; Tan, B.; Guo, Z.; Li, B.; Li, H. The temporal evolution mechanism of structure and function of oxidized soy protein aggregates. *Food Hydrocoll.* **2022**, *15*, 100382. [CrossRef] [PubMed]

Disclaimer/Publisher's Note: The statements, opinions and data contained in all publications are solely those of the individual author(s) and contributor(s) and not of MDPI and/or the editor(s). MDPI and/or the editor(s) disclaim responsibility for any injury to people or property resulting from any ideas, methods, instructions or products referred to in the content.

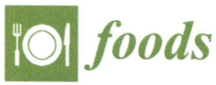

Article

The Molecular Mechanism of Yam Polysaccharide Protected H_2O_2-Induced Oxidative Damage in IEC-6 Cells

Mingyue Shen, Ruixin Cai, Zhedong Li, Xiaodie Chen and Jianhua Xie *

State Key Laboratory of Food Science and Technology, Nanchang University, Nanchang 330047, China
* Correspondence: jhxie@ncu.edu.cn; Tel.: +86-0791-8830-4347

Abstract: Oxidative stress is involved in maintaining homeostasis of the body, and an in-depth study of its mechanism of action is beneficial for the prevention of chronic illnesses. This study aimed to investigate the protective mechanism of yam polysaccharide (CYP) against H_2O_2-induced oxidative damage by an RNA-seq technique. The expression of genes and the function of the genome in the process of oxidative damage by H_2O_2 in IEC-6 cells were explored through transcriptomic analysis. The results illustrated that H_2O_2 damaged cells by promoting cell differentiation and affecting tight junction proteins, and CYP could achieve cell protection via restraining the activation of the MAPK signaling pathway. RNA-seq analysis revealed that H_2O_2 may damage cells by promoting the IL-17 signaling pathway and the MAPK signaling pathway and so forth. The Western blot showed that the pretreatment of CYP could restrain the activation of the MAPK signaling pathway. In summary, this study demonstrates that the efficacy of CYP in modulating the MAPK signaling pathway against excessive oxidative stress, with a corresponding preventive role against injury to the intestinal barrier. It provides a new perspective for the understanding of the preventive role of CYP on intestinal damage. These findings suggest that CYP could be used as oxidation protectant and may have potential application prospects in the food and pharmaceutical industries.

Keywords: intestinal barrier; yam polysaccharide; RNA-seq; oxidative damage; signaling pathways

Citation: Shen, M.; Cai, R.; Li, Z.; Chen, X.; Xie, J. The Molecular Mechanism of Yam Polysaccharide Protected H_2O_2-Induced Oxidative Damage in IEC-6 Cells. *Foods* **2023**, *12*, 262. https://doi.org/10.3390/foods12020262

Academic Editor: Antonio Cilla

Received: 30 November 2022
Revised: 31 December 2022
Accepted: 3 January 2023
Published: 6 January 2023

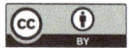

Copyright: © 2023 by the authors. Licensee MDPI, Basel, Switzerland. This article is an open access article distributed under the terms and conditions of the Creative Commons Attribution (CC BY) license (https://creativecommons.org/licenses/by/4.0/).

1. Introduction

Oxidative stress is a response of the body's cells and tissues to stimuli that increase reactive oxygen species and free radicals, resulting in the dysregulation of the intracellular oxidative–oxidative system [1]. When oxidative stress occurs in cells, the expressions of superoxide dismutase, catalase, and glutathione peroxidase in the body are significantly altered. Meanwhile, the harmful superoxide anion generated is catalyzed to H_2O_2, which is further decomposed into water and molecular oxygen [2,3]. Oxidative stress also disrupts the intestinal environmental balance and changes intestinal permeability, giving rise to intestinal damage and triggering a range of intestinal diseases [4]. Stress response can induce intestinal cells to produce ROS metabolites in quantity, lipid peroxidation, protein denaturation, cell apoptosis, and, ultimately, resulting in intestinal mucosal damage and inflammatory intestinal diseases [5].

Irritation of the gastrointestinal tract by multiple factors can lead to gastrointestinal dysfunction, which is one of the most vulnerable systems [6]. The intestinal barrier is considered to be the first line of defense against host invasion by pathogens [7]. Imbalances in the gut microbiome and impaired intestinal mucosal barrier have been linked to damage from inflammation, oxidative stress, and various systemic diseases, such as inflammatory bowel disease (IBD), irritable bowel syndrome (IBS), liver fibrosis, diabetic nephropathy, lupus nephritis, and sepsis [8,9]. H_2O_2 is naturally present in various cells of the body and also stimulates cells by oxidative stress that occurs with the body, and excess H_2O_2 will disrupt the oxidative–antioxidant balance within the cells, giving rise to the production of ROS [10], altering the permeability of intestinal cells, as well as decreasing the intestinal barrier function [9]. There are many studies investigating the activation of related proteins on intracellular signaling pathways via Western blot technique, but there are few reports on the expression of intracellular tight junction proteins in intestinal epithelial cells in response to some stimuli, and the intracellular signaling pathway activation pathways are still not clear.

Polysaccharides extracted from yams by water extraction and alcohol precipitation methods have biological effects, such as antitumor, antioxidant, and modulating immune activity [11,12]. In vitro antioxidant activity of floral mushroom polysaccharides showed that they scavenged 79.46% and 74.18% of DPPH and hydroxyl radicals (OH), respectively [13]. The effect of yam polysaccharides on I-type diabetic mice has also been reported, and after treatment with yam polysaccharides, the reactive oxygen species and malondialdehyde (MDA) content in diabetic mice were reduced, indicating that yam polysaccharides have antioxidant effects in diabetic mice, thus validly guarding against multifarious complications of diabetes [14]. In addition, yam polysaccharides can reduce DPPH radicals, hydroxyl radicals, and superoxide radicals' production so as to promote endometrial epithelial cell proliferation [15,16]. However, the recent studies on the antioxidant activity of yam polysaccharides mainly focused on the scavenging ability of free radicals in vitro, while the role of oxidative damage at the cellular level is still less and the mechanism of action has not been reported. Therefore, to explore the protective effect of yam polysaccharides against oxidative damage from the cellular level is need.

RNA-Sequencing (RNA-seq) is regarded as a new method to analyze gene functions and interactions at the histological level, and the current RNA-seq method can determine the expression levels of all most genes, which has been broadly used in frontier fields, such as molecular biology [17,18]. Wang et al. [19] analyzed the resistance of periplaneta Americana peptide to human ovarian granulosa cell apoptosis under hydrogen peroxide poisoning, and RNA-seq analysis showed that activation of IL-6 trans-signaling pathway in retinal endothelial cells caused gene expression changes. In addition, the combined RNA-seq and cytobiology techniques illustrated that Cyclocarya paliurus polysaccharide has protective effects against H_2O_2-induced oxidative damage in L02 cells and regulates mitochondrial function, oxidative stress, and PI3K/Akt and MAPK signaling pathways [20].

This study aimed to probe the underlying molecular mechanism of CYP against H_2O_2-induced oxidative lesions and the protective role on the gut barrier by transcriptomic sequencing technology based on the IEC-6 cell model.

2. Materials and Methods

2.1. Reagents

Fresh yams (Dioscoreae Rhizoma) were purchased from Jiujiang, Jiangxi, China. Fetal bovine serum (FBS) was obtained from Viva cell Biosciences Ltd. (Shanghai, China). Dulbecco's modified eagle medium (DMEM) was purchased from Solarbio (Beijing, China). Antibodies were gained from Cell Signaling Technology (USA). The IEC-6 cell line was purchased from the Cell Bank of the Chinese Academy of Sciences (Shanghai, China).

2.2. Preparation of CYP

We weighed 300 g of yam powder and added 6 L of ultrapure water in the ratio of 1:20. Then, we stirred while heating at 80 °C, centrifuged, and concentrated the mixture to 1/10 of the original volume. Then, we added 95% ethanol and precipitated the mixture 4 °C overnight. The next day, the precipitate was redissolved and treated with glycosylase, α-amylase, and papain after adjusting the pH of the solution to 4.5 and 6.5, respectively. Finally, the Sevage method was used to deproteinization, followed by dialysis in a dialysis bag (retention capacity of 8000–14,000 Da). The dialyzed solution was lyophilized after secondary alcohol precipitation with anhydrous ethanol to obtain the crude polysaccharide [21,22]. The contents of carbohydrate, uronic acid, and protein were 33.62%, 34.95%, and 5.26%, respectively, and the molecular weight was 20.89 kDa [23].

2.3. Cell Culture

IEC-6 cells in good growth condition were taken and inoculated in 6-well plates at a cell density of 2×10^5 cells/mL for subsequent experiments. Cells were pretreated with different concentrations of CYP for 24 h after cell apposition, and the polysaccharide samples were incubated with the configured H_2O_2 solution for 4 h. Groups were divided as follows: Blank control group—cells were cultured daily with medium containing 10% FBS; Model group—cells were cultured with medium containing 10% FBS and treated with 300 µmol/L H_2O_2 solution on the last day; Low-concentration polysaccharide group—treated with 200 µg/mL of yam polysaccharide solution for 24 h, followed by 300 µmol/L of H_2O_2 solution; Medium-concentration polysaccharide group—treated with 400 µg/mL of yam polysaccharide solution for 24 h, followed by 300 µmol/L of H_2O_2 solution; and High-concentration polysaccharide group—treated with 800 µg/mL of yam polysaccharide solution for 24 h, followed by 300 µmol/L of H_2O_2 solution.

2.4. RNA-Seq Analysis

Total RNA was collected and purified from cell samples using the Trizol reagent kit (Invitrogen, Carlsbad, CA, USA) on the grounds of the manufacturer's certificate, and subsequent library preparation and sequencing was performed at Shanghai Personal Biotechnology (Shanghai, China). RNA-seq libraries were identified using an Agilent 2100 Bioanalyzer (Agilent Technologies, Palo Alto, CA, USA) to evaluate the quality of the RNA. Appropriate libraries were sequenced on the Illumina NextSeq500 platform (Illumina, San Diego, CA, USA).

Read Count values were statistically compared to each gene using HTSeq as the benchmark for gene expression. DESeq was used to analyze the difference of gene expression, and $|\log2$ fold change$| > 1$ and $p < 0.05$ were selected as the condition of screening differentially expressed genes (DEGs). In Gene Ontology (GO) analysis, topGO was used to map the DEGs to their specific directed acyclic graphs (DAGs) structure, and the intensity of the color depended on the enrichment fraction. Then, the P-value was estimated by a super geometric allocation method to calculate the p-value (significant enrichment is defined as $p < 0.05$) to recognize GO terms that were apparently enriched in differential genes in comparison with the entire genomic background, and thus determined the primary biological effect exercised by the differential genes. KEGG enrichment analysis was executed with the cluster-profiler where the gene list and gene number of each pathway were estimated through the differential genes annotated in the KEGG pathway, and then the P-value was calculated by the hypergeometric allocation method (the criterion for significant enrichment was $p < 0.05$) to pick out the target genes. The KEGG pathways that are significantly enriched in differential genes contrast with the gross genomic background are then used to identify the major biological functions executed via the differential genes.

2.5. Inhibition of MAPKs Using Specific Inhibitors

PD98059 is a potent and selective ERK inhibitor that specifically inhibits MAPK kinase activation in both in vivo and in vitro experiments [24,25]. In order to judge if the activating effect of CYP on IEC-6 cells is via the MAPK signaling pathway, the PD98059 inhibitor was added to DMEM medium and configured as a 10 µM solution. The configured ERK inhibitor solution was added an hour prior to the addition of H_2O_2 damage to the cells. The proteins in the cells were extracted at the end of H_2O_2 damage and Western blot was applied to estimate the expression of the relevant proteins.

2.6. Western Blot Analysis

Western and IP Cell Lysis Solution were used for lysing cells at $-20\ °C$ and then the lysate was transferred to an EP tube and centrifuged (4 °C, 10,000 r/min, 8 min.) After centrifugation, the supernatant was collected and the protein concentration was estimated with the BCA kit in line with the procedure, followed by the addition of SDS-PAGE loading buffer (6×) and denaturation at 95 °C for 5 min. After the electrophoresis, the gel was cut out at the destination position according to the molecular weight, indicated by the marker. The electrode was covered and sent to the membrane transfer apparatus to transfer the membrane at 25 V for 7 min. After the transfer, the protein strips were cut according to the experimental purpose, submerged in the blocking solution (5% BSA), and shaken at room temperature for 1 h. The target primary antibody was selected for overnight incubation, and the secondary antibody was added after three washes with TBST for 15 min each time on the next day. Eventually, target protein bands were captured and photographed by chemiluminescence imaging system.

2.7. Statistical Analysis

All experimental values are from at least three tinning sessions and data were expressed as mean ± standard deviation (SD). Differences among data mean values were tested for statistical significance at the $p < 0.05$ level using One-way ANOVA analysis of variance by SPSS 17.0 (SPSS Inc., Chicago, IL, USA).

3. Results and Discussion

3.1. Purity and Quality of Isolated RNA

The quality of the resulting RNA was evaluated by agarose gel electrophoresis. The total RNA electrophoresis bands of the samples were clear, with a total of three bands, from large to small, 28S, 18S, and 5S, with decreasing brightness. The 28S band was brighter than the 18S band (Figure 1), which was twice as bright, while 5S was very light, in normal condition, without obvious trailing and smears, with good RNA integrity and no significant degradation of mRNA. The results mentioned met the requirements of the subsequent experiments and could be carried out in the next step.

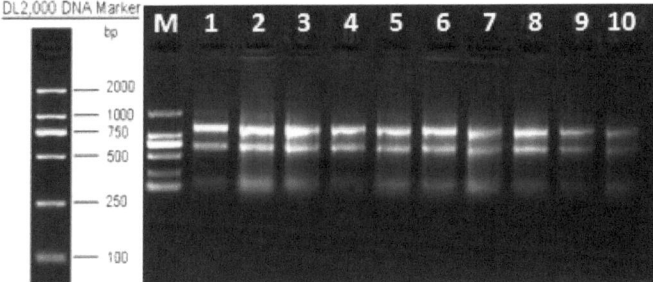

Figure 1. Determination of total RNA quality.

3.2. Expression Difference Result Statistics

RNA-seq is broadly applied to study molecular mechanisms associated with the pharmacological activity of natural drugs' polysaccharides [26,27]. Figure 2A shows the differential gene values in the form of bar graphs. In the blank control group compared with the CYP group, it identified 2637 gene sequences and the up-regulated genes consisted of 1563 and the down-regulated ones were 1074; in the model group compared with the CYP group, it identified 1407 differentially expressed genes, of which the up-regulated genes consisted of 358 and the down-regulated ones were 1049; in comparison to blank and model groups, there were 3712 differential gene sequences, of which 2630 were upwardly adjusted and 1082 were downgraded. The heat map shown in Figure 2B is expressed at the gene level, with one sample in each column, with red for highly expressed genes and blue for low-expressed genes. Due to the similarity of gene expression mode, gene sequence samples can be clustered for analysis. It can be seen that the correlation coefficients are greater than 0.9 for samples within the same group and less than 0.8 for samples between different groups (Figure 2C), indicating good sample parallelism between groups. On the basis of results of the one-way analysis of variance (ANOVA), the Wayne plot was able to calculate the number of unique differential genes shared between the comparable groups. The number of genes differing among the comparison groups and the overlapping relationship among the comparison groups were indicated. In the Venn diagram (Figure 2D), it can be seen that there are the same 417 differentially expressed genes in the three two-by-two comparisons.

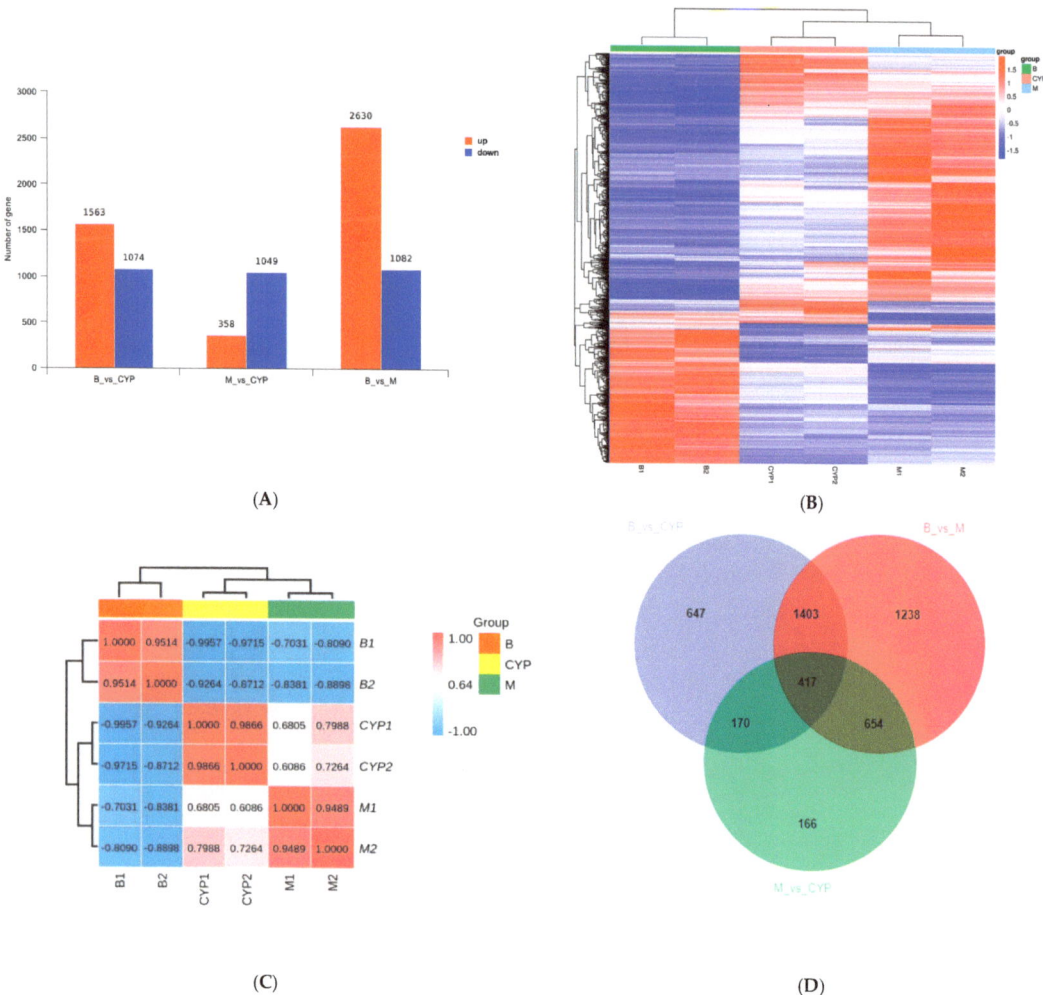

Figure 2. Changes in the mRNA expression profile of IEC-6 cells induced by H_2O_2 after CYP pre-treatment. (**A**) Statistics of differentially expressed genes between groups. (**B**) DEGs thermogram representation between groups. (**C**) Correlation test between groups. (**D**) Venn diagram between groups.

3.3. Functional Prediction Analysis by GO Enrichment

GO enrichment analysis starts by mapping all DEGs into each term of the GO database, using the whole genome as the background, subsequently calculating the *P*-value by hypergeometric distribution algorithm to determine the GO term, which is prominently captured in differential genes within the whole genome background, thereby ascertaining the biological effect represented by the differential genes [28]. The regulatory role of CYP on IEC-6 cells is still unclear at the transcriptome level. Figure 3B–D showed the classification of biological processes (BP), molecular functions (MF), and cellular components (CC) on the grounds of sequencing analysis, respectively. GO function analysis revealed 26 BP terms, 20 MF terms, and 18 CC terms in the DEGs.

The functional groups that changed significantly in terms of model group and control group were the development of anatomical structures, course of development, development of multicellular organisms, cell differentiation, processes of cell development, system development, positive regulation of biological processes, and protein binding. The functional groups that changed significantly in the CYP group were the development of multicellular organisms, system development, development of anatomical structures, course of development, regulatory signals, regulation of cell communication, the developmental processes, cell differentiation, development of animal organs, regulation of responses to stimuli, regulation of signal transduction, negative regulation of biochemical reactions, movement in motor cells or subcellular components, protein binding, positive regulation of biochemical reactions, signal transduction regulation, and cell differentiation. The functional groups that changed remarkably in the CYP group compared to the model group were the development of anatomical structures, cell developmental processes, system development, development of multicellular organisms, cell differentiation, regulation of multicellular biological processes, bio-adhesion, cell adhesion, cell surface receptor signaling pathways, regulation of cell differentiation, regulation of multicellular biological development, and metal ion transport activity across membranes (Figure 3A). The above sequencing data indicates that CYP can regulate the mechanism of oxidative damage in IEC-6 cells.

3.4. Signaling Pathway Analysis by KEGG Enrichment

The KEGG database integrates genomic, biochemical information, and signal pathways condition in one, using the pathway mapping process to link the genome to life as a reference [19]. To identify H_2O_2-induced signaling pathways activated by IEC-6 cells, the quantity of DEGs in the KEGG analysis were calculated. KEGG analysis was confirmed with bubble plots showing the top 20 canonical pathways.

The pathways that changed significantly in the model group compared to the control group were IL-17 signaling pathway, tumor necrosis factor, MAPK, and cAMP signaling pathways, cytokine receptor interactions, endocrine resistance and atherosclerosis, TGF-beta pathway, and FoxO. The pathways that changed more significantly in CYP were tumor necrosis factor, neuro glioma, MAPK, p53, PI3K-Akt, IL-17, cytokine–cytokine receptor interaction, HIF-1, FoxO, calcium signaling pathways, cellular senescence, and cell cycle. The functional groups that changed remarkably in the CYP group in comparison to the model group were tumor necrosis factor signaling pathway, IL-17 signaling pathway, protein digestion and absorption, cytokine–cytokine receptor interaction, cGMP-PKG signaling pathway, and mineral uptake. The MAPK pathway was significantly changed in the control group compared with both the model group and CYP group (Figure 4). Therefore, the above results indicated that CYP may make sense in protecting cells from oxidative damage by affecting MAPK signaling pathway subsequent validation from the MAPK pathway as proposed.

3.5. Effect of ERK Inhibitor on MAPK Pathway of H_2O_2-Induced Oxidative Damage in IEC-6 Cells

Our preceding study has illustrated that the phosphorylated expression of three proteins, JNK, ERK, and P38, in the MAPK pathway activated by H_2O_2 was significantly reduced in the presence of CYP, which was able to inhibit the activation of the MAPK pathway [23]. In consequence, to bear out that activating the MAPK signaling pathway in RNA-seq results, ERK inhibitor (PD98059) was added before treating the cells with H_2O_2. Compared with the H_2O_2 group, pretreatment with ERK inhibitor was effective in reducing the ratios of p-ERK to ERK, p-P38 to P38, and p-JNK to JNK, and the phosphorylation content of both JNK and ERK proteins' gray value was declined by the co-treatment of ERK inhibitor with CYP, but not as strongly as CYP alone (Figure 5). Our results indicated that the combination of ERK inhibitor with CYP did not have an enhanced inhibitory effect, which may be due to the negative effect of the addition of PD98059 on the protective effect of CYP. According to the above results, CYP has a similar effect to ERK inhibitors in declining the expression of protein phosphorylation and inhibiting the activation of MAPK pathway.

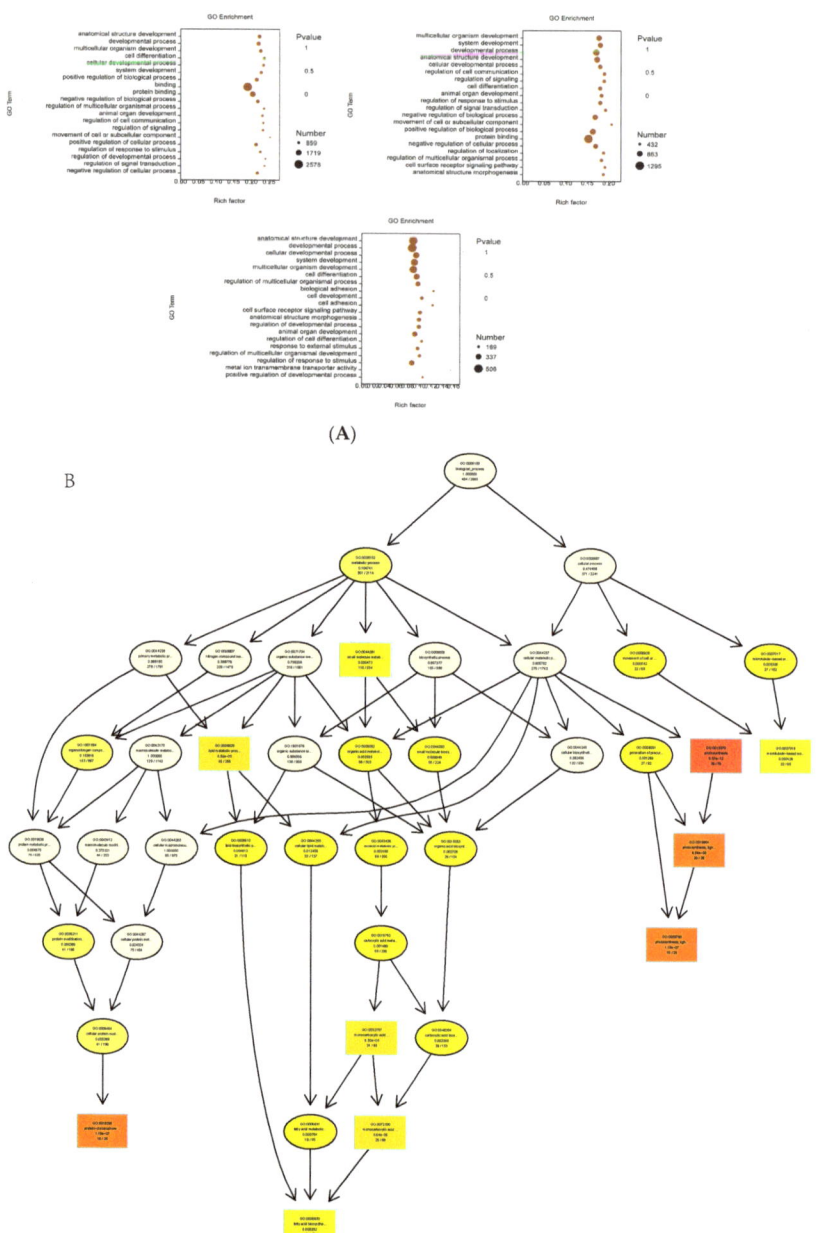

Figure 3. Cont.

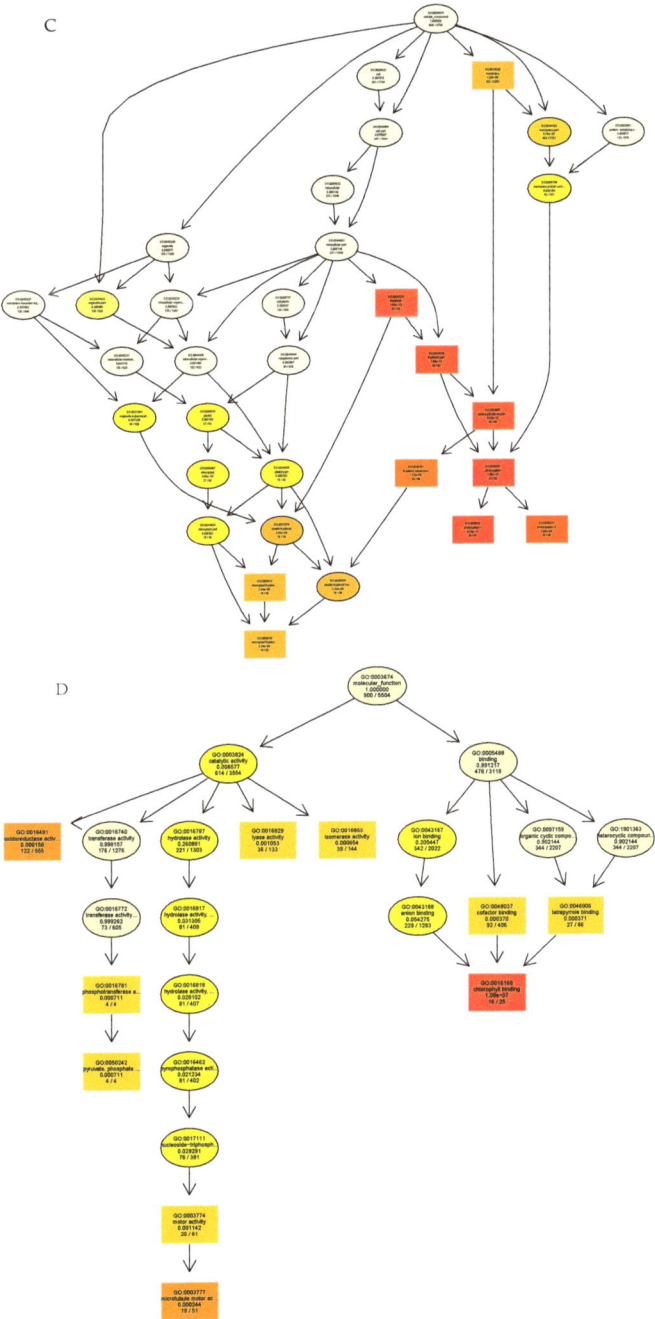

Figure 3. GO enrichment analyses of DEGs identified in H_2O_2-stimulated IEC-6 cells. (**A**) GO enrichment analyses of DEGs. The x-axis represents the number of DEGs and the y-axis represents the enriched GO terms. The size of the point indicates the number of DEGs enriched in the pathway, and the redder the color, the more significant the enrichment result is. (**B**–**D**) Thumbnails view of directed acyclic graphs (DEGs) on BP, CC, and MF.

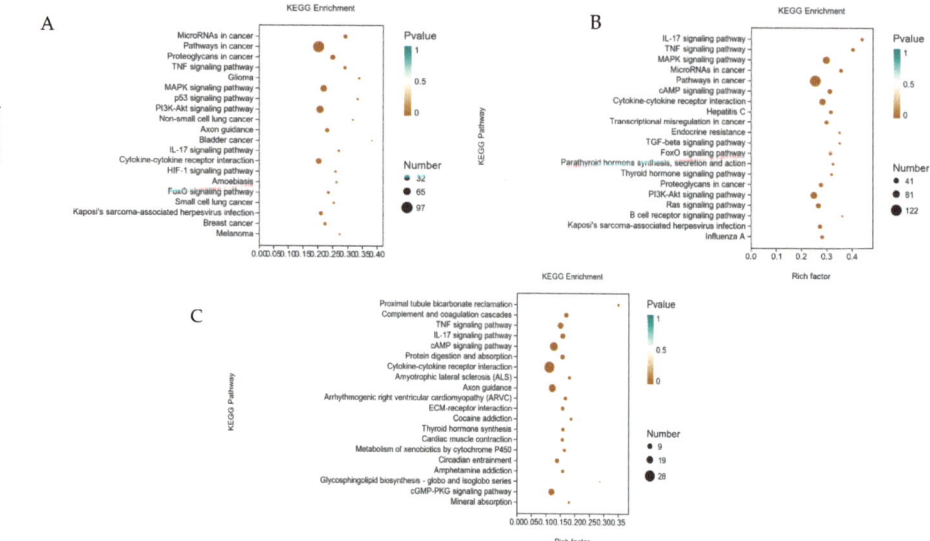

Figure 4. Enrichment analysis diagram of KEGG in H_2O_2-stimulated IEC-6 cells. (**A**) Control group, (**B**) Model group. (**C**) CYP group. The top 20 classical pathways obtained through KEGG enrichment are shown in the figure.

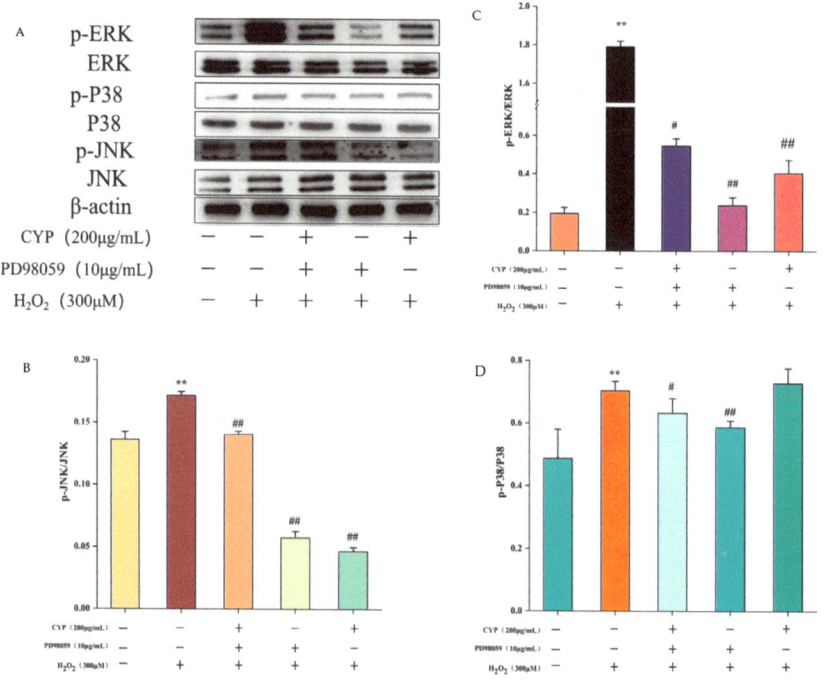

Figure 5. Effect of ERK inhibitor on H_2O_2-induced IEC-6 cell injury through MAPK pathway. (**A**) Western blot showing the protein expression of ERK, p-ERK, p38, p-p38, JNK and p-JNK. (**B–D**) The quantification of JNK, p-JNK, ERK, p-ERK, p38, and p-p38 expression. Results shown are expressed as means ± SD (n = 3). # $p < 0.05$, ## $p < 0.01$ compared with normal group, ** $p < 0.01$ compared with H_2O_2 group alone.

3.6. Effect of CYP on Intestinal Tight Junction Proteins ZO-1, Occludin, and Claudin-1

Intestinal tight junction proteins have a positive impact on protecting intestinal cells as a barrier for intestinal mucosal cells [29]. The, ZO-1, Claudin-1, and Occludin expressions were decreased after H_2O_2 treatment compared with the control group (Figure 6), indicating that H_2O_2 treatment impaired the intestinal barrier function. After pretreatment with CYP at 200 μg/mL, the expression of all three tight junction proteins was up-regulated to some extent, whereas when the concentration of CYP was increased to 400 μg/mL, the expression of Occludin showed a decrease, and when soaring again to 800 μg/mL, the expression content of ZO-1 and Claudin-1 was lower than that of the control group. The results illustrated that the gut mucosal barrier of IEC-6 cells can be protected under low concentration of CYP treatment, but too-high concentration of CYP can have a negative effect.

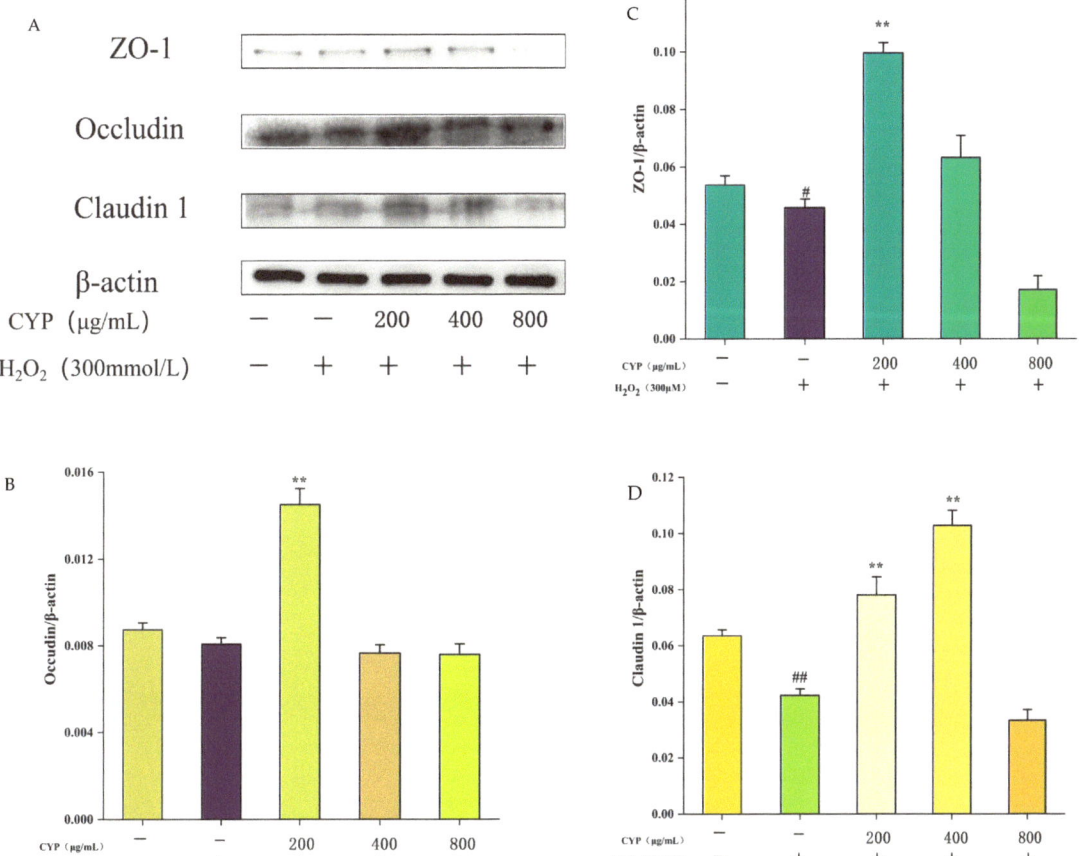

Figure 6. Effects of CYP on ZO-1, Occludin, and Claudin-1 levels of H_2O_2-induced IEC-6 cells. (**A**) Western blot showing the protein expression of ZO-1, Occludin and Claudin-1 in IEC-6. (**B–D**) The quantification of Occludin, ZO-1, and Claudin-1 expression. Results shown are expressed as means ± SD (n = 3). # $p < 0.05$, ## $p < 0.01$ compared with normal group, ** $p < 0.01$ compared with H_2O_2 group alone.

4. Discussion

The protective mechanism of yam polysaccharides in opposition to H_2O_2-induced oxidative lesions in IEC-6 cells was investigated based on RNA-seq technology, while the protective efficacy of CYP against H_2O_2-induced injury in IEC-6 cells was explored in the MAPK pathway, and the effect of combined use of ERK inhibitors on MAPK pathway was further selected to validate the effect of CYP based on the results of KEGG enrichment analysis.

RNA sequencing is a method that allows the evaluation of a complete set of organisms' transcribed genes, non-coding RNAs, and their transcriptomes [27]. Therefore, we used sequencing to screen all transcripts of CYP against H_2O_2-induced oxidative damage in IEC-6 cells. In this study, the expression of differential genes was detected via using RNA-seq technology and further classified based on the information from the differential gene analysis to analyze which functions these genes are referred to. Experimental results illustrated that there are many differentially expressed genes in both CYP and model groups versus the control group, manifesting a large number of genes expressed after H_2O_2 stimulation of cells with pretreatment of CYP. GO database provides biological annotation of sample genes in the light of effect, biological pathway, and cellular localization [19,30]. GO enrichment analysis showed that the functional groups were significantly changed during this process with cell differentiation and development of multicellular organisms and so on, indicating that CYP can influence the physiological function of IEC-6 cells. In addition, in comparison to GO analysis, KEGG enrichment analysis possesses a mighty graphical representation, which could utilize diagrammatic form instead of text material to demonstrate a range of signal pathways, offering more intuitionistic and all-sided information. For the sake of investigating the signaling pathway of CYP affecting IEC-6 cells, we found that MAPK and IL-17 signaling pathways were remarkably enriched.

Enzymes in the MAPK signaling pathway jointly regulate cell growth, differentiation, environmental stress adaptation, inflammatory response, and other important cell physiology [31]. The functional groups that are significantly changed from inside the GO enrichment analysis are cell differentiation, which coincides with the function of the MAPK pathway. The MAPK signaling pathway is mainly activated through the sequence of MAPK kinase, phosphorylation-activated MAPK kinase, and MAPK (transmission of downstream information) activation to complete [25]. To keep off mutual interference, the MAPK cascade is split into fixed modules using scaffold proteins. Among mammals, the MAPK signaling cascade is usually classified into four subgroups: the extracellular signal-regulated protein kinase 1 and 2 (ERK1/2) cascade, the c-Jun N-terminal kinase (JNK) cascade, the p38 MAPK cascade, and the ERK5 cascade [32,33]. These subgroups are connected to signaling pathways with various biochemical actions. For example, ERK1/2 gains command of cell growth and differentiation [34], JNK is correlated with stress, p38 MAPK is relevant to immune regulation and inflammatory response [35], and ERK5 is associated with multifarious diseases, especially cardiovascular disease and cancer [36].

Western blot protein bands indicated that pretreatment with CYP inhibited the phosphorylated expression of three proteins in the pathway and suppressed MAPK pathway activation. Further validation with the combination of ERK inhibitors showed that CYP exerted an inhibitory effect on the phosphorylated expression of the related proteins in the MAPK pathway and that the effect was similar to that of ERK inhibitors. This indicates that CYP can inhibit the MAPK pathway and, thus, reduce the oxidative damage in cells. Consistent with our results, polysaccharides from Agrocybe cylindracea residue mitigate the liver and colon injury in type II diabetes through p38 MAPK signaling pathway [37]. Maintaining the integrity of the intestinal mucosal barrier is essential to protecting the host from gut microbes, food antigens, and toxins. Huang et al. [38] investigated the effects of CYP and SCYP on intestinal microbiota in vitro study. Consequently, it is speculated that CYP may affect the gut barrier. The present study found that low concentration of CYP can promote the expression of intestinal compact junction protein, which plays a role in protecting the intestinal tract.

5. Conclusions

To sum up, our study demonstrated that cells differentiated and protein binding genes changed significantly according to the sequencing results and CYP-regulated MAPK signaling pathways with ERK inhibitor to prevent excessive oxidative stress responses and protect the intestinal barrier by affecting intestinal proteins (Figure 7). Indeed, this is the first comprehensive study of the potential protective mechanism of CYP, which provides an original perspective for incisive understanding of the protective role of CYP on the gut, and likewise offers a theoretical foundation for the CYP-relevant products' development.

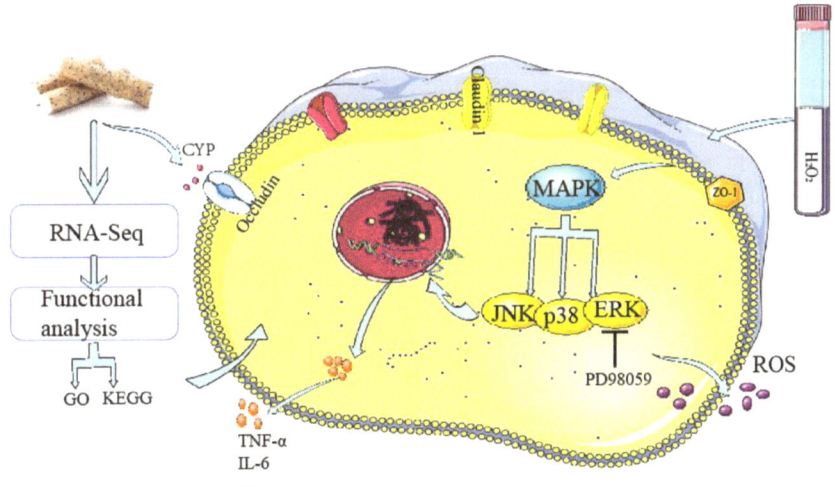

Figure 7. Schematic of mechanism in CYP on H_2O_2-induced oxidative damage in IEC-6 cell.

Author Contributions: Conceptualization, R.C. and Z.L.; methodology, R.C., J.X. and M.S.; formal analysis, X.C. and Z.L.; resources, J.X. and M.S.; data curation, Z.L. and R.C.; writing—original draft preparation, R.C.; writing—review and editing, X.C. and M.S. All authors have read and agreed to the published version of the manuscript.

Funding: This research work was financially supported by the National Natural Science Foundation of China (81960708).

Institutional Review Board Statement: Not applicable.

Informed Consent Statement: Not applicable.

Data Availability Statement: The data used to support the findings of this study can be made available by the corresponding author upon request.

Acknowledgments: The authors gratefully acknowledge the financial supports by the National Natural Science Foundation of China (81960708).

Conflicts of Interest: The authors declare no conflict of interest.

References

1. Zou, Y.; Fan, F.; Fang, Y.; Li, P.; Xia, J.; Shen, X.; Liu, Q.; Hu, Q. Neuroprotective Effect of Alkylresorcinols from Wheat Bran in HT22 Cells: Correlation with in vitro Antioxidant Activity. *eFood* **2021**, *2*, 13–20. [CrossRef]
2. Valko, M.; Leibfritz, D.; Moncol, J.; Cronin, M.T.D.; Mazur, M.; Telser, J. Free radicals and antioxidants in normal physiological functions and human disease. *Int. J. Biochem. Cell Biol.* **2007**, *39*, 44–84. [CrossRef] [PubMed]
3. Yun, B.; King, M.; Draz, M.S.; Kline, T.; Rodriguez-Palacios, A. Oxidative reactivity across kingdoms in the gut: Host immunity, stressed microbiota and oxidized foods. *Free. Radic. Biol. Med.* **2022**, *178*, 97–110. [CrossRef]
4. Moloney, J.N.; Cotter, T.G. ROS signalling in the biology of cancer. *Semin. Cell Dev. Biol.* **2018**, *80*, 50–64. [CrossRef] [PubMed]

5. Sarmiento-Salinas, F.L.; Perez-Gonzalez, A.; Acosta-Casique, A.; Ix-Ballote, A.; Diaz, A.; Treviño, S.; Rosas-Murrieta, N.H.; Millán-Perez-Peña, L.; Maycotte, P. Reactive oxygen species: Role in carcinogenesis, cancer cell signaling and tumor progression. *Life Sci.* **2021**, *284*, 119942. [CrossRef]
6. Chopyk, D.M.; Grakoui, A. Contribution of the Intestinal Microbiome and Gut Barrier to Hepatic Disorders. *Gastroenterology* **2020**, *159*, 849–863. [CrossRef]
7. Kataoka, K. The intestinal microbiota and its role in human health and disease. *Med. Invest.* **2016**, *63*, 27–37. [CrossRef] [PubMed]
8. Camara-Lemarroy, C.R.; Metz, L.; Meddings, J.B.; Sharkey, K.A.; Yong, V.W. The intestinal barrier in multiple sclerosis: Implications for pathophysiology and therapeutics. *Brain* **2018**, *141*, 1900–1916. [CrossRef] [PubMed]
9. Medini, F.; Bourgou, S.; Lalancette, K.; Snoussi, M.; Mkadmini, K.; Coté, I.; Abdelly, C.; Legault, J.; Ksouri, R. Phytochemical analysis, antioxidant, anti-inflammatory, and anticancer activities of the halophyte Limonium densiflorum extracts on human cell lines and murine macrophages. *South Afr. J. Bot.* **2015**, *99*, 158–164. [CrossRef]
10. Wang, Y.; Xie, M.; Ma, J.; Fang, Y.; Yang, W.; Ma, N.; Fang, D.; Hu, Q.; Pei, F. The antioxidant and antimicrobial activities of different phenolic acids grafted onto chitosan. *Carbohydr. Polym.* **2019**, *225*, 115238. [CrossRef]
11. Hao, W.; Chen, Z.; Yuan, Q.; Ma, M.; Gao, C.; Zhou, Y.; Zhou, H.; Wu, X.; Wu, D.; Farag, M.A.; et al. Ginger polysaccharides relieve ulcerative colitis via maintaining intestinal barrier integrity and gut microbiota modulation. *Int. J. Biol. Macromol.* **2022**, *219*, 730–739. [CrossRef]
12. Feng, T.; Yang, X.; Kong, Q.; Lu, J. Editorial: Food Bioactive Polysaccharides and Their Health Functions. *RSC Adv.* **2021**, *8*, 632. [CrossRef] [PubMed]
13. Wang, J.H.; Xu, J.L.; Zhang, J.C.; Liu, Y.; Sun, H.J.; Zha, X. Physicochemical properties and antioxidant activities of polysaccharide from floral mushroom cultivated in Huangshan Mountain. *Carbohydr. Polym.* **2015**, *131*, 240–247. [CrossRef] [PubMed]
14. Xing, W.H.; Hou, J.L.; Han, H.P.; Wu, C.Z.; Zhang, L.Q. Effects of Yam Polysaccharide on Blood Glucose and Serum Antioxidant Capacity in Type I Diabetic Mice. *Food Res. Dev.* **2014**, *35*, 17.
15. Ju, Y.; Xue, Y.; Huang, J.; Zhai, Q.; Wang, X.H. Antioxidant Chinese yam polysaccharides and its pro-proliferative effect on endometrial epithelial cells. *Int. J. Biol. Macromol.* **2014**, *66*, 81–85. [CrossRef]
16. Shao, Y.; Kang, Q.; Zhu, J.; Zhao, C.C. Antioxidant properties and digestion behaviors of polysaccharides from Chinese yam fermented by Saccharomyces boulardii. *LWT* **2022**, *154*, 112752. [CrossRef]
17. Ahmed, W. RNA-seq resolving host-pathogen interactions: Advances and applications. *Ecol. Genet. Genom.* **2020**, *15*, 100057. [CrossRef]
18. Ding, X.; Yu, Q.; Hou, K.; Hu, X.; Wang, Y.; Chen, Y.; Xie, J.; Nie, S.; Xie, M. Indirectly stimulation of DCs by Ganoderma atrum polysaccharide in intestinal-like Caco-2/DCs co-culture model based on RNA-seq. *J. Funct. Foods* **2020**, *67*, 103850. [CrossRef]
19. Wang, Q.; Fu, R.; Cheng, H.; Li, Y.; Sui, S. Analysis of the resistance of small peptides from Periplaneta americana to hydrogen peroxide-induced apoptosis in human ovarian granular cells based on RNA-seq. *Gene* **2022**, *813*, 146120. [CrossRef]
20. Chen, X.; Wang, X.; Shen, M.; Chen, Y. Combined RNA-seq and molecular biology technology revealed the protective effect of Cyclocarya paliurus polysaccharide on H2O2-induced oxidative damage in L02 cells thought regulating mitochondrial function, oxidative stress and PI3K/Akt and MAPK signaling pathways. *Food Res. Int.* **2022**, *155*, 111080.
21. Hao, B.H.; Yang, X.; Ma, Y. Study on deproteinization in extraction of polysaccharides from Patentillaunserina by Sevage. *Sci. Technol. Food Ind.* **2011**, *32*, 254–258.
22. Huang, G.; Chen, F.; Yang, W.; Huang, H. Preparation, deproteinization and comparison of bioactive polysaccharides. *Trends Food Sci. Technol.* **2021**, *109*, 564–568. [CrossRef]
23. Li, Z.; Xiao, W.; Xie, L.; Chen, Y.; Yu, Q.; Zhang, W.; Shen, M. Isolation, Characterization and Antioxidant Activity of Yam Polysaccharides. *Foods* **2022**, *11*, 800. [CrossRef] [PubMed]
24. Taguchi, K.; Kaneko, N.; Okudaira, K.; Matsumoto, T.; Kobayashi, T. Endothelial dysfunction caused by circulating microparticles from diabetic mice is reduced by PD98059 through ERK and ICAM-1. *Eur. J. Pharmacol.* **2021**, *913*, 174630. [CrossRef]
25. Liang, Y.-J.; Yang, W.-X. Kinesins in MAPK cascade: How kinesin motors are involved in the MAPK pathway? *Gene* **2019**, *684*, 1–9. [CrossRef]
26. Su, X.; Zhao, M.; Fu, X.; Ma, X.; Xu, W.; Hu, S. Immunomodulatory activity of purified polysaccharides from Rubus chingii Hu fruits in lymphocytes and its molecular mechanisms. *J. Funct. Foods* **2021**, *87*, 104785. [CrossRef]
27. Zhao, M.; Hou, J.; Zheng, S.; Ma, X.; Fu, X.; Hu, S.; Zhao, K.; Xu, W. Peucedanum praeruptorum Dunn polysaccharides regulate macrophage inflammatory response through TLR2/TLR4-mediated MAPK and NF-kappaB pathways. *Biomed Pharm.* **2022**, *152*, 113258. [CrossRef] [PubMed]
28. Flynn, A.R.; Chang, H.Y. Long Noncoding RNAs in Cell-Fate Programming and Reprogramming. *Cell Stem Cell* **2014**, *14*, 752–761. [CrossRef]
29. Yu, J.; Zhao, J.; Xie, H.; Cai, M.; Yao, L.; Li, J.; Han, L.; Chen, W.; Yu, N.; Peng, D. Dendrobium huoshanense polysaccharides ameliorate ulcerative colitis by improving intestinal mucosal barrier and regulating gut microbiota. *J. Funct. Foods* **2022**, *96*, 105231. [CrossRef]
30. Xu, W.; Du, A.; Hu, S. Transcriptome analysis of bovine lymphocytes stimulated by Atractylodis macrocephalae Koidz. polysaccharides in vitro. *Vet. Immunol. Immunopathol.* **2018**, *196*, 30–34. [CrossRef]

31. Abdelzaher, W.Y.; Bahaa, H.A.; Elkhateeb, R.; Atta, M.; Fawzy, M.A.; Ahmed, A.F.; Rofaeil, R.R. Role of JNK, ERK, and p38 MAPK signaling pathway in protective effect of sildenafil in cyclophosphamide-induced placental injury in rats. *Life Sci.* **2022**, *293*, 120354. [CrossRef] [PubMed]
32. Hoang, V.T.; Yan, T.J.; Cavanaugh, J.E.; Flaherty, P.T.; Beckman, B.S.; Burow, M.E. Oncogenic signaling of MEK5-ERK5. *Cancer Lett.* **2017**, *392*, 51–59. [CrossRef] [PubMed]
33. Wu, J.; Chien, C.-C.; Yang, L.-Y.; Huang, G.-C.; Cheng, M.-C.; Lin, C.-T.; Shen, S.-C.; Chen, Y.-C. Vitamin K3-2,3-epoxide induction of apoptosis with activation of ROS-dependent ERK and JNK protein phosphorylation in human glioma cells. *Chem. -Biol. Interact.* **2011**, *193*, 3–11. [CrossRef] [PubMed]
34. Montes-Alvarado, J.B.; Barragán, M.; Larrauri-Rodríguez, K.A.; Perez-Gonzalez, A.; Delgado-Magallón, A.; Millán-Perez-Peña, L.; Rosas-Murrieta, N.H.; Maycotte, P. ERK activation modulates invasiveness and Reactive Oxygen Species (ROS) production in triple negative breast cancer cell lines. *Cell. Signal.* **2023**, *101*, 110487.
35. Ding, H.; Wang, F.; Su, L.; Zhao, L.; Hu, B.; Zheng, W.; Yao, S.; Li, Y. Involvement of MEK5/ERK5 signaling pathway in manganese-induced cell injury in dopaminergic MN9D cells. *J. Trace Elem. Med. Biol.* **2020**, *61*, 126546. [CrossRef] [PubMed]
36. Kim, H.-Y.; Park, S.-Y.; Choung, S.-Y. Enhancing effects of myricetin on the osteogenic differentiation of human periodontal ligament stem cells via BMP-2/Smad and ERK/JNK/p38 mitogen-activated protein kinase signaling pathway. *Eur. J. Pharmacol.* **2018**, *834*, 84–91. [CrossRef]
37. Sun, W.; Zhang, Y.; Jia, L. Polysaccharides from Agrocybe cylindracea residue alleviate type 2-diabetes-induced liver and colon injuries by p38 MAPK signaling pathway. *Food Biosci.* **2022**, *47*, 101690. [CrossRef]
38. Huang, R.; Xie, J.; Liu, X.; Shen, M. Sulfated modification enhances the modulatory effect of yam polysaccharide on gut microbiota in cyclophosphamide-treated mice. *Food Res. Int.* **2021**, *145*, 110393. [CrossRef]

Disclaimer/Publisher's Note: The statements, opinions and data contained in all publications are solely those of the individual author(s) and contributor(s) and not of MDPI and/or the editor(s). MDPI and/or the editor(s) disclaim responsibility for any injury to people or property resulting from any ideas, methods, instructions or products referred to in the content.

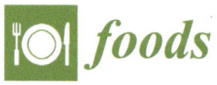 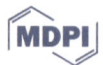

Article

Characterization of Novel Exopolysaccharides from *Enterococcus hirae* WEHI01 and Its Immunomodulatory Activity

Kaiying Jia [†], Min Wei [†], Yao He, Yujie Wang, Hua Wei and Xueying Tao *

State Key Laboratory of Food Science and Technology, Nanchang University, Nanchang 330047, China
* Correspondence: 1027txy@163.com or taoxueying@ncu.du.cn; Tel.: +86-791-8833-4578; Fax: +86-791-8833-3708
† These authors contributed equally to this work.

Abstract: Exopolysaccharide (EPS) from probiotic *Enterococcus hirae* WEHI01 was isolated and purified by anion exchange chromatography and gel chromatography, the results of which show that the EPS consists of four fractions, namely I01-1, I01-2, I01-3, and I01-4. As the main purification components, I01-2 and I01-4 were preliminarily characterized for their structure and their immunomodulatory activity was explored. The molecular weight of I01-2 was 2.28×10^4 Da, which consists mainly of galactose, and a few other sugars including glucose, arabinose, mannose, xylose, fucose, and rhamnose, while the I01-4 was composed of galactose only and has a molecular weight of 2.59×10^4 Da. Furthermore, the results of an evaluation of immunomodulatory activity revealed that I01-2 and I01-4 could improve the viability of macrophage cells, improve phagocytosis, boost NO generation, and encourage the release of cytokines including TNF-α and IL-6 in RAW 264.7 macrophages. These results imply that I01-2 and I01-4 could improve macrophage-mediated immune responses and might be useful in the production of functional food and medications.

Keywords: *Enterococcus hirae* WEHI01; exopolysaccharide; immunomodulatory properties

Citation: Jia, K.; Wei, M.; He, Y.; Wang, Y.; Wei, H.; Tao, X. Characterization of Novel Exopolysaccharides from *Enterococcus hirae* WEHI01 and Its Immunomodulatory Activity. *Foods* 2022, 11, 3538. https://doi.org/10.3390/foods11213538

Academic Editor: Lovedeep Kaur and Souhail Besbes

Received: 27 September 2022
Accepted: 4 November 2022
Published: 7 November 2022

Publisher's Note: MDPI stays neutral with regard to jurisdictional claims in published maps and institutional affiliations.

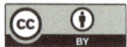

Copyright: © 2022 by the authors. Licensee MDPI, Basel, Switzerland. This article is an open access article distributed under the terms and conditions of the Creative Commons Attribution (CC BY) license (https://creativecommons.org/licenses/by/4.0/).

1. Introduction

Exopolysaccharides (EPSs) are peculiar polymers of extracellular high-molecular-weight which can be produced by a variety of microorganisms (e.g., bacteria, fungi, and microalgae) [1]. EPSs isolated from lactic acid bacteria (LAB) are generally recognized as safe (GRAS) and are crucial natural additives in the food, cosmetic, and pharmaceutical industries [2,3]. EPS-producing LAB strains have great commercial potential due to their capability to enhance the rheology, texture, and mouthfeel of food [4–7]. Growing evidence demonstrated that EPSs from LAB possess various beneficial physiological effects including antioxidant [8], antimicrobial [9], antitumor [10], immunomodulatory [11], anti-biofilm [12], anti-viral [13], and cholesterol-lowering activities [14].

A growing number of publications demonstrated the immune-modulating effects of LAB-derived EPSs. Nikolic et al. reported that the EPS of *Lactobacillus paraplantarum* BGCG11 induced a significant immunoreaction [15]. The EPS of *Lactobacillus plantarum* JKL0142 could stimulate the immune activity of immunosuppressed mice macrophages [16]. Other reports demonstrated that LAB-derived EPSs increased particular cellular and humoral immune responses to antigens by promoting T/B-lymphocyte proliferation and boosting macrophage phagocytic activity, promoting the production of NO and cytokines [11,17,18]. In addition, the immunomodulatory activities of EPS are involved with their physicochemical properties such as their molecular weight and composition of monosaccharides [19].

Among EPS-producing LAB strains, in addition to the most studied *Lactobacillus* and *Bifidobacterium*, some *Enterococcus* strains are also known for their potential probiotic properties and desirable physical and chemical properties, and are preferred for use in many commercial probiotic feed additives to poultry and cattle [20,21]. Daillere et al. showed that the anti-tumor efficacy of cyclophosphamide relies on two gut commensal species, *Enterococcus hirae* and *Barnesiella intestinihominis* [22]. Hamid et al. found that adding *E. hirae* UPM02 to the diet of hybrid catfish successfully influenced immune responses and improved the expression of the immunity-related genes [23]. Recently, EPS from probiotic *Enterococcus* has also received more and more attention, on which most reports have focused on the EPS's physicochemical characterization [24], antioxidant [25], antibiofilm [26] and anti-adhesion of the pathogen [27], but little is known about the immunomodulatory activity of EPS from probiotic enterococci. Our previous studies showed that the probiotic strain *E. hirae* WEHI01 isolated from healthy infants' feces [28] was proven to alleviate inflammation, improve type 2 diabetes, regulate intestinal flora [29], and lower cholesterol [30] in rats. However, as an important component, the EPS of *E. hirae* WEHI01 has not yet been investigated, and its structure and function are still unknown.

In the host defense systems, macrophages are the bridge between innate and adaptive immunity [31]. Activated macrophages directly neutralize xenobiotics through phagocytosis and kill cancer cells and pathogenic microorganisms by secreting proinflammatory cytokines, including IL-1β, TNF-α, IL-6, and cytotoxic molecules NO [32,33]. Therefore, macrophages are considered to be crucial target cells in immunomodulatory effects.

In the present study, we purified EPS from *E. hirae* WEHI01 by using anion exchange chromatography and gel chromatography and characterized the primary structure by using Absolute Molecular Weight Analyzer, Fourier-transform infrared (FT-IR), and gas chromatography–mass spectrometry (GC-MS). Furthermore, we investigated the immunomodulatory activity of EPS fractions using a murine macrophage RAW 264.7 cell. This study aimed to reveal the primary structure of EPS from *E. hirae* WEHI01 and its capacity for immune regulation.

2. Materials and Methods

2.1. Materials and Reagents

The Cell Bank of the Chinese Academy of Sciences (Beijing, China) provided the murine macrophage cell line RAW 264.7 for use in research. Trimethylchlorosilane, hexamethyldisilane, pyridine, and trifluoroacetic acid (TFA) were obtained from Aladdin Biological Technology Co., Ltd. (Shanghai, China). Rhamnose, arabinose, xylose, fucose, mannose, glucose, and galactose were purchased from YuanYe Bio-Technology Co., Ltd. (Shanghai, China). Lipopolysaccharides (LPSs), Brain Heart Infusion (BHI), Mw cut-off 8000–14,000 Da MWCO membranes (MD34), and 0.1% neutral red stain solution were bought from Solarbio Life Science and Technology Co. Ltd. (Beijing, China). Bovine calf serum was purchased from Sigma Chemical Co., Ltd. (Saint Louis, MO, USA). ELISA kits for the analysis of TNF-α and IL-6 were purchased from Neobioscience Technology Co., Ltd. (Shenzhen, China). Cell Counting Kit-8 (CCK-8) was purchased from Beyotime Biotechnology Co. Ltd. (Shanghai, China). A kit for measuring nitric oxide (NO) was purchased from Nanjing Jiancheng Bioengineering Institute (Nanjing, China).

2.2. The Culture of Strain

The EPS-producing probiotic bacteria were previously isolated from healthy infant's feces and named *E. hirae* WEHI01 [28], and cultured in BHI under anaerobic conditions at 37 °C.

2.3. Extraction, Production and Purification of EPS

Briefly, *E. hirae* WEHI01 was cultured in BHI for 20 h at 37 °C under anaerobic conditions, then underwent centrifugation at $9000 \times g$ for at least 5 min to collect supernatant and precipitated by mixing with two volumes of pre-cooled absolute ethyl alcohol. The precipitation was then collected by centrifugation ($10,000 \times g$, 20 min) and re-dissolved in Milli-Q water [27]. After deproteinized by Sevag reagent [34], dialysis of crude EPS against milli-Q water and lyophilized. To determine the yields of EPS, the supernatant (50 mL) was collected at different time intervals ranging from 0 to 50 h for EPS extraction. Using glucose as a standard, the EPS contents were determined by the phenol-sulfuric acid method and the absorbance was measured at 490 nm.

The purification of crude EPS according to our previous method, and the use of the phenol-sulfuric acid technique to determine the amount of carbohydrates in the eluate (2.0 mL/tube) [35]. Peak fractions were concentrated and further fractionated by a Superdex G-200 column (10 mm × 300 mm) and then eluted with 0.2 M NH_4HCO_3. The EPS fractions eluted in one peak were pooled together and dialyzed against ultrapure water, and finally concentrated by freeze-dried (SCIENTZ-10N, Ningbo SCIENTZ Biotechnology Co., LTD, China) for further analyses.

2.4. Structure Characterization of EPS

2.4.1. Purity and Molecular Weight

The UV spectrum of I01-2 and I01-4 (0.1 mg/mL) was obtained on a U-3900 UV/VIS Spectrophotometer over a range of 200–600 nm. The homogeneity and molecular weight of EPS were determined using PL aquagel-OH MIXED (7.5 mm × 300 mm, 8 μm) (Aglient, Santa Rosa, CA, USA) equipped with Differential Refractometer (BI-DNDC/GPC, Brookhaven Inc., New York, NY, USA) and Molecular Weight Analyzer (BI-MwA, Brookhaven Inc., New York, NY, USA) according to our previous report [27].

2.4.2. FT-IR Spectroscopy Analysis

FT-IR was recorded using the KBr-disks method [36] with the FT-IR spectrophotometer (Nicolet Nexus 470, Thermo Nicolet Co., Madison, WI, USA). The EPS measurement range was 400–4000 cm^{-1}, as previously reported [37].

2.4.3. Analysis of Monosaccharide Composition

With a slight modification based on our previously reported method [38], the monosaccharide composition was analyzed by GC-MS after acetylation. Firstly, I01-2, I01-4, and standard sugars were hydrolyzed with 2.0 M TFA at 110 °C for 4 h. The TFA residue was then removed by washing the hydrolysate twice with methanol and drying it under nitrogen. The product was then reduced with $NaBH_4$, and acetylated with acetic anhydride (AC_2O). To create the derivatives, chloroform was used to extract the substance. Then, the acetate derivatives were analyzed through GC-MS apparatus (Shimadzu GCMS-QP 2010, Japan) equipped with an RXI-5 SIL MS chromatographic column (30 m × 0.25 mm × 0.25 μm) (J&W Scientific, Folsom, CA, USA). The GC-MS operation was performed under the following conditions: Helium (carrier gas) at a constant flow velocity of 1.0 mL/min, injection temperature: 250 °C, initial column temperature: 120 °C and holding for 5 min, increasing to 250 °C at a rate of 3 °C/min, and holding at 250 °C for 5 min.

2.5. Immunocompetence Assays

2.5.1. Cell Culture and Its Viability Assay

The murine macrophage cell line RAW 264.7 was cultured in DMEM supplemented with 10% bovine calf serum at 37 °C in an atmosphere of 5% CO_2. Cells in 96-well plates (5.0×10^4 cells/well) were treated with various concentrations (50, 100, 200, 400, 800. and 1000 μg/mL) of I01-2 and I01-4 for 24 h. Additionally, the proliferation of RAW 264.7 was detected by CCK-8 according to the manufacturer's protocol. The absorbance was measured at 450 nm by a microplate reader (Varioskan Flash, Thermo Scientific, Waltham, MA, USA). Cell viability was calculated using the following equation:

$$\text{Cell viability (\%)} = \frac{A_2}{A_1} \times 100$$

where A_1 is the absorbance of the blank group, and A_2 is the absorbance of cells after treatment with EPS.

2.5.2. Phagocytosis Assay and Morphology Observation

The phagocytic capacity of RAW 264.7 cells was evaluated by neutral red uptake assay [39]. The intervention of RAW 264.7 cells was made with various concentrations of I01-2, I01-4, and LPS (1 μg/mL) for 24 h in a 96-well plate. After washing the cells twice with Hanks, add 100 μL of 0.1% neutral red stain solution to each well. After incubation at 37 °C for another 3 h, the cells were washed three times with Hanks and then lysed by adding 200 μL lysate (anhydrous ethanol and acetic acid in a 1:1 ratio) to incubate for 1 h at room temperature. The absorbance at 540 nm was measured with a microplate reader. An optical microscope (Olympus, Tokyo, Japan) was used to observe the morphology.

2.5.3. NO and Cytokines Secretion

Briefly, I01-2, I01-4, or LPS were incubated with RAW 264.7 cells in 6-well plates (1.0×10^6 cells/well) for 12 h [40], and the quantities of NO, TNF-α and IL-6 in the supernatants were measured using commercial kits in accordance with the manufacturer's instructions.

2.5.4. Gene Expression Analysis by RT-qPCR

RAW 264.7 cells were handled as described above in 6-well plates. Following the manufacturer's instructions, total RNA was obtained using the MiniBEST Universal RNA Extraction Kit. PrimeScript ™ RT Reagent Kit with g DNA Eraser was used by the directions to create single-strand cDNA. Using SYBR Premix Ex Taq II kit quantitative real-time PCR (qPCR) was carried out to examine the transcription level of *iNOS*, *TNF-α*, and *IL-6* genes. The qPCR was run using the following cycling profile: preheating at 95 °C for 5 min, followed by 40 cycles of 95 °C for 30 s, 60 °C for 30 s, and 72 °C for 30 s. The $2^{-\Delta\Delta Ct}$ method was used to analyze real-time PCR, which was carried out in triplicate. The *β-actin* gene served as a reference gene. Table 1 contains a list of the primers used.

Table 1. Primers used for qPCR.

Genes	Forward Primer (5'-3')	Reverse Primer (5'-3')
iNOS	GCGAAAGGTCATGGCTTCAC	TCTTCCAAGGTGCTTGCCTT
TNF-α	CGAGTGACAAGCCTGTAGCC	ACAAGGTACAACCCATCGGC
IL-6	GTCCTTCCTACCCCAATTTCCA	CGCACTAGGTTTGCCGAGTA
β-actin	GCTCCTCCTGAGCGCAAGTA	CAGCTCAGTAACAGTCCGCC

2.6. Statistical Analysis

At least three different replications of the experiment's findings were made and all data were then presented as mean ± SD. Independent one-way ANOVA tests were utilized for statistical analysis in the Origin 2022 software (OriginLab, Northampton, MA, USA).

3. Results and Discussion

3.1. Extraction and Purification of EPS

EPS reached a maximum value of 606 mg/L, while the cell counts maintained 10.26 log CFU/mL at 30 h. The rough EPS was isolated from *E. hirae* WEHI01 and purified by chromatography. As shown in Figure 1A, four fractions (I01-1, I01-2, I01-3, and I01-4) were obtained by a HiTrap Q HP column and calculated by the number of crude EPS, the recovery rates of I01-1, I01-2, I01-3, and I01-4 were 12.2%, 21.6%, 8.1%, and 15.9%, respectively. The major fractions I01-2 and I01-4 were further purified by Sephadex G-200 gel permeation chromatography, and the result showed that each eluting peak was a separate fraction (Figure 1B,C), which was used for subsequent analysis. I01-1 is a neutral polysaccharide and the other three purified components are acidic polysaccharides. Similar results were observed in our previous study that the EPS from *E. faecium* WEFA23 was also composed of four fractions [27].

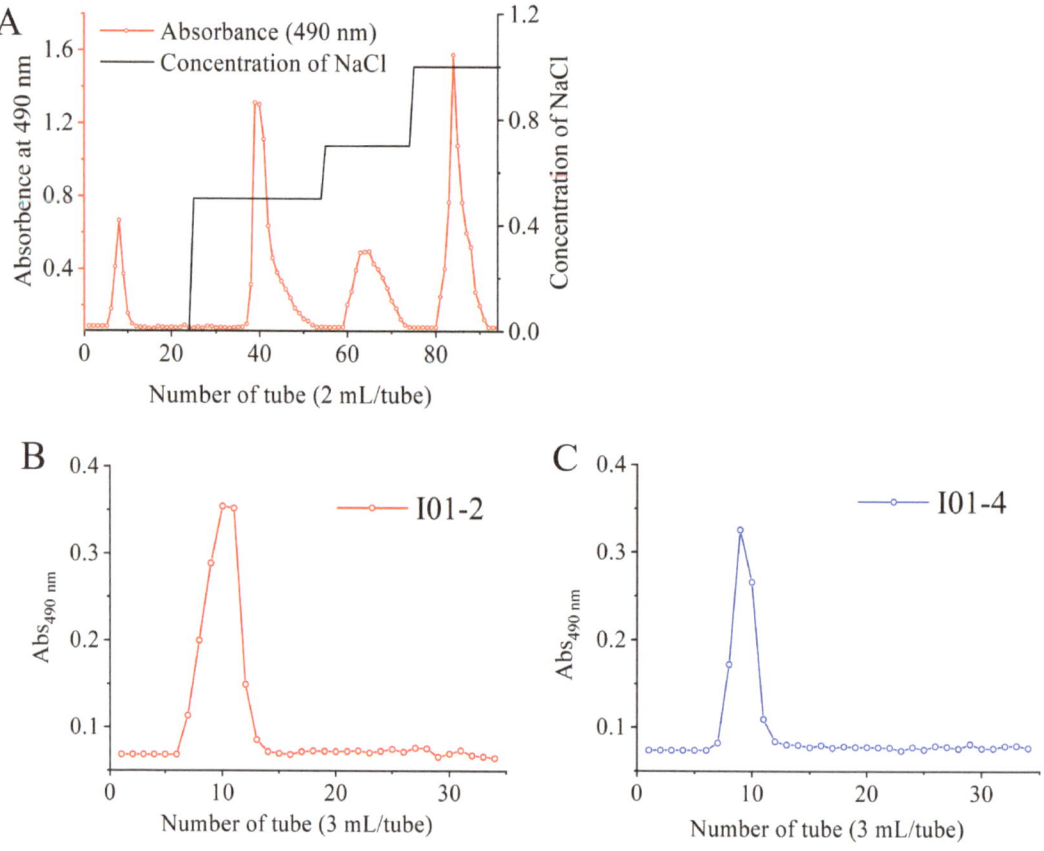

Figure 1. Elution profile of *E. hirae* WEHI01 crude EPS on HiTrap Q HP chromatography column with NaCl solutions (0, 0.5, 0.7, and 1 M) (**A**) and elution profile of I01-2 (**B**) and I01-4 (**C**) on Sephadex G-200 gel chromatography column with 0.2 M NH_4HCO_3 (**B**). –○–, 490 nm for the detection of carbohydrate.

3.2. Mw and Monosaccharides Composition of I01-2 and I01-4

An Absolute Molecular Weight Analyzer was used to confirm the homogeneity and establish the average molecular weight distribution of I01-2 and I01-4. The curve of I01-2 and I01-4 were unimodal symmetrical peaks, as shown in Figure 2A,B. This indicates that the two fractions after purification were homogeneous, and the molecular weight of I01-2 and I01-4 was calculated to be 2.28×10^4 and 2.59×10^4 Da, respectively. By using GC-MS, the monosaccharide compositions of I01-2 and I01-4 were examined and their retention times were compared to reference sugar standards. As shown in Figure 2C, I01-2 was composed of galactose, glucose, arabinose, mannose, xylose, fucose, and rhamnose with a molar ratio of 1:0.296:0.262:0.120:0.08:0.08:0.048. However, the I01-4 fraction was composed of galactose only.

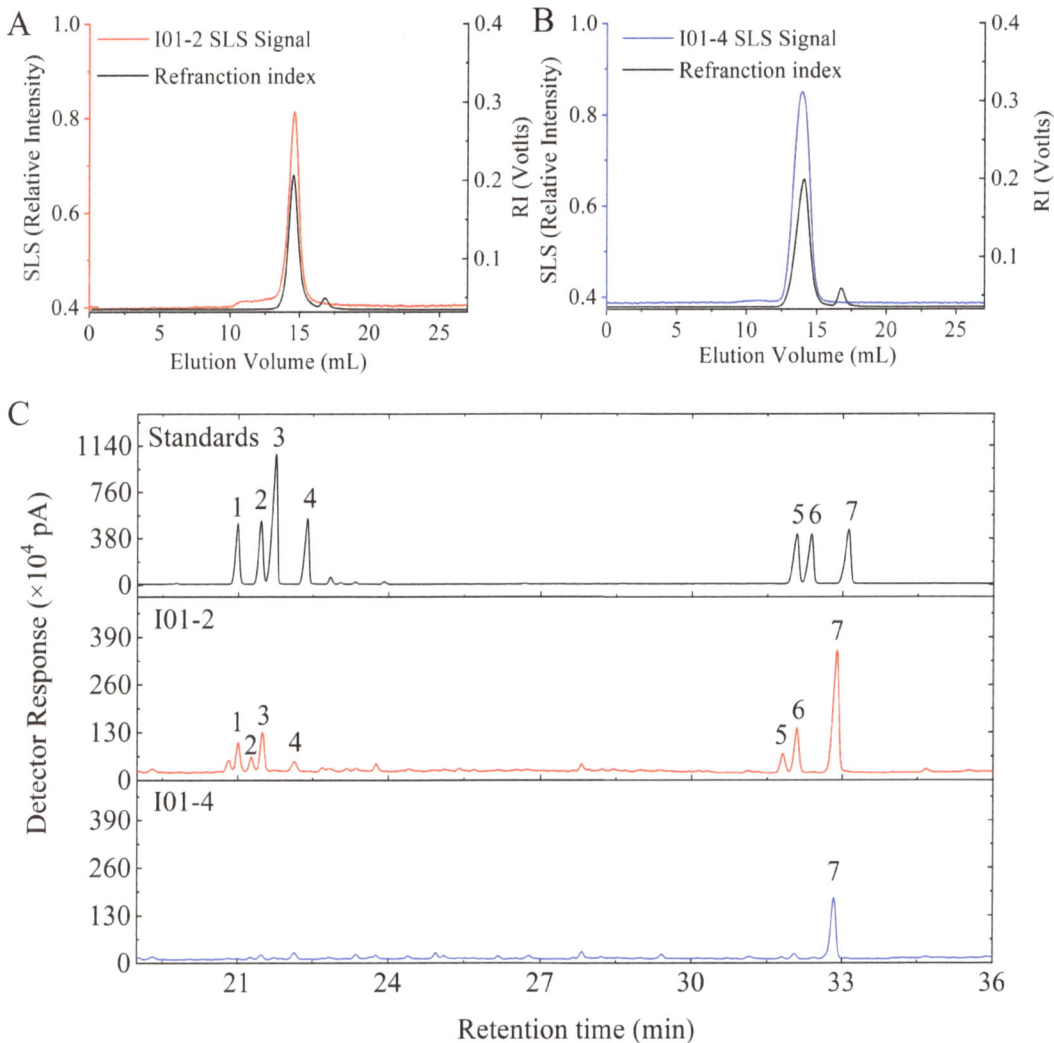

Figure 2. SEC-LLS analysis of I01-2 (**A**) and I01-4 (**B**) and GC chromatograms of the monosaccharide composition (**C**).

3.3. FT-IR Spectrum Analysis of I01-2 and I01-4

The FT-IR spectrum of I01-2 and I01-4 is shown in Figure 3. I01-2 and I01-4 exhibited intense and broad peaks around 3415 and 3423 cm^{-1}, respectively, which were assigned to the O-H stretching vibrations' absorption peaks of sugar compounds [41]. The peaks at 2934 and 2917 cm^{-1} were due to the C-H stretching vibration [42]. The carbonyl absorption peak is a strong C=O stretching absorption band in the 1900–1600 cm-1 region, and I01-2 and I01-4 each have an absorption peak at 1653 and 1632 cm^{-1}, respectively, corresponding to the characteristic peak of C=O and indicating the presence of uronic acid [43]. Moreover, the absorption peaks at 1416 was attributed to the stretching vibrations of carboxylic groups (COO-), which indicated that the purified I01-4 was acidic polysaccharides, and the locations of these peaks was similar to the study of *Sibiraea laevigata (L.) Maxim* polysaccharides by FT-IR [44]. The 1260 cm^{-1} of I01-4 were assigned to O-H deformation vibrations [45]. The band between 1600 cm^{-1} and 1650 cm^{-1}, which is assigned to the bending vibration of the coordinated water molecule, should be classified as a water band [46]. In addition, the absorption peaks at approximately 845 and 1090 cm^{-1} indicate the presence of the glycosidic bonds of both α and β configurations in I01-4 [47].

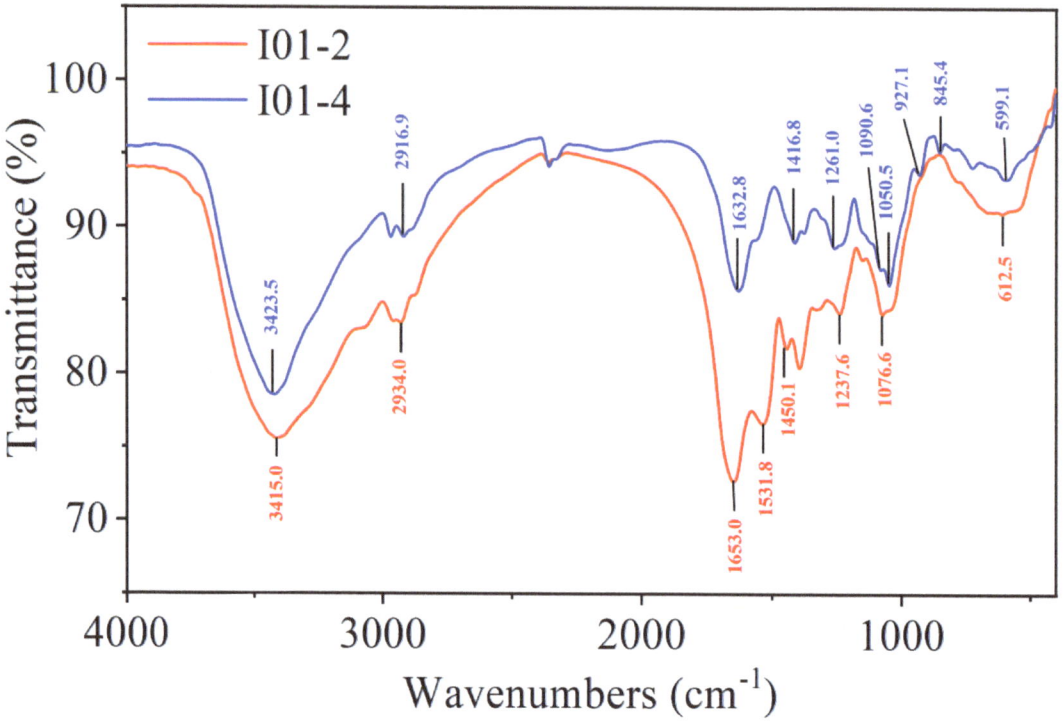

Figure 3. FT-IR spectra of I01-2 and I01-4 in the range of 400–4000 cm^{-1}.

3.4. Immunomodulatory Activities of I01-2 and I01-4 on RAW264.7 Cells

3.4.1. Effect of I01-2 and I01-4 on Cell Viability of RAW264.7

Macrophages considered the crucial target cells for immunomodulatory effects, play a crucial role in the host's first-line defense against various infections and cancer [48,49]. In the current study, the macrophage RAW 264.7 cell was used to evaluate the immunomodulatory activity of I01-2 and I01-4. By using the CCK-8 assay, the impact of I01-2 and I01-4 on cell viability was assessed. In Figure 4, I01-2 and I01-4 at concentrations of 50–1000 μg/mL exhibited non-toxicity to RAW 264.7 cells. On the other hand, both I01-2 and I01-4 increased the proliferation of RAW264.7 cells. The largest boosting effects for I01-2 and I01-4, respectively, were at 800 g/mL and 200 g/mL, reaching a maximum of 173.10% and 196.6%, respectively. Remarkably, the proliferation effect of I01-4 was obviously stronger than that of I01-2 at 50–400 μg/mL. Our result was in agreement with previous reports that EPS0142 (50–1000 μg/mL) from *L. plantarum* JLK0142 had no toxicity on RAW 264.7 cells [16] and EPS (5–1000 μg/mL) from *L. plantarum* NTU 102 promoted the cell viability of RAW 264.7 macrophages [50].

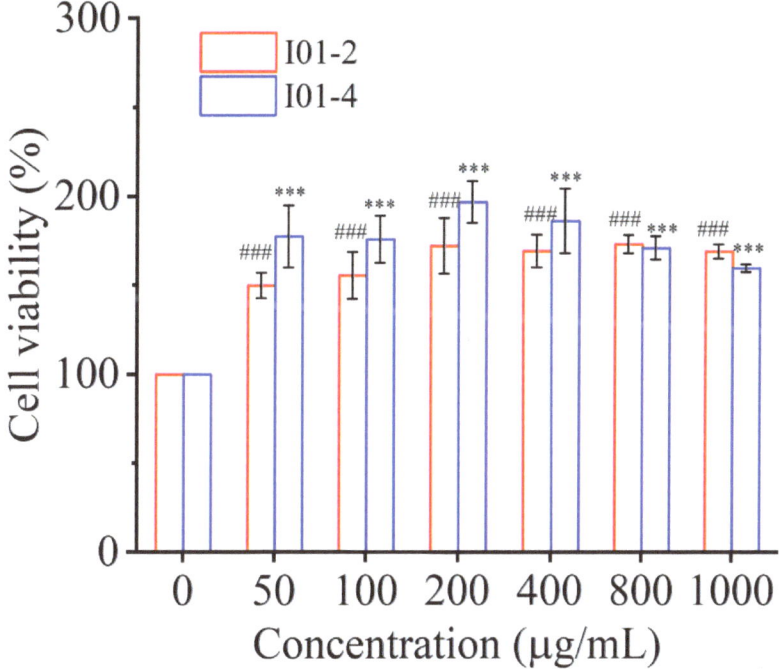

Figure 4. The effect of I01-2 and I01-4 on the viability of RAW 264.7 cells. Data were expressed as mean ± SEM. *** $p < 0.001$ (vs. I01-4 at concentrations of 0 μg/mL), ### $p < 0.001$ (vs. I01-2at concentrations of 0 μg/mL).

3.4.2. Effects of I01-2 and I01-4 on Phagocytosis of RAW 264.7 Cells

Phagocytosis is one of macrophage activation's most distinguishing features [51]. Macrophages become antigen-presenting cells after phagocytic uptake and interplay with lymphocytes to modulate the adaptive immune response [52,53]. The effect of I01-2 and I01-4 on macrophage phagocytosis was measured by neutral red uptake assay in the present study. In contrast to the control, LPS dramatically increased the phagocytosis of RAW 264.7 cells, as seen in Figure 5. As for I01-2 and I01-4, the phagocytosis of RAW 264.7 cells was significantly higher than that of the negative control (0 μg/mL), with the strongest phagocytosis at a concentration of 50 μg/mL and 200 μg/mL, respectively. This result indicates that I01-2 and I01-4 enhanced the pinocytosis of RAW 264.7 cells, which was consistent with a previous report that EPS from *Lactobacillus* significantly improved the phagocytosis of RAW 264.7 cells [11,16,54].

3.4.3. Effects of I01-2 and I01-4 on the RAW264.7 Cells' Morphology

An inverted fluorescent microscope was employed to observe the RAW264.7 cells to determine whether I01-2 and I01-4 had any impact on their morphology. As shown in Figure 6, the RAW264.7 cells in the blank control group were round in shape and showed to be aggregated and growing under a white light 20× objective lens, whereas the cell morphology markedly changed to polygonal and dendritic when treated with LPS. Similarly, after treatment with I01-2 and I01-4, the morphology of RAW264.7 cells also showed concentration-dependent dendritic changes, and the morphological changes of RAW264.7 caused by I01-2 were more significant than those of I01-4.

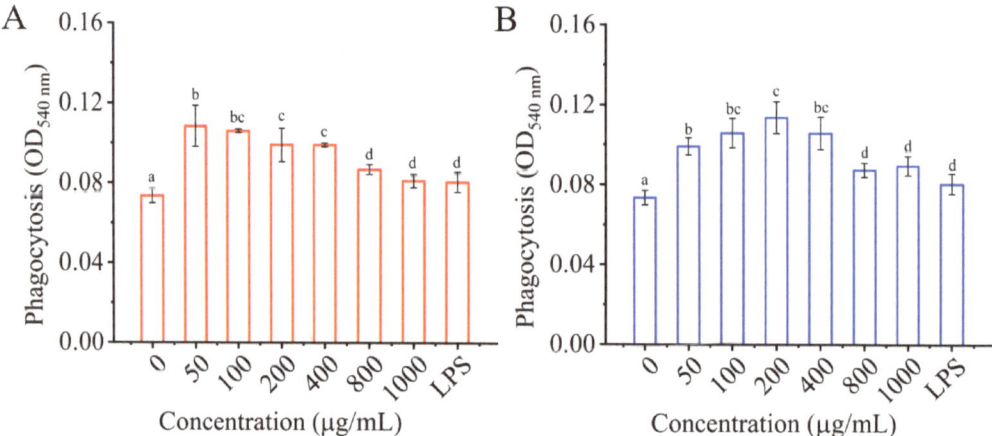

Figure 5. The effect of I01-2 (**A**) and I01-4 (**B**) on the phagocytosis of RAW 264.7 cells. The group was incubated with medium (0 μg/mL of I01-2 and I01-4) as a negative control and LPS (1.0 μg/mL) treatment as a positive control. Different superscript letters (a–d) indicate significant differences ($p < 0.05$) between the groups.

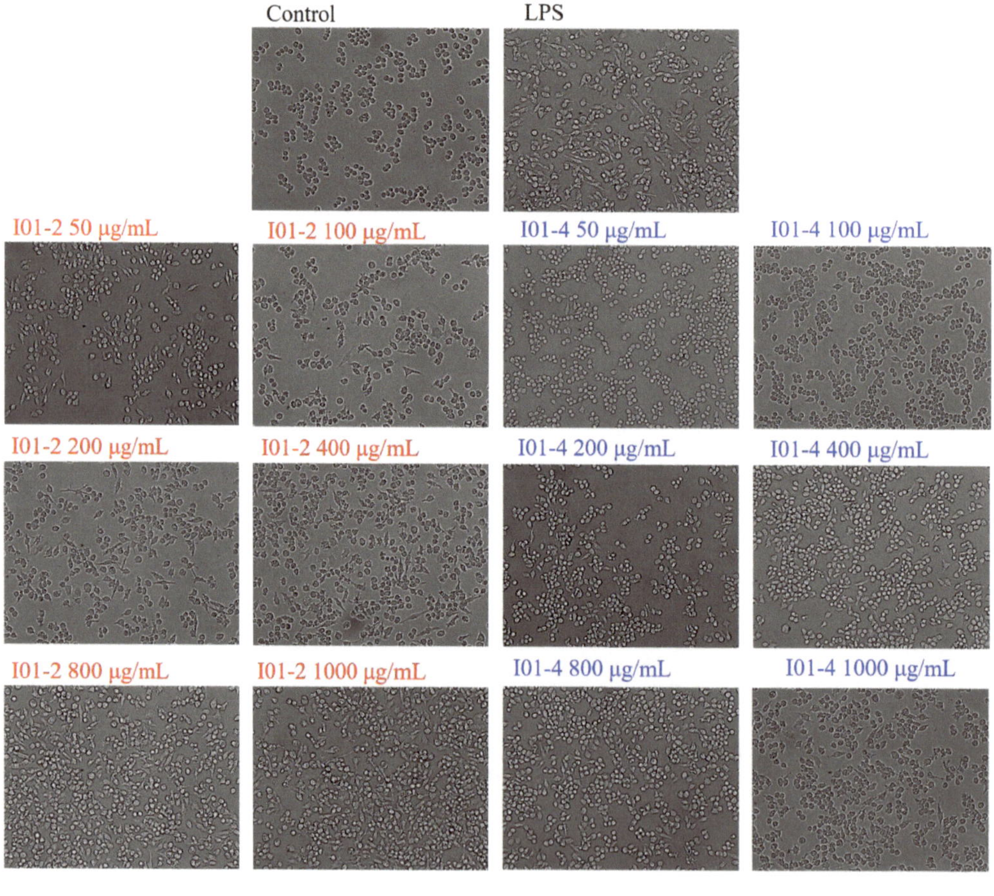

Figure 6. The effect of I01-2 and I01-4 on the morphology of RAW264.7 cells.

3.4.4. Effects of I01-2 and I01-4, Respectively, on the Generation of NO and the Secretion of IL-6 and TNF-α

Macrophages play a potential immunoregulatory role through the production of various mediators and cytokines and are therefore a significant part of host defense systems. While iNOS is a crucial NOS isoform that triggers NO synthesis, NO is an intracellular messenger molecule that plays a role in immunological responses and controls a diverse range of physiological processes, including the regulation of apoptosis [55–58]. Therefore, another indicator of macrophage activation in this investigation was the level of NO production. As can be seen from the data in Figure 7A,B, cells without EPS secreted a bit of NO, whereas I01-2 and I01-4 improved the production of NO at 50–400 μg/mL of I01-2 and 100–800 μg/mL of I01-4 in a dose-dependent manner, and reached the maximum of 85.67 and 59.12 μmol/L, respectively. Notably, however, excessive NO generation is hazardous and may cause apoptosis in macrophages [59]. As a result, we hypothesized that the decreased cell viability and phagocytic capacity of I01-2 and I01-4 with an increase in concentration from 400 μg/mL or 1000 μg/mL, respectively, might be caused by an excessive build-up of NO in macrophages. Additionally, the NO levels in groups receiving EPS treatments were weaker than those in the group receiving LPS treatments, indicating that the EPS effects were more moderate than that of LPS [60].

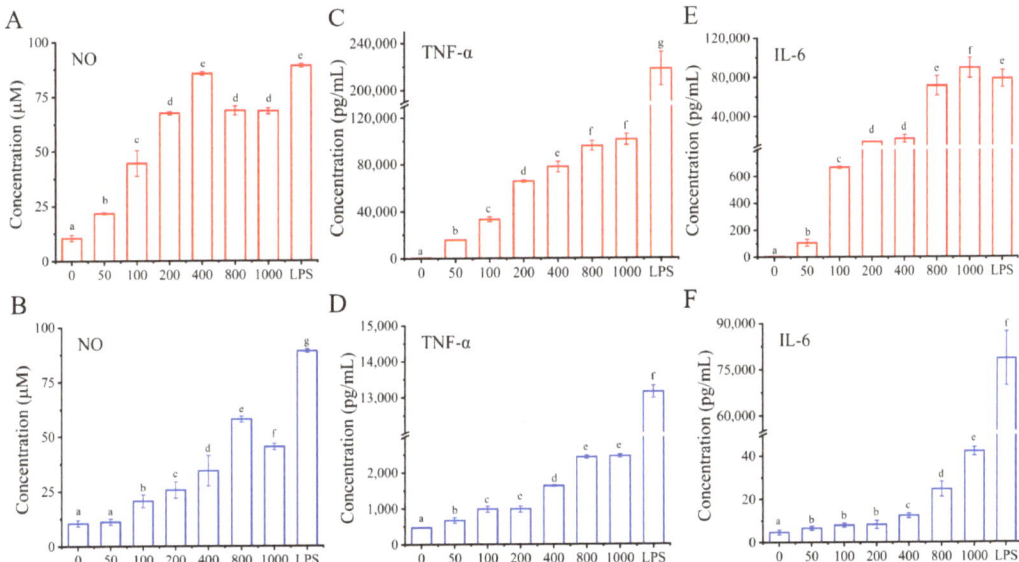

Figure 7. The effect of I01-2 and I01-4 on the production of NO (**A**,**B**), TNF-α (**C**,**D**), and IL-6 (**E**,**F**) in RAW 264.7 cells, respectively. The group incubated with medium only (0 μg/mL of I01-2 and I01-4) was used as a control. Different superscript letters (a–g) indicate significant differences ($p < 0.05$) between the groups.

Activated macrophages can also produce a variety of cytokines other than NO that regulate cellular and humoral immune responses. TNF-α is a pleiotropic cytokine that regulates a wide spectrum of physiological processes, including cell proliferation, differentiation, apoptosis, and inflammation, and it is required for macrophage function [61,62]. However, IL-6 plays a key role in response signaling, which is associated with inflammatory regulation and antigen-presenting [63]. As shown in Figure 7C–F, the control group secreted a basal level of TNF-α and IL-6, while the intervention of I01-2 and I01-4 at all tested concentrations (50–1000 μg/mL) resulted in a remarkable ($p < 0.05$) increase in a dose-dependent manner, in which I01-2 showed better immune activity than I01-4—and its IL-6 and TNF-α contents reached maximums of 8.64×10^4 and 1.01×10^5 pg/mL, respectively, which were 1977 and 41 times those of I01-4, respectively. Similar results have been found that *L. plantarum* NTU 102-EPS exhibited strong immunomodulatory activities at the level of TNF-α and IL-6 [50] as EPS from *L. helveticus* LZ-R-5 enhanced the immunological activity by stimulating the secretion of TNF-α, IL-1β, and IL-6 in RAW264.7 [11]. However, EPS from *L. rhamnosus* KL37 could induce the release of IL-10 in RAW 264.7 cells [64].

Previous studies have confirmed that the activation of macrophages is regulated by immune-related genes [65]. To confirm the effects of I01-2 and I01-4 on the mRNA expression of cytokines in this study, RT-qPCR was used to detect the gene transcription level of *iNOS*, *TNF-α*, and *IL-6*. In Figure 8A–F, the mRNA levels of *iNOS*, *TNF-α* and *IL-6* also showed a significant increase in cells treated with I01-2, I01-4, or LPS when compared to the control group, which was consistent with the NO, TNF-α, and IL-6 secretion levels. It was also found that the EPS from *L. plantarum* RS20D could up-regulate pro-inflammatory cytokines at the mRNA level [66]. Furthermore, all I01-2 and I01-4 treated groups had lower levels of *iNOS*, *TNF-α*, and *IL-6* at the mRNA level than that of the LPS-treated group ($p < 0.05$), which is consistent with the results corresponding to NO production, TNF-α, and IL-6 secretion. Studies demonstrated a relationship between the structural traits of polysaccharides and their biological activity, including the chemical make-up, molecular weight, conformation, glycosidic linkages, and degree of branching [39]. The structure of EPS, in terms of functional groups and glycosidic bonds, is very intimately related to their immunomodulatory activities [26]. A high level of immunomodulatory action was noted in some acidic, galactose-rich EPS, according to several publications [57,67,68]. Hidalgo-Cantabrana et al. reported that EPSs with a negative charge and/or small size can operate as mild stimulators of immune cells and that the galactose content of EPSs may enhance their immunomodulatory effects on the macrophages [69,70]. In our study, I01-2 exhibited an immunomodulatory activity superior to that of I01-4, which may also be due to their differences in monosaccharide composition. All of these findings suggested that I01-2 and I01-4 could cause macrophages to produce more NO, TNF-α, and IL-6, therefore improving the immunological activity, which might play a protective role in host defense against infections or cancer.

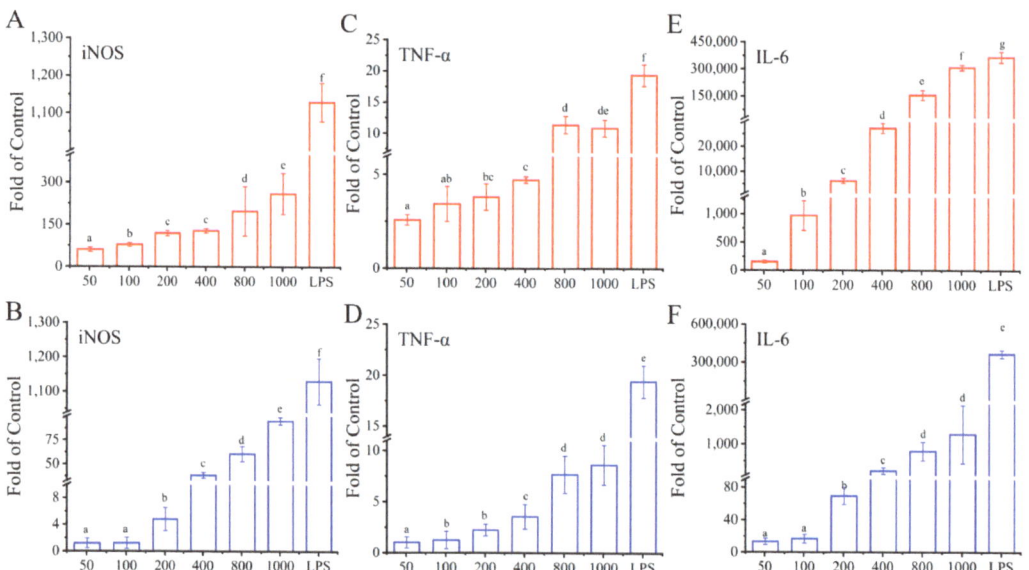

Figure 8. The effects of I01-2 and I01-4 on mRNA levels of *iNOS* (**A**,**B**), *TNF-α* (**C**,**D**), *IL-6* (**E**,**F**) in RAW 264.7 cells, respectively. Different superscript letters (a–g) indicate significant differences ($p < 0.05$) between the groups.

4. Conclusions

In the present study, the production, purification, characterization, and immunomodulatory activity of EPS from *E. hirae* WEHI01 were investigated in vitro. I01-2 and I01-4, which were major fractions therein, were described for their preliminary structure and in vitro immunomodulatory activities. I01-2 and I01-4 are acidic polysaccharides with molecular weights of 2.28×10^4 and 2.59×10^4 Da, respectively. The composition of I01-2 was mainly composed of galactose and a few other sugars, namely galactose, glucose, arabinose, mannose, xylose, fucose, and rhamnose, while galactose only constituted I01-4. Additionally, I01-2 and I01-4 also showed strong immunomodulatory action by accelerating macrophage phagocytosis, producing more NO, and encouraging the release of TNF-α and IL-6 in RAW 264.7 cells. According to all of these findings, I01-2 and I01-4 demonstrated immunomodulatory action and might have positive effects on the production of functional foods and medications.

Author Contributions: K.J. and M.W. helped with the planning and execution of this study, the analysis of the findings, and the manuscript writing. The research data were interpreted with help from Y.H. and Y.W., whilst X.T. and H.W. helped with the research project's planning, X.T. assisted with editing the manuscript and the results from the analysis. All authors have read and agreed to the published version of the manuscript.

Funding: The National Natural Science Foundation of China (grant no. NSF 32060030, Beijing, China) provided funding for this project.

Data Availability Statement: The data used to support the findings of this study can be made available by the corresponding author upon request.

Conflicts of Interest: The authors declare no conflict of interest.

References

1. Freitas, F.; Torres, C.A.; Reis, M.A. Engineering aspects of microbial exopolysaccharide production. *Bioresour. Technol.* **2017**, *245*, 1674–1683. [CrossRef] [PubMed]
2. Lynch, K.M.; Coffey, A.; Arendt, E.K. Exopolysaccharide producing lactic acid bacteria: Their techno-functional role and potential application in gluten-free bread products. *Food Res. Int.* **2018**, *110*, 52–61. [CrossRef] [PubMed]
3. Buksa, K.; Kowalczyk, M.; Boreczek, J. Extraction, purification and characterisation of exopolysaccharides produced by newly isolated lactic acid bacteria strains and the examination of their influence on resistant starch formation. *Food Chem.* **2021**, *362*, 130221. [CrossRef]
4. Lynch, K.M.; McSweeney, P.L.; Arendt, E.K.; Uniacke-Lowe, T.; Galle, S.; Coffey, A. Isolation and characterisation of exopolysaccharide-producing Weissella and Lactobacillus and their application as adjunct cultures in Cheddar cheese. *Int. Dairy J.* **2014**, *34*, 125–134. [CrossRef]
5. Tiwari, S.; Kavitake, D.; Devi, P.B.; Shetty, P.H. Bacterial exopolysaccharides for improvement of technological, functional and rheological properties of yoghurt. *Int. J. Biol. Macromol.* **2021**, *183*, 1585–1595. [CrossRef] [PubMed]
6. Bachtarzi, N.; Kharroub, K.; Ruas-Madiedo, P. Exopolysaccharide-producing lactic acid bacteria isolated from traditional Algerian dairy products and their application for skim-milk fermentations. *LWT* **2019**, *107*, 117–124. [CrossRef]
7. Saadat, Y.R.; Khosroushahi, A.Y.; Gargari, B.P. A comprehensive review of anticancer, immunomodulatory and health beneficial effects of the lactic acid bacteria exopolysaccharides. *Carbohydr. Polym.* **2019**, *217*, 79–89. [CrossRef]
8. Zhang, Z.; Liu, Z.; Tao, X.; Wei, H. Characterization and sulfated modification of an exopolysaccharide from Lactobacillus plantarum ZDY2013 and its biological activities. *Carbohydr. Polym.* **2016**, *153*, 25–33. [CrossRef]
9. Ayyash, M.; Abu-Jdayil, B.; Itsaranuwat, P.; Galiwango, E.; Tamiello-Rosa, C.; Abdullah, H.; Esposito, G.; Hunashal, Y.; Obaid, R.S.; Hamed, F. Characterization, bioactivities, and rheological properties of exopolysaccharide produced by novel probiotic Lactobacillus plantarum C70 isolated from camel milk. *Int. J. Biol. Macromol.* **2019**, *144*, 938–946. [CrossRef]
10. Jiang, B.; Tian, L.; Huang, X.; Liu, Z.; Jia, K.; Wei, H.; Tao, X. Characterization and antitumor activity of novel exopolysaccharide APS of Lactobacillus plantarum WLPL09 from human breast milk. *Int. J. Biol. Macromol.* **2020**, *163*, 985–995. [CrossRef]
11. You, X.; Li, Z.; Ma, K.; Zhang, C.; Chen, X.; Wang, G.; Yang, L.; Dong, M.; Rui, X.; Zhang, Q.; et al. Structural characterization and immunomodulatory activity of an exopolysaccharide produced by Lactobacillus helveticus LZ-R-5. *Carbohydr. Polym.* **2020**, *235*, 115977. [CrossRef]
12. Sarikaya, H.; Aslim, B.; Yuksekdag, Z. Assessment of anti-biofilm activity and bifidogenic growth stimulator (BGS) effect of lyophilized exopolysaccharides (l-EPSs) from *Lactobacilli* strains. *Int. J. Food Prop.* **2016**, *20*, 362–371. [CrossRef]

13. Biliavska, L.; Pankivska, Y.; Povnitsa, O.; Zagorodnya, S. Antiviral Activity of Exopolysaccharides Produced by Lactic Acid Bacteria of the Genera Pediococcus, Leuconostoc and Lactobacillus against Human Adenovirus Type 5. *Medicina* **2019**, *55*, 519. [CrossRef] [PubMed]
14. Yılmaz, T.; Şimşek, Ö. Potential Health Benefits of Ropy Exopolysaccharides Produced by *Lactobacillus plantarum*. *Molecules* **2020**, *25*, 3293. [CrossRef] [PubMed]
15. Nikolic, M.; López, P.; Strahinic, I.; Suárez, A.; Kojic, M.; Fernández-García, M.; Topisirovic, L.; Golic, N.; Ruas-Madiedo, P. Characterisation of the exopolysaccharide (EPS)-producing Lactobacillus paraplantarum BGCG11 and its non-EPS producing derivative strains as potential probiotics. *Int. J. Food Microbiol.* **2012**, *158*, 155–162. [CrossRef]
16. Wang, J.; Wu, T.; Fang, X.; Min, W.; Yang, Z. Characterization and immunomodulatory activity of an exopolysaccharide produced by Lactobacillus plantarum JLK0142 isolated from fermented dairy tofu. *Int. J. Biol. Macromol.* **2018**, *115*, 985–993. [CrossRef]
17. Khalil, M.A.; Sonbol, F.I.; Al-Madboly, L.A.; Aboshady, T.A.; Alqurashi, A.S.; Ali, S.S. Exploring the therapeutic potentials of exopolysaccharides derived from lactic acid bacteria and bifidobacteria: Antioxidant, antitumor, and periodontal regeneration. *Front. Microbiol.* **2022**, *13*, 803688. [CrossRef]
18. Park, H.-R.; Hwang, D.; Suh, H.-J.; Yu, K.-W.; Kim, T.Y.; Shin, K.-S. Antitumor and antimetastatic activities of rhamnogalacturonan-II-type polysaccharide isolated from mature leaves of green tea via activation of macrophages and natural killer cells. *Int. J. Biol. Macromol.* **2017**, *99*, 179–186. [CrossRef]
19. Hidalgo-Cantabrana, C.; Nikolic, M.; López, P.; Suárez, A.; Miljkovic, M.; Kojic, M.; Margolles, A.; Golic, N.; Ruas-Madiedo, P. Exopolysaccharide-producing Bifidobacterium animalis subsp. lactis strains and their polymers elicit different responses on immune cells from blood and gut associated lymphoid tissue. *Anaerobe* **2014**, *26*, 24–30. [CrossRef]
20. Lodemann, U.; Hübener, K.; Jansen, N.; Martens, H. Effects of *Enterococcus faecium* NCIMB 10415 as probiotic supplement on intestinal transport and barrier function of piglets. *Arch. Anim. Nutr.* **2006**, *60*, 35–48. [CrossRef]
21. Awad, W.; Ghareeb, K.; Böhm, J. Intestinal Structure and Function of Broiler Chickens on Diets Supplemented with a Synbiotic Containing Enterococcus faecium and Oligosaccharides. *Int. J. Mol. Sci.* **2008**, *9*, 2205–2216. [CrossRef] [PubMed]
22. Daillère, R.; Vétizou, M.; Waldschmitt, N.; Yamazaki, T.; Isnard, C.; Poirier-Colame, V.; Duong, C.P.M.; Flament, C.; Lepage, P.; Roberti, M.P.; et al. Enterococcus hirae and Barnesiella intestinihominis Facilitate Cyclophosphamide-Induced Therapeutic Immunomodulatory Effects. *Immunity* **2016**, *45*, 931–943. [CrossRef] [PubMed]
23. Hamid, N.H.; Daud, H.M.; Kayansamruaj, P.; Abu Hassim, H.; Yusoff, S.M.; Abu Bakar, S.N.; Srisapoome, P. Short- and long-term probiotic effects of Enterococcus hirae isolated from fermented vegetable wastes on the growth, immune responses, and disease resistance of hybrid catfish (Clarias gariepinus × Clarias macrocephalus). *Fish Shellfish Immunol.* **2021**, *114*, 1–19. [CrossRef] [PubMed]
24. Jayamanohar, J.; Devi, P.B.; Kavitake, D.; Rajendran, S.; Priyadarisini, V.B.; Shetty, P.H. Characterization of α-D-glucan produced by a probiont Enterococcus hirae KX577639 from feces of south Indian Irula tribals. *Int. J. Biol. Macromol.* **2018**, *118*, 1667–1675. [CrossRef] [PubMed]
25. Bhat, B.; Bajaj, B.K. Hypocholesterolemic and bioactive potential of exopolysaccharide from a probiotic Enterococcus faecium K1 isolated from kalarei. *Bioresour. Technol.* **2018**, *254*, 264–267. [CrossRef]
26. Ferreira, S.S.; Passos, C.P.; Madureira, P.; Vilanova, M.; Coimbra, M.A. Structure–function relationships of immunostimulatory polysaccharides: A review. *Carbohydr. Polym.* **2015**, *132*, 378–396. [CrossRef]
27. Jia, K.; Tao, X.; Liu, Z.; Zhan, H.; He, W.; Zhang, Z.; Zeng, Z.; Wei, H. Characterization of novel exopolysaccharide of Enterococcus faecium WEFA23 from infant and demonstration of its in vitro biological properties. *Int. J. Biol. Macromol.* **2018**, *128*, 710–717. [CrossRef]
28. Zhang, F.; Jiang, M.; Wan, C.; Chen, X.; Chen, X.; Tao, X.; Shah, N.P.; Wei, H. Screening probiotic strains for safety: Evaluation of virulence and antimicrobial susceptibility of enterococci from healthy Chinese infants. *J. Dairy Sci.* **2016**, *99*, 4282–4290. [CrossRef]
29. Wei, M.; Gu, E.; Luo, J.; Zhang, Z.; Xu, D.; Tao, X.; Shah, N.P.; Wei, H. Enterococcus hirae WEHI01 isolated from a healthy Chinese infant ameliorates the symptoms of type 2 diabetes by elevating the abundance of Lactobacillales in rats. *J. Dairy Sci.* **2020**, *103*, 2969–2981. [CrossRef]
30. Zhang, F.; Qiu, L.; Xu, X.; Liu, Z.; Zhan, H.; Tao, X.; Shah, N.P.; Wei, H. Beneficial effects of probiotic cholesterol-lowering strain of Enterococcus faecium WEFA23 from infants on diet-induced metabolic syndrome in rats. *J. Dairy Sci.* **2017**, *100*, 1618–1628. [CrossRef]
31. Panda, S.; Ding, J.L. Natural Antibodies Bridge Innate and Adaptive Immunity. *J. Immunol.* **2014**, *194*, 13–20. [CrossRef] [PubMed]
32. Zhang, M.; Yan, M.; Yang, J.; Li, F.; Wang, Y.; Feng, K.; Wang, S.; Lin, N.; Wang, Y.; Yang, B. Structural characterization of a polysaccharide from Trametes sanguinea Lloyd with immune-enhancing activity via activation of TLR4. *Int. J. Biol. Macromol.* **2022**, *206*, 1026–1038. [CrossRef] [PubMed]
33. Cheng, X.-D.; Wu, Q.-X.; Zhao, J.; Su, T.; Lu, Y.-M.; Zhang, W.-N.; Wang, Y.; Chen, Y. Immunomodulatory effect of a polysaccharide fraction on RAW 264.7 macrophages extracted from the wild Lactarius deliciosus. *Int. J. Biol. Macromol.* **2019**, *128*, 732–739. [CrossRef]
34. Zhang, H.-L.; Cui, S.-H.; Zha, X.-Q.; Bansal, V.; Xue, L.; Li, X.-L.; Hao, R.; Pan, L.-H.; Luo, J.-P. Jellyfish skin polysaccharides: Extraction and inhibitory activity on macrophage-derived foam cell formation. *Carbohydr. Polym.* **2014**, *106*, 393–402. [CrossRef] [PubMed]

35. Xie, Y.; Zhou, R.-R.; Xie, H.-L.; Yu, Y.; Zhang, S.-H.; Zhao, C.-X.; Huang, J.-H.; Huang, L.-Q. Application of near infrared spectroscopy for rapid determination the geographical regions and polysaccharides contents of Lentinula edodes. *Int. J. Biol. Macromol.* **2018**, *122*, 1115–1119. [CrossRef] [PubMed]
36. Li, C.; Fu, X.; Luo, F.; Huang, Q. Effects of maltose on stability and rheological properties of orange oil-in-water emulsion formed by OSA modified starch. *Food Hydrocoll.* **2012**, *32*, 79–86. [CrossRef]
37. Liu, C.; Zhang, D.; Shen, Y.; Tao, X.; Liu, L.; Zhong, Y.; Fang, S. DPF2 regulates OCT4 protein level and nuclear distribution. *Biochim. Biophys. Acta* **2015**, *1853*, 3279–3293. [CrossRef]
38. Liu, J.; Zhang, C.; Wang, Y.; Yu, H.; Liu, H.; Wang, L.; Yang, X.; Liu, Z.; Wen, X.; Sun, Y.; et al. Structural elucidation of a heteroglycan from the fruiting bodies of Agaricus blazei Murill. *Int. J. Biol. Macromol.* **2011**, *49*, 716–720. [CrossRef]
39. Yu, Y.; Shen, M.; Wang, Z.; Wang, Y.; Xie, M.; Xie, J. Sulfated polysaccharide from Cyclocarya paliurus enhances the immunomodulatory activity of macrophages. *Carbohydr. Polym.* **2017**, *174*, 669–676. [CrossRef]
40. Zhang, M.; Wang, G.; Lai, F.; Wu, H. Structural Characterization and Immunomodulatory Activity of a Novel Polysaccharide from *Lepidium meyenii*. *J. Agric. Food Chem.* **2016**, *64*, 1921–1931. [CrossRef]
41. Wang, Y.; Li, C.; Liu, P.; Ahmed, Z.; Xiao, P.; Bai, X. Physical characterization of exopolysaccharide produced by Lactobacillus plantarum KF5 isolated from Tibet Kefir. *Carbohydr. Polym.* **2010**, *82*, 895–903. [CrossRef]
42. Wang, X.; Shao, C.; Liu, L.; Guo, X.; Xu, Y.; Lü, X. Optimization, partial characterization and antioxidant activity of an exopolysaccharide from Lactobacillus plantarum KX041. *Int. J. Biol. Macromol.* **2017**, *103*, 1173–1184. [CrossRef] [PubMed]
43. Isfahani, F.M.; Tahmourespour, A.; Hoodaji, M.; Ataabadi, M.; Mohammadi, A. Characterizing the new bacterial isolates of high yielding exopolysaccharides under hypersaline conditions. *J. Clean. Prod.* **2018**, *185*, 922–928. [CrossRef]
44. Yang, X.H.; Yang, J.T.; Liu, H.H.; Ma, Z.R.; Guo, P.H.; Chen, H.; Gao, D.D. Extraction, structure analysis and antioxidant activity of Sibiraea laevigata (L.) Maxim polysaccharide. *Int. J. Food Prop.* **2022**, *25*, 2267–2285. [CrossRef]
45. Wang, Y.; Mao, F.; Wei, X. Characterization and antioxidant activities of polysaccharides from leaves, flowers and seeds of green tea. *Carbohydr. Polym.* **2012**, *88*, 146–153. [CrossRef]
46. Liu, J.; Luo, J.; Ye, H.; Sun, Y.; Lu, Z.; Zeng, X. Production, characterization and antioxidant activities in vitro of exopolysaccharides from endophytic bacterium Paenibacillus polymyxa EJS-3. *Carbohydr. Polym.* **2009**, *78*, 275–281. [CrossRef]
47. Kozarski, M.; Klaus, A.; Niksic, M.; Jakovljevic, D.; Helsper, J.P.; Van Griensven, L.J. Antioxidative and immunomodulating activities of polysaccharide extracts of the medicinal mushrooms Agaricus bisporus, Agaricus brasiliensis, Ganoderma lucidum and Phellinus linteus. *Food Chem.* **2011**, *129*, 1667–1675. [CrossRef]
48. Wang, G.; Zhu, L.; Yu, B.; Chen, K.; Liu, B.; Liu, J.; Qin, G.; Liu, C.; Liu, H.; Chen, K. Exopolysaccharide from Trichoderma pseudokoningii induces macrophage activation. *Carbohydr. Polym.* **2016**, *149*, 112–120. [CrossRef]
49. Wang, S.; Liu, R.; Yu, Q.; Dong, L.; Bi, Y.; Liu, G. Metabolic reprogramming of macrophages during infections and cancer. *Cancer Lett.* **2019**, *452*, 14–22. [CrossRef]
50. Liu, C.-F.; Tseng, K.-C.; Chiang, S.-S.; Lee, B.-H.; Hsu, W.-H.; Pan, T.-M. Immunomodulatory and antioxidant potential of Lactobacillus exopolysaccharides. *J. Sci. Food Agric.* **2011**, *91*, 2284–2291. [CrossRef]
51. Li, C.; Li, X.; You, L.; Fu, X.; Liu, R.H. Fractionation, preliminary structural characterization and bioactivities of polysaccharides from Sargassum pallidum. *Carbohydr. Polym.* **2017**, *155*, 261–270. [CrossRef] [PubMed]
52. Feng, L.; Yin, J.; Nie, S.; Wan, Y.; Xie, M. Fractionation, physicochemical property and immunological activity of polysaccharides from Cassia obtusifolia. *Int. J. Biol. Macromol.* **2016**, *91*, 946–953. [CrossRef] [PubMed]
53. Schepetkin, I.A.; Quinn, M.T. Botanical polysaccharides: Macrophage immunomodulation and therapeutic potential. *Int. Immunopharmacol.* **2006**, *6*, 317–333. [CrossRef] [PubMed]
54. Xu, Y.; Cui, Y.; Wang, X.; Yue, F.; Shan, Y.; Liu, B.; Zhou, Y.; Yi, Y.; Lü, X. Purification, characterization and bioactivity of exopolysaccharides produced by Lactobacillus plantarum KX041. *Int. J. Biol. Macromol.* **2019**, *128*, 480–492. [CrossRef]
55. Wen, Z.-S.; Xiang, X.-W.; Jin, H.-X.; Guo, X.-Y.; Liu, L.-J.; Huang, Y.-N.; OuYang, X.-K.; Qu, Y.-L. Composition and anti-inflammatory effect of polysaccharides from Sargassum horneri in RAW264.7 macrophages. *Int. J. Biol. Macromol.* **2016**, *88*, 403–413. [CrossRef]
56. Alderton, W.K.; Cooper, C.E.; Knowles, R.G. Nitric oxide synthases: Structure, function and inhibition. *Biochem. J.* **2001**, *357*, 593–615. [CrossRef]
57. Wang, W.; Zou, Y.; Li, Q.; Mao, R.; Shao, X.; Jin, D.; Zheng, D.; Zhao, T.; Zhu, H.; Zhang, L.; et al. Immunomodulatory effects of a polysaccharide purified from Lepidium meyenii Walp. on macrophages. *Process Biochem.* **2016**, *51*, 542–553. [CrossRef]
58. Wang, M.; Zhu, P.; Zhao, S.; Nie, C.; Wang, N.; Du, X.; Zhou, Y. Characterization, antioxidant activity and immunomodulatory activity of polysaccharides from the swollen culms of Zizania latifolia. *Int. J. Biol. Macromol.* **2017**, *95*, 809–817. [CrossRef]
59. Nie, C.; Zhu, P.; Ma, S.; Wang, M.; Hu, Y. Purification, characterization and immunomodulatory activity of polysaccharides from stem lettuce. *Carbohydr. Polym.* **2018**, *188*, 236–242. [CrossRef]
60. Zheng, D.; Zou, Y.; Cobbina, S.J.; Wang, W.; Li, Q.; Chen, Y.; Feng, W.; Zou, Y.; Zhao, T.; Zhang, M.; et al. Purification, characterization and immunoregulatory activity of a polysaccharide isolated from Hibiscus sabdariffa L. *J. Sci. Food Agric.* **2016**, *97*, 1599–1606. [CrossRef]
61. Habijanic, J.; Berovic, M.; Boh, B.; Plankl, M.; Wraber, B. Submerged cultivation of Ganoderma lucidum and the effects of its polysaccharides on the production of human cytokines TNF-α, IL-12, IFN-γ, IL-2, IL-4, IL-10 and IL-17. *New Biotechnol.* **2015**, *32*, 85–95. [CrossRef] [PubMed]

62. Aggarwal, B.B. Signalling pathways of the TNF superfamily: A double-edged sword. *Nat. Rev. Immunol.* **2003**, *3*, 745–756. [CrossRef] [PubMed]
63. Mihara, M.; Hashizume, M.; Yoshida, H.; Suzuki, M.; Shiina, M. IL-6/IL-6 receptor system and its role in physiological and pathological conditions. *Clin. Sci.* **2011**, *122*, 143–159. [CrossRef] [PubMed]
64. Ciszek-Lenda, M.; Nowak, B.; Śróttek, M.; Gamian, A.; Marcinkiewicz, J. Immunoregulatory potential of exopolysaccharide from Lactobacillus rhamnosus KL37. Effects on the production of inflammatory mediators by mouse macrophages. *Int. J. Exp. Pathol.* **2011**, *92*, 382–391. [CrossRef] [PubMed]
65. Wang, L.; Nie, Z.-K.; Zhou, Q.; Zhang, J.-L.; Yin, J.-J.; Xu, W.; Qiu, Y.; Ming, Y.-L.; Liang, S. Antitumor efficacy in H22 tumor bearing mice and immunoregulatory activity on RAW 264.7 macrophages of polysaccharides from Talinum triangulare. *Food Funct.* **2014**, *5*, 2183–2193. [CrossRef] [PubMed]
66. Zhu, Y.; Wang, X.; Pan, W.; Shen, X.; He, Y.; Yin, H.; Zhou, K.; Zou, L.; Chen, S.; Liu, S. Exopolysaccharides produced by yogurt-texture improving Lactobacillus plantarum RS20D and the immunoregulatory activity. *Int. J. Biol. Macromol.* **2018**, *121*, 342–349. [CrossRef]
67. Georgiev, Y.N.; Ognyanov, M.H.; Kiyohara, H.; Batsalova, T.G.; Dzhambazov, B.M.; Ciz, M.; Denev, P.N.; Yamada, H.; Paulsen, B.S.; Vasicek, O.; et al. Acidic polysaccharide complexes from purslane, silver linden and lavender stimulate Peyer's patch immune cells through innate and adaptive mechanisms. *Int. J. Biol. Macromol.* **2017**, *105*, 730–740. [CrossRef]
68. Wang, M.; Zhao, S.; Zhu, P.; Nie, C.; Ma, S.; Wang, N.; Du, X.; Zhou, Y. Purification, characterization and immunomodulatory activity of water extractable polysaccharides from the swollen culms of Zizania latifolia. *Int. J. Biol. Macromol.* **2018**, *107*, 882–890. [CrossRef]
69. Hidalgo-Cantabrana, C.; Lopez-Suarez, P.; Gueimonde, M.; Reyes-Gavilan, C.D.L.; Suarez-Diaz, A.M.; Margolles, A.; Ruas-Madiedo, P. Immune Modulation Capability of Exopolysaccharides Synthesised by Lactic Acid Bacteria and Bifidobacteria. *Probiotics Antimicrob. Proteins* **2012**, *4*, 227–237. [CrossRef]
70. Chen, Y.-C.; Wu, Y.-J.; Hu, C.-Y. Monosaccharide composition influence and immunomodulatory effects of probiotic exopolysaccharides. *Int. J. Biol. Macromol.* **2019**, *133*, 575–582. [CrossRef]

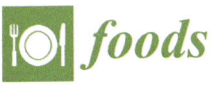

Article

Effect of Hydrothermal Treatment on the Structure and Functional Properties of Quinoa Protein Isolate

Xingfen He [1], Bin Wang [2], Baotang Zhao [2], Yuecheng Meng [1], Jie Chen [1,*] and Fumin Yang [2,*]

[1] School of Food Science and Biotechnology, Zhejiang Gongshang University, Hangzhou 310018, China
[2] College of Food Science and Engineering, Gansu Agricultural University, Lanzhou 730070, China
* Correspondence: chenjie@zjgsu.edu.cn (J.C.); yfumin@gsau.edu.cn (F.Y.); Tel.: +86-13588805519 (J.C.); +86-13893337478 (F.Y.)

Abstract: The aim of this study was to investigate the effects of hydrothermal treatment at different temperatures and times on the structure and functional properties of quinoa protein isolate (QPI). The structure of QPI was investigated by analyzing changes in the intrinsic fluorescence spectrum, ultraviolet (UV) spectrum, and Fourier transform infrared spectrum. The solubility, water/oil-holding capacity, emulsifying activity, and emulsion stability of QPI were studied, as were the particle size and the thermogravimetric properties of QPI. The results showed that the average particle size of QPI gradually increased with the increase in hydrothermal treatment time and temperature, and reached a maximum value of 121 °C for 30 min. The surface morphology also became rough and its thermal stability also increased. The endogenous fluorescence and UV spectral intensity at 280 nm decreased gradually with increasing hydrothermal treatment time and temperature, and reduced to the minimum values at 121 °C for 30 min, respectively. After hydrothermal treatment, the secondary structure of QPI tended to be disordered. The functional properties of QPI after treatment were all superior to those of the control. The results of this study might provide a basis for the processing and utilization of QPI.

Keywords: quinoa (*Chenopodium quinoa* Willd); protein isolate; hydrothermal treatment; structure; functional properties

1. Introduction

Chenopodium quinoa Willd is a kind of quasi-grain. Its protein content is 12.0–23.0%, which is higher than rice, maize and barley [1]. Quinoa protein isolate (QPI) is rich in all the essential amino acids needed by the human body, with a balanced amino acid content, and is easily absorbed by the human body [2]. Quinoa protein is mainly composed of 37% 11S globulin and 35% 2S albumin; disulfide bonds are the key to stabilizing the protein structure, while gluten and gliadin are less so [3]. In addition, 11S globulin is a hexamer composed of a 22–23 kDa basic group and a 32–39 kDa acidic group [4]. 2S Albumin is a heterodimer linked by about 30–40 and 60–90 residues via disulfide bonds (Mw 8–9 kDa) [5]. Compared with most grain proteins, QPI is closer to milk and meat, and is a sustainable high-quality plant protein. In recent years, QPI has gradually become a research hotspot due to its good functional and physicochemical properties that could be used in the food industry [6]. Studies have shown that the emulsifying activity and emulsion stability of QPI are higher than those of wheat protein and soybean protein [7]. QPI has strong water and oil-holding capacities which are higher than those of oats, soybeans, and wheat proteins [8–10].

The structure and functional properties of protein determine its application scope in food processing. The commonly used modification methods in the food industry include ultrasound, high pressure, pH and heat treatment, among which heat treatment has attracted wide attention due to its simple operation and low cost [11–15]. Heat treatment causes thermal denaturation through the destruction of covalent bonds, which increases the exposure of hydrophobic and thiol (SH) groups, and has a substantial impact on the functional properties of food proteins such as solubility, foaming, and emulsifying properties [11]. Heat treatment and alkali treatment can improve the performance of rice protein [16]. Ultrasonic heat treatment reduced the relative content of α-helix and β-sheet in soybean protein secondary structure, and increased the relative content of random coil, resulting in loose tertiary structure [17]. Heat treatment significantly affects the conformation of *Cuminum cyminum* protein, resulting in a surface hydrophobicity increase [15]. Heat treatment at 85 °C for 15 s increased the particle size, turbidity, zeta potential, and surface hydrophobicity of goat milk proteins, further improving their functional properties [18]. Studies also have shown that heat treatment has an effect on the structural and functional properties of faba bean protein [19], protein isolate from *Stauntonia brachyanthera* seeds [20], and sunflower protein [21]. Up to the present, there are few reports indicating the potential effect of heat treatment on QPI. Previous studies have shown that different kinds of heat treatments significantly affected the structural and functional properties of QPI [22]. In addition, the degree of aggregation of QPI can be changed by adjusting the hydrothermal treatment conditions [23]. The water retention capacity improved considerably in the heat-modified and frozen QPI [24]. Mir et al. (2021) have investigated the effects of heat treatment at 80, 90, and 100 °C for 15 and 30 min on the functional properties of QPI [25]. However, the aims of present study are to analyze the effects of the ordinary hydrothermal treatment and simulated autoclaving hydrothermal treatment on the new variety "Longli-1" quinoa protein isolate. We focused on the effects of ordinary hydrothermal treatment and simulated autoclaving on the secondary and tertiary structure of QPI and their effects on functional properties, which are important for processing. The results of this study provide some valuable information for the application of quinoa protein in a variety of foods.

The aims of this study were to (1) determine the changes in the particle size of quinoa protein under different temperature and time hydrothermal treatments; (2) investigate the effects of hydrothermal treatment conditions on the thermal stability of quinoa protein; (3) study how hydrothermal treatment affects the secondary and tertiary structure of quinoa protein; and (4) measure the different functional properties of quinoa protein after hydrothermal treatments.

2. Materials and Methods

2.1. Materials

The "Longli-1" quinoa was kindly supplied by Gansu Academy of Agricultural Sciences (Lanzhou, China). After mechanical shelling, quinoa was packed in woven bags and the samples were stored at room temperature (22 ± 3 °C, RH 55–60%) for 7 d. Sodium dodecyl sulfate (SDS) and phosphate buffer saline were purchased from Shanghai Yuanye Biological Technology Co., Ltd., (Shanghai, China). Edible soybean oil was purchased from a local supermarket.

2.2. Isolation of QPI

The quinoa seeds were crushed and passed through a 60-mesh sieve. The quinoa powder was defatted (petroleum ether, 30–60 °C) 3 times and placed in a fume hood to air dry. The defatted quinoa flour and deionized water were mixed in a ratio of 1:20 g·mL^{-1} and the suspension was then prepared. This suspension was adjusted to pH 10, stirred for 2 h in a water bath at 47 °C, and centrifugated (5000 rpm, 15 min) to take the supernatant. The pH of the supernatant was adjusted to 4.5 (1 M HCl) and the precipitate was collected by centrifugation (5000 rpm, 15 min, 4 °C). The precipitate was reconstituted and washed with deionized water 5 times. The washed precipitate was redissolved in phosphate buffer saline solution at pH 7.0 and placed in a dialysis bag with a molecular retention of 8 kDa. Then the dialysis bag was placed in primary water for dialysis for 48 h (4 °C), and the water was replaced every 3 h. The suspension was vacuum freeze-dried (LyoQuest-85, Telstar Lab, Madrid, Spain) to obtain QPI [26].

2.3. Hydrothermal Treatment of QPI

A 5% QPI solution was prepared using phosphate buffer saline and treated at different temperatures of 25, 60, 70, 80, 90, 100, and 121 °C for 5, 10, 20, and 30 min (60–100 °C was carried out in a water bath, HH-4, Guohua Electric Co., Ltd., Shanghai, China, 121 °C was carried out in an autoclave, MLS-3750, SANYO Corporation, Osaka, Japan), and then quickly cooled. (25 °C in the text refers to QPI without hydrothermal treatment, i.e., natural QPI, which is recorded as control.) The hydrothermally treated QPI solution was vacuum freeze-dried (LyoQuest-85, Telstar Lab, Madrid, Spain) to obtain freeze-dried QPI [27].

2.4. Structural Properties of QPI

2.4.1. Particle Size

Laser particle size analyzer (Bettersize 2600, Dandong Better Instruments Co., Ltd., Dandong, China) was used to measure the particle size of the QPI. The measurement temperature was 25 °C, the refractive index of the sample and the dispersant were 1.46 and 1.33, respectively, and the refractive index was 1.20–1.40% when measured. The QPI was added to cuvette dropwise till the refractive index reached between 5.00% and 10.0% [28].

2.4.2. Thermogravimetric Characteristics

The thermogravimetric analysis of QPI was determined by TGA (TGA 550, TA Instruments Co., Ltd., New Castle, DE, USA). Freeze-dried QPI (5–10 mg) was placed in a platinum–rhodium alloy tray, the scan rate was set to 50 °C/min, and the temperature range was 50 to 700 °C. TGA was performed on QPI under nitrogen atmosphere [29].

2.4.3. Intrinsic Fluorescence Spectrum

Intrinsic fluorescence of QPI was determined using a Fluorescence spectrophotometer (F-4700, Hitachi High-Tech Science Co., Ltd. Naka Office, Naka, Japan). Freeze-dried QPI was mixed with phosphate buffer saline to prepare 0.15 mg/mL QPI solutions (the solution was filtered through a 0.45 μm aqueous filter). The setting parameters were: excitation wavelength 290 nm, emission spectrum was recorded in the range of 300–460 nm, and excitation and emission slits were both 5 nm [30].

2.4.4. Ultra-Violet (UV) Spectrum

Freeze-dried QPI was mixed with phosphate buffer saline to prepare 1 mg/mL QPI solutions (the solution was filtered through a 0.45 μm aqueous filter), and performed UV spectrum scanning (UV-2450, Shimadzu Instruments Co., Ltd., Tokyo, Japan). The scanning wavelength and scanning rate were set to 200–400 nm and 2 nm/s, respectively [31].

2.4.5. FTIR

FTIR of freeze-dried QPI was characterized using an FTIR spectrum (FTIR920, Tianjin Tuopu Instrument Co., Ltd., Tianjin, China). The freeze-dried QPI and KBr were mixed uniformly at a ratio of 1:200, then pulverized and compressed for determination. The measurement temperature was the ambient temperature (25 °C), the wave number, resolution and wave number accuracy were set to 400–4000 cm^{-1}, 4 cm^{-1} and 0.01 cm, respectively, and the number of scans was 64 times [32].

2.5. Determination of Functional Properties of QPI

2.5.1. Solubility

The freeze-dried QPI was dissolved in phosphate buffer saline pH 7 (0.500%), magnetically stirred at ambient temperature (25 °C) for 20 min, and then centrifuged (4000 rpm, 20 min) [33].

The solubility of QPI was expressed as follows:

$$\text{Solubility}/\% = \frac{\text{Protein content in supernatant}}{\text{Total protein content in the sample}} \times 100 \quad (1)$$

The protein content in the supernatant, i.e., the content of soluble protein, was determined by the Coomassie brilliant blue method (CCB) [34]. The specific steps were as follows: Coomassie brilliant blue G-250 was used for color development, and bovine serum albumin (BSA) was used as the reference substance. The content of soluble protein was determined by visible spectrophotometry at the detection wavelength of 595 nm (2700, UV–Vis Spectrophotometer, Co., Ltd. Shimadzu, Tokyo, Japan). The standard curve used was Y = 0.0009X + 0.1834 (R^2 = 0.9898). The total protein content was determined by Kjeldahl method (total nitrogen × 6.38). In this method, 0.5 g freeze-dried quinoa protein powder was used as a sample for determination.

2.5.2. Water-Holding Capacity (WHC) and Oil-Holding Capacity (OHC)

Freeze-dried QPI (0.5 g) was placed in a dry centrifuge tube and mixed with 10 mL of deionized water. The mixture was magnetically stirred at 25 °C for 30 min and then centrifuged (4000 rpm, 30 min). After decanting the supernatant, the centrifuge tube was tilted (45°) for 30 min to remove excess water. The total mass of the centrifuge tube and sediment was recorded. The water-holding capacity (WHC) was calculated using the equation:

$$\text{WHC}/\% = \frac{m_2 - m_1}{0.5} \times 100 \tag{2}$$

where m_1 is the mass of freeze-dried QPI and centrifuge tube (g), m_2 is the mass of sediment and centrifuge tube (g).

Freeze-dried QPI (0.5 g) was placed in a dry centrifuge tube and mixed with 3 mL of soybean oil. The mixture was vortexed at room temperature (25 °C) for 30 min and then centrifuged (4000 rpm, 30 min). After decanting the supernatant, the centrifuge tube was tilted (45°) for 30 min to remove excess oil. The mass of the sediment is recorded. The oil-holding capacity (OHC) was calculated as follows:

$$\text{OHC}/\% = \frac{m_2 - m_1}{0.5} \times 100 \tag{3}$$

where m_1 is the mass of QPI (g), and m_2 is QPI's sediment (g) [35].

2.5.3. Emulsifying Activity (EA) and Emulsion Stability (ES)

A mixed solution of 24 mL hydrothermal treatment QPI solution (1.00%, w/v) and 8 mL soybean oil was whipped with a high-speed shearing dispersing emulsifier (FA25, FLUKO Equipment Shanghai Co., Ltd., Shanghai, China) at 10,000 rpm for 5 min at 25 °C. The emulsion (0.05 mL) and 5 mL of sodium dodecyl sulfate (SDS) solution (0.100%) were mixed and immediately shaken to mix. The absorbance of the emulsion after being placed for 0 min and 10 min were measured at a wavelength of 500 nm with 0.100% SDS solution as a control. The emulsifying activity (EA) was calculated using the equation:

$$\text{EA}\left(m^2/g\right) = \frac{2 \times 2.303 \times A_0 \times DF}{C \times \rho \times \theta \times 10000} \tag{4}$$

where A_0, DF, ρ, and θ are the absorbance value of the sample, dilution factor (100), optical path (1 cm), and oil volume fraction (0.25), respectively.

The emulsion stability (ES) was calculated as follows:

$$\text{ES}/\% = \frac{EA_{10}}{EA} \times 100 \tag{5}$$

where EA_{10} is the emulsifying activity (m^2/g) at 10 min after being placed [36].

2.6. Data Analysis

The indicators involved in the test were measured three times. All data were calculated using Excel 2007 (Microsoft, Redmond, WA, USA) to calculate the mean and standard deviation, Origin 8.5 (Origin Lab, Northampton, MA, USA) was used for graphing, SPSS 17.0 (International Business Machines, Armonk, NY, USA) was used for one-way ANOVA, and Peak Fit V4.12 (Reachsoft, Beijing, China) was used for fitting analysis of infrared spectra.

3. Results and Discussion

3.1. Structural Properties of QPI

3.1.1. Particle Size

The functional properties of proteins are affected by protein particle size [37]. The results showed that compared with the control, the particle size distribution of QPI after hydrothermal treatment became wider, and the overall distribution shifted to the right with the increase in hydrothermal treatment time and temperature, and 121 °C had the most significant effect on it (Figure 1A–D). The volumetric mean particle size $D_{[4,3]}$ of QPI gradually increased with increasing hydrothermal treatment time and temperature, and the effect was most significant of 121 °C, reaching a maximum at 121 °C for 30 min, which was 3.31 times higher than the control ($p < 0.05$) (Table 1). $D_{[5,0]}$ can reflect to some extent the aggregation of proteins, a key factor in the evaluation of protein quality [36]. $D_{[5,0]}$ of QPI increased with increasing hydrothermal treatment time and temperature, reaching a maximum at hydrothermal treatment conditions of 121 °C for 30 min, which was significantly higher than the control by 3.93 times ($p < 0.05$) (Table 1).

Table 1. Effects of different hydrothermal treatment conditions on $D_{[4,3]}$ and $D_{[5,0]}$, nm. A–F indicates the significant differences between different temperatures and a–c indicates the significant differences between different times ($p < 0.05$).

Size (nm)	Temperature (°C)	Time (min)			
		5	10	20	30
$D_{[4,3]}$	25	11.54 ± 1.10 [Ea]	11.54 ± 1.10 [Fa]	11.54 ± 1.10 [Ea]	11.54 ± 1.10 [Fa]
	60	13.57 ± 0.53 [Db]	14.23 ± 0.99 [Eab]	14.35 ± 0.59 [Dab]	15.67 ± 1.09 [Ea]
	70	14.78 ± 0.65 [Db]	16.13 ± 0.53 [Db]	16.44 ± 1.10 [Cb]	18.61 ± 0.96 [Da]
	80	16.76 ± 0.64 [Cc]	18.84 ± 0.98 [Cb]	21.09 ± 0.79 [Ba]	22.01 ± 0.77 [Ca]
	90	18.11 ± 0.45 [Cb]	20.59 ± 1.11 [BCb]	21.24 ± 0.61 [Bb]	21.64 ± 1.30 [Ca]
	100	20.20 ± 0.31 [Bc]	21.87 ± 0.48 [Bb]	20.52 ± 0.46 [Bc]	24.47 ± 0.74 [Ba]
	121	34.49 ± 0.41 [Ac]	143.02 ± 0.49 [Ab]	49.58 ± 0.41 [Aa]	49.69 ± 0.87 [Aa]
$D_{[5,0]}$	25	7.37 ± 0.52 [Da]	7.37 ± 0.52 [Da]	7.37 ± 0.52 [Da]	7.37 ± 0.52 [Ea]
	60	10.90 ± 0.40 [Cb]	9.62 ± 0.54 [Cc]	10.04 ± 0.43 [Cbc]	12.94 ± 0.62 [Da]
	70	9.69 ± 0.44 [Cc]	10.37 ± 0.45 [Cbc]	10.92 ± 0.34 [Cb]	11.95 ± 0.62 [Da]
	80	9.85 ± 0.36 [Cb]	10.36 ± 0.46 [Cb]	14.60 ± 0.30 [Ba]	15.49 ± 0.35 [Ca]
	90	9.84 ± 0.13 [BCd]	13.05 ± 0.44 [Bc]	14.87 ± 0.37 [Bb]	15.72 ± 0.35 [Ca]
	100	12.33 ± 0.28 [Bd]	13.94 ± 0.36 [Bc]	15.03 ± 0.18 [Bb]	17.87 ± 0.61 [Ba]
	121	24.51 ± 0.42 [Ac]	30.55 ± 0.39 [Ab]	36.16 ± 0.16 [Aa]	36.36 ± 0.65 [Aa]

We also found that the average particle size of QPI increased with the increase in temperature, and the degree of particle size inhomogeneity also increased, which is similar to the results from the study of the influence of heating on the particle size of lotus (*Nelumbo nucifera* Gaertn.) seed protein. The results showed that all heat treatments resulted in a significant increase in protein particle size compared to native QPI [38]. Previous studies showed that the particle size of rice gluten increased gradually during heat treatment [39]. The possible reasons may be due to hydrothermal treatment, which causes the 7S and 11S globulins in the protein to cross-link through disulfide bonds to form aggregates and the intact 11S globulin monomers to readily form covalent aggregates, leading to an increase in the particle size of the protein [40]. It is suggested that the hydrothermal treatment causes changes such as cross-linking or aggregation between protein molecules, generating a large number of aggregates, and the degree of protein aggregation increases during the heat treatment, which is consistent with the findings of Wang et al., (2020) [22]. In addition, similar results were found in a study on the effect of heat treatment on the particle size of sunflower protein isolates [21]. This suggests that hydrothermal treatment causes QPI to form aggregates leading to a significant increase in its particle size. However, the results are in contradiction with the results of Mir et al., (2021) who observed a reverse kind of trend whereby the particle size of all QPI samples after heat treatment was smaller than that of native QPI [25]. Among all the heat-treated QPI, the decrease in QPI particle size was the highest at 80 °C for 30 min, and the decrease in QPI particle size was the lowest at 100 °C for 30 min. However, in our results hydrothermal treatment significantly increased the particle size of QPI. The possible reasons for this may be due to the quinoa used in this study is a new variety, Longli-1, which is cultivated in China. Studies have shown that the chemical composition and amino acid profile of different varieties of grains are different, which has a great impact on the physicochemical properties of proteins, therefore affecting the degree of aggregation and particle size [41,42].

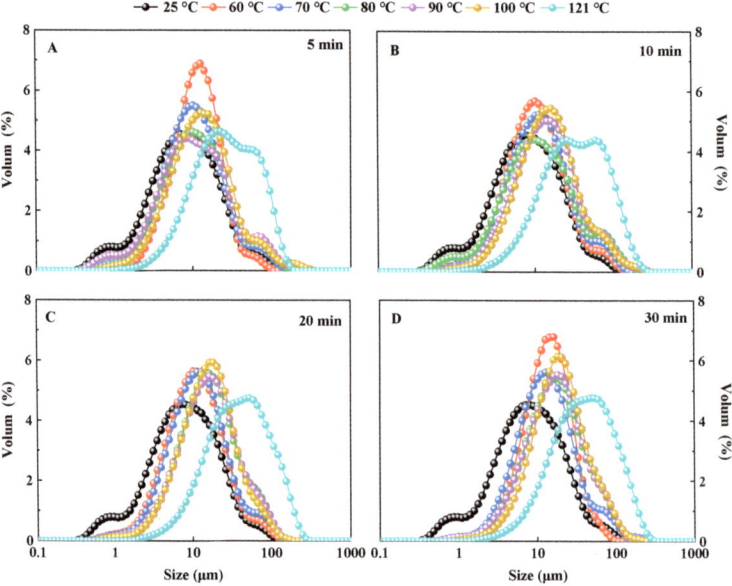

Figure 1. Effects of hydrothermal treatment of 5 min (**A**), 10 min (**B**), 20 min (**C**), 30 min (**D**) on particle size distribution of QPI.

3.1.2. Thermogravimetric Characteristics

The effect of hydrothermal treatment on the thermal stability of QPI was investigated by thermogravimetric analysis of QPI. The results showed that different temperatures had significant effects on the thermogravimetric properties of QPI. The thermal degradation of QPI was divided into three stages, the first stage was from 50 to 200 °C; the weight loss in this stage was due to the evaporation of residual water and the degradation of low molecular weight volatiles. The second stage was from 200 to 400 °C. As the temperature increased further, both non-covalent and covalent bonds in QPI broke, including covalent peptide bonds, disulfide bonds, O-O and O-N, resulting in the complete breakdown of the QPI protein backbone and the release of various gases, such as CO, CO_2, and NH_3 [43]. The third stage was from 400 to 700 °C, during which the slope of the TGA curve changed, the weight loss slowed down, and the degradation of the control began at about 200 °C, while the degradation of the QPI hydrothermally treated at 121 °C began at about 230 °C. This showed that the QPI after heat treatment had higher thermal stability, and when the heat treatment temperature was 121 °C, the thermal stability of QPI was the highest (Figure 2A).

In all three degradation stages, the weight loss of QPI was lower after hydrothermal treatment compared to the control. A similar phenomenon was also found in phosphate-modified peanut protein isolates [44] and protein concentrate of an edible seaweed named *Kappaphycus alvarezii* (Doty) Doty [45]. Similar trends were observed when Malik and Saini investigated the thermogravimetric properties of heat-treated sunflower protein [46].

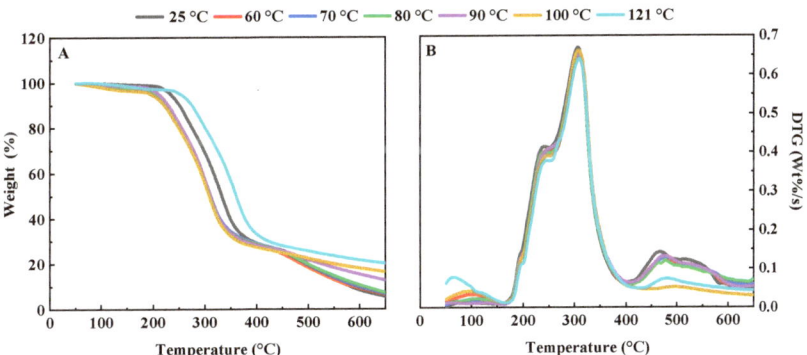

Figure 2. Effects of different hydrothermal treatment temperatures on thermogravimetric (**A**) and derivative thermogravimetric curve (**B**) of QPI.

The derivative thermogravimetric (DTG) curve of QPI showed a unimodal change with a distinct peak (Figure 2B). Corresponding to TGA curve analysis, this peak was mainly caused by the breakage of both non-covalent bonds and covalent bonds in QPI. QPI obtained the maximum decomposition rate at the DTG peak [23]. The decomposition rate of the control was the highest and the decomposition rate of QPI treated at 121 °C was the smallest, which was consistent with the results of TGA. Similar results were reported by Zhang et al., (2019) [47]. The possible reasons for this may be due to hydrothermal treatment of QPI led to protein defolding and subsequent cross-linking of denatured protein molecules, resulting in higher thermal stability [21]. In conclusion, hydrothermal treatment increased the thermal stability of QPI. In addition, Mir et al., (2021) also found that the thermal stability of QPI was significantly improved after heat treatment by a DSC study of quinoa protein [25]. This is consistent with our results in this study.

3.1.3. Intrinsic Fluorescence Spectrum

The QPI after hydrothermal treatment had the same peak shape as the control (Figure 3A–D). However, the hydrothermal treatment significantly affected its maximum absorption wavelength and its corresponding maximum fluorescence intensity. The maximum absorption wavelength of QPI increased gradually with the increase in hydrothermal treatment time and temperature, and reached the maximum when the hydrothermal treatment condition was 121 °C for 20 min, which was 2.25% higher than that of the control (Figure 3E). The maximum fluorescence intensity of QPI decreased gradually with the increase of hydrothermal treatment time and temperature, and dropped to the lowest when the hydrothermal treatment condition was 121 °C for 30 min, which was lower than that of control by 55.3% (Figure 3F). This was probably because hydrothermal treatment increased the hydrophobicity of the QPI and subsequently enhanced the intermolecular hydrophobic interactions of the exposed tryptophan residues, resulting in a decrease in intrinsic fluorescence intensity [21]. A similar phenomenon was observed in the study of heat treatment on sunflower protein isolates near an isoelectric point [46]. However, the results are in contradiction with the results of Chao et al., (2018) who observed a reverse kind of trend whereby the 100 °C pretreated cowpea protein isolates had an increased fluorescence intensity at pH 7.0 when compared to the untreated protein [48]. A plausible reason is that the QPI used in this work had higher surface hydrophobicity, which could enhance protein–protein interactions as compared to the cowpea proteins.

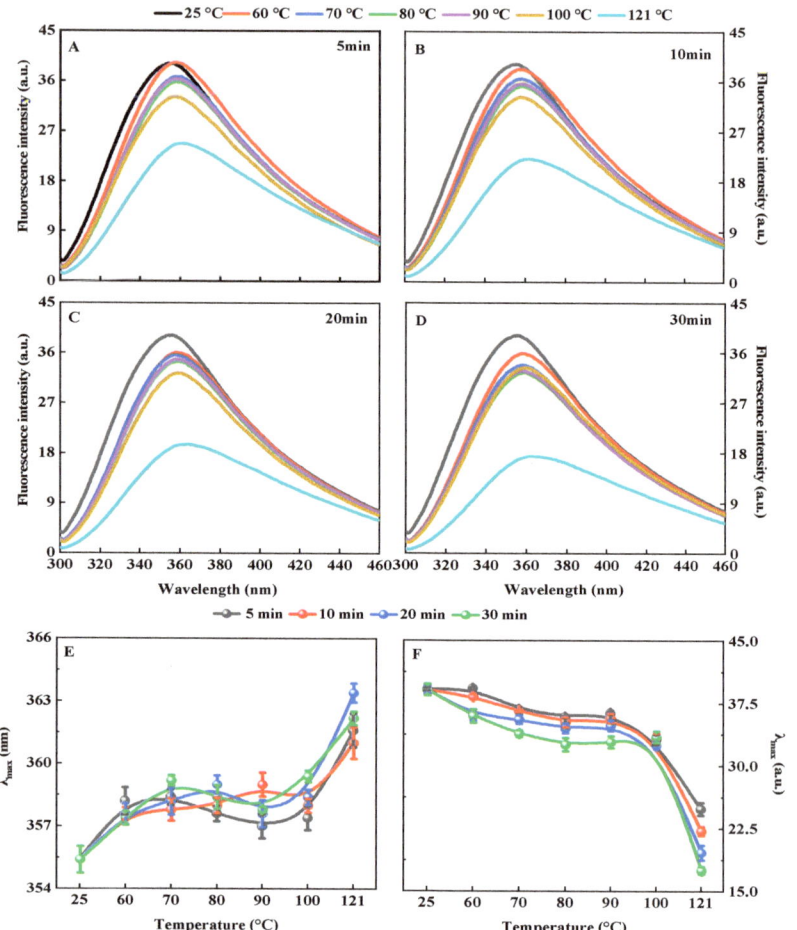

Figure 3. Effects of hydrothermal treatment of 5 min (**A**), 10 min (**B**), 20 min (**C**), and 30 min (**D**) on endogenous fluorescence spectrum, maximum absorption wavelength (**E**), and maximum fluorescence intensity (**F**) of QPI.

In addition, this study found that hydrothermal treatment at 121 °C for 20 min had the most significant effect on the endogenous fluorescence intensity of tryptophan in QPI, and the maximum endogenous fluorescence emission wavelength was significantly red-shifted (increased from 355.4 nm to 363.4 nm), which was 2.25% higher than that of the control. This result indicated that the degree of denaturation of QPI was greater at this time, the tertiary structure of QPI was destroyed, and tryptophan residues were gradually exposed on the protein surface. At the same time, some amide groups initially located on the main peptide chain of the protein were exposed [49]. A similar phenomenon was observed in the study of heat treatment on the tertiary structure of salt-soluble proteins of Pacific oyster (*Crassostrea gigas*) [50]. This suggests that hydrothermal treatment could alter the tertiary structure of QPI.

3.1.4. Ultra-Violet (UV) Spectrum

In this study, we found that the hydrothermally treated QPI had the same UV absorption peak shape as the control, but its absorption peak intensity decreased with the increase in hydrothermal treatment temperature and time (Figure 4A–D). This is probably because the tyrosine or tryptophan content of QPI decreases during the hydrothermal treatment [51]. The minimum absorption peaks at 220 nm and 280 nm were observed in QPI hydrothermally treated at 121 °C for 30 min, which were 5.07% and 6.35% lower than the control, respectively ($p < 0.05$) (Figure 4E,F). Furthermore, the wavelength of the maximum absorption peak near 220 nm was blueshifted by 6 nm compared to the control. This is probably due to the aggregation of the microstructure of QPI by high-temperature treatment, where the color-emitting groups are wrapped and the UV-absorbing groups are reduced [52]. It was shown that hydrothermal treatment reduced the tyrosine, phenylalanine and tryptophan in QPI and the framework structure of QPI was changed. However, the result was inconsistent with the report of He et al., (2014). They observed that the UV absorption peak intensity of rapeseed protein increased after heat treatment [53]. In addition, when compared to the native rapeseed protein, the near-UV CD spectra peak at 262 nm underwent a red shift of 3–5 nm after heat treatment. The possible reasons for this may be due to the difference in the type and quantity of amino acids contained in rapeseed protein and QPI.

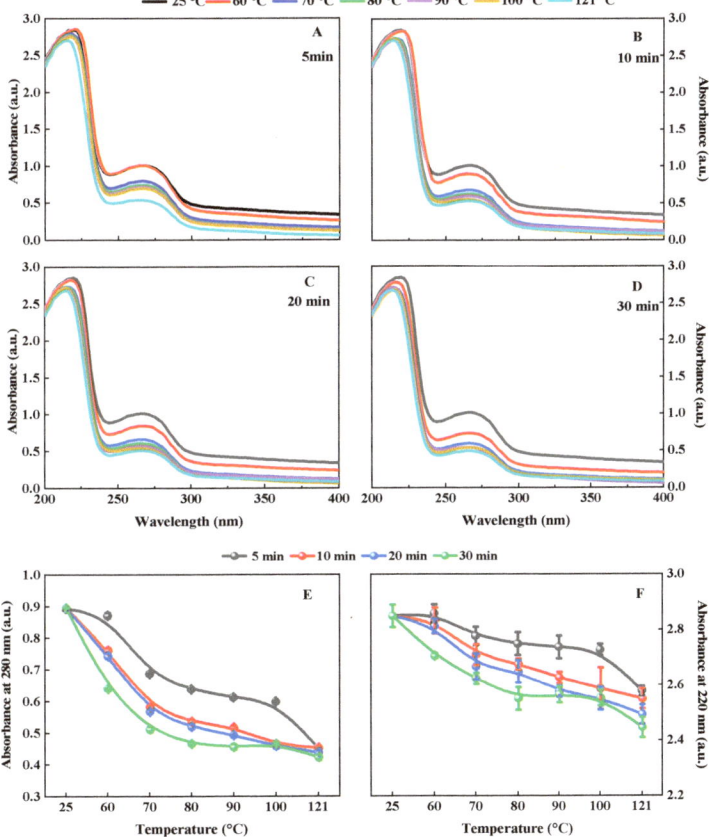

Figure 4. Effects of hydrothermal treatment of 5 min (**A**), 10 min (**B**), 20 min (**C**), and 30 min (**D**) on the UV absorption spectrum of QPI and the absorption value at wavelengths of 280 nm (**E**) and 220 nm (**F**), respectively.

3.1.5. Fourier Transform Infrared Spectrum (FTIR)

Conformational information on protein secondary structure could be efficiently analyzed by FTIR [54]. Figure 5A–D showed the original infrared spectra of QPI for different hydrothermal treatment conditions. Previous studies have shown that the FTIR region of the amide I band corresponds to the secondary structure in proteins as follows: 1610–1640 cm^{-1} belongs to β-sheet, 1660–1670 cm^{-1} belongs to β-turn, 1650–1658 cm^{-1} belongs to α-helix, and 1640–1650 cm^{-1} belongs to random coil [31]. The deconvolution and curve-fitting of the amide I region of QPI to obtain its second derivative spectrum (Figure S1). The relative content of each secondary structure was obtained according to the second derivative spectrum of the amide I band of QPI (Figure 5E–H).

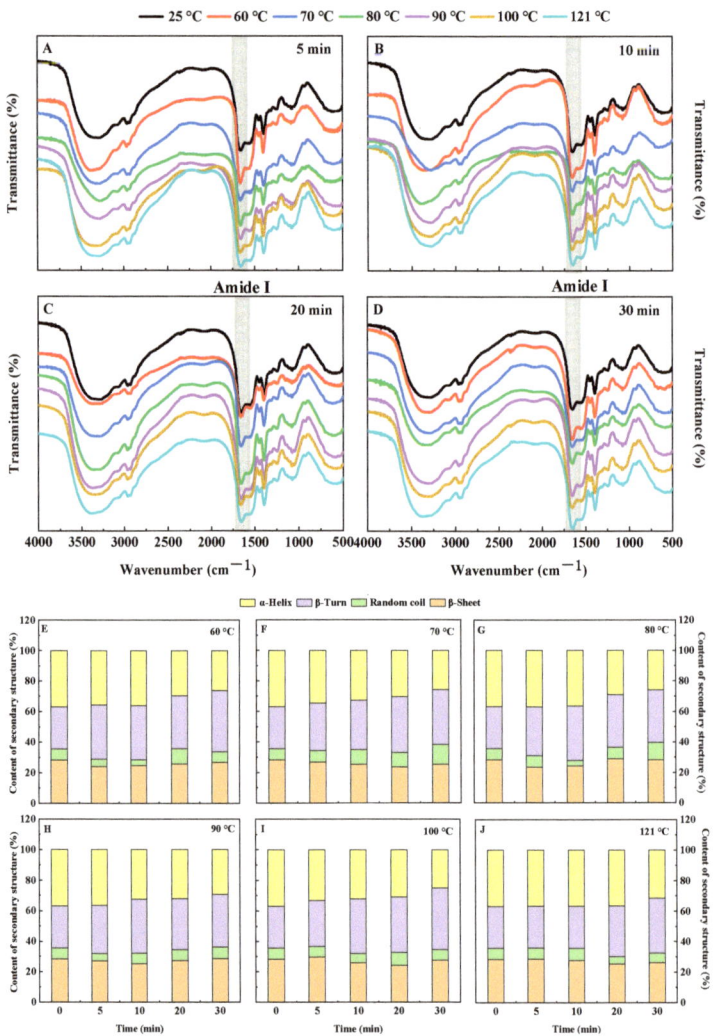

Figure 5. Effects of hydrothermal treatment of 5 min (**A**), 10 min (**B**), 20 min (**C**), and 30 min (**D**) on the Fourier infrared spectrum of QPI, 60 °C (**E**), 70 °C (**F**), 80 °C (**G**), 90 °C (**H**), 100 °C (**I**) and 121 °C (**J**) on the relative content of the secondary structure of QPI.

The relative contents of α-helix, β-sheet, β-turn, and random coil in the secondary structure of QPI all changed significantly after hydrothermal treatment ($p < 0.05$). When the temperature was kept constant, the relative contents of α-helix in the QPI secondary structure gradually decreased with the increase in heat treatment time, while the relative contents of β-turn showed the opposite trend. In addition, the changing trends of the relative contents of β-sheets and random coils were irregular with the increase of heat treatment time. However, the relative contents of β-sheet in the QPI after hydrothermal treatment were lower than the control. In addition, when the temperature was lower than 100 °C and the hydrothermal treatment was performed for 30 min, the relative contents of random coils of QPI were greater than that of the control (Figure 5E–H). This is probably due to the destruction of the hydrogen bonds between adjacent peptide chains in the QPI during the heating process, resulting in the unfolding of the most compact α-helix in the protein molecule and the β-sheet aggregated inside the protein [55]. The relative content of α-helix in the protein gradually decreased with the heating time, which is consistent with our results. Moreover, similar results were found in the study of the effect of heat treatment on the secondary structure of camelina seeds protein isolates [56].

The results of this study indicated that the α-helix and β-sheet of QPI were transformed into β-turn and random coil. This structural change might be related to the denaturation of molecules in QPI under hydrothermal treatment [46]. The protein molecules that are denatured have their internal hydrogen bonds broken, and the protein molecules are unfolded, while the α-helix and β-sheet structures mainly use hydrogen bonds as the force, so the breakdown of hydrogen bonds leads to a decrease in the content of both [57]. Furthermore, β-turn and random coil may be transformed from more ordered structural units, and the β-sheet between the molecules of the thermal aggregates is also easily transformed into β-turn, which leads to an increase in the relative content of β-turn and random coil [58]. It is inferred that β-turn and random coil play an important role in the formation of thermal aggregates. Moreover, the findings of this study are consistent with the results of Mir et al., (2021) [25]. In the study of the secondary structure changes of QPI after heat treatment by circular dichroism, they found that the secondary structure of native and heat–treated QPI was dominated by α-helix and β-sheet, and heat treatment led to the destruction of α-helix in the secondary structure of QPI.

3.2. Determination of Functional Properties of QPI

3.2.1. Solubility

Solubility, as the basis for other functional properties of proteins, is one of the most important functional properties of proteins and has a very close relationship with emulsification, foaming, and other properties of proteins. It also accurately reflects the degree of aggregation of proteins and whether their internal structure is denatured [27]. It is generally believed that proteins aggregate after heat treatment, thereby reducing solubility. However, some studies have shown that moderate heat treatment could improve the solubility of proteins [59]. In this study, we found that when the heat treatment time was kept constant, the solubility of QPI showed a trend of first increasing and then decreasing in the range of 60–121 °C, and reached a maximum of 90 °C for 30 min, which was higher than that of the control by 33.4% ($p < 0.05$). Previous studies showed that the solubility of soybean proteins after treatment at 85 °C was higher than those of samples treated at 55 °C [60]. This is probably due to the fact that poorly water-soluble proteins expose more hydrophilic groups after proper heat treatment, and these groups can subsequently interact with water, leading to a higher water solubility [61].

When the temperature was 100 °C and 121 °C, the solubility of QPI decreased slowly with the increase in hydrothermal treatment time, and finally reduced to the minimum at 121 °C for 30 min (Figure 6). Similar results were reported by Lv et al., (2017) [62]. The possible reason for this may be that the high temperature causes the protein to form a large number of insoluble aggregates. This is consistent with the findings of Yu et al. (2021) on the effect of heat treatment on the solubility of soybean protein. This suggests that high–temperature treatment can reduce protein solubility [63]. In addition, the results indicated that the solubility of QPI extracted by alkali-soluble acid precipitation ranged from 28.34% to 78.46%, while the solubility of the native QPI was 44.12%. This may be due to differences in extraction pH, which lead to changes in the interaction between the protein and water, resulting in different solubility [6].

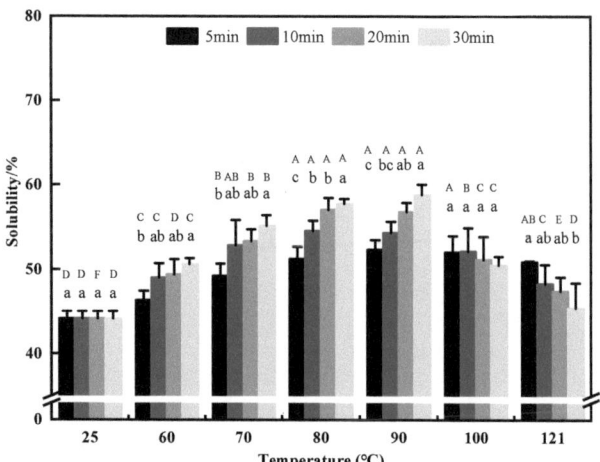

Figure 6. Effects of different hydrothermal treatment conditions on the solubility. A–F indicates the significant differences between different temperatures and a–c indicates the significant differences between different times ($p < 0.05$).

3.2.2. Water-Holding Capacity (WHC) and Oil-Holding Capacity (OHC)

WHC and OHC are the ability of a substance to bind water and oil under limited water and oil conditions [64]. In this study, it was found that the WHC and OHC of QPI after hydrothermal treatment were significantly higher than those of the control, and the WHC and OHC of QPI increased first and then decreased with the increase in temperature. In the range of 60–90 °C, the WHC and OHC of QPI increased gradually with the increase in hydrothermal treatment time and reached a maximum of 90 °C and 30 min, which were 12.50% and 14.18% higher than those of the control, respectively ($p < 0.05$) (Table 2). Previous studies found that the WHC and OHC of peanut seed albumin increased gradually with the increase in heat treatment temperature from 15 to 55 °C [65]. In addition, different heat treatments significantly increased the WHC of guar proteins [66]. This is probably due to the fact that the spatial structure of the protein is opened after heating, which allows some polar groups inside to be transferred to the surface, therefore increasing its WHC and OHC [67]. Furthermore, the findings of this study are consistent with the results of Cerdan et al., (2019) who observed that the WHC and OHC of the heat-treated QPI were 2-fold and 10-fold higher than those of the native QPI, respectively [24]. However, such an increase is much higher than the results of this study, which may be because they used a method of vacuum drying at 35 °C is different from the method in this study.

The WHC and OHC of QPI decreased gradually with the increase in hydrothermal treatment time when the temperature was higher than 90 °C, and the minimum values of 145% and 157% were reached when the heat treatment conditions were 121 °C for 30 min, respectively. It was also found that excessive temperature could significantly reduce its WHC and OHC in the study of heat–treated sunflower protein [20]. This is probably due to the complete denaturation of the protein at high temperature, leading to the exposure of the hydrophobic groups hidden inside, which leads to the reduction in WHC and OHC. Moreover, the OHC of the QPI in this study was slightly higher than that in the previous report [29], which is probably due to the different quinoa varieties used, and the protein content and composition were different. In this study, the trends of WHC and OHC of QPI were found to be in good agreement with solubility. Therefore, we speculate that the WHC and OHC of QPI might be related to its solubility.

Table 2. Effects of different hydrothermal treatment conditions on the water–holding capacity and oil–holding capacity, %. A–E indicates the significant differences between different temperatures and a–c indicates the significant differences between different times ($p < 0.05$).

Capacity (%)	Temperature (°C)	Time (min)			
		5	10	20	30
water	25	143.53 ± 2.30 [Da]	143.53 ± 2.30 [Aa]	143.53 ± 2.30 [Ea]	143.53 ± 2.30 [Ea]
	60	144.80 ± 0.95 [Da]	145.33 ± 3.97 [Aa]	145.87 ± 1.52 [Da]	146.07 ± 1.08 [Da]
	70	147.40 ± 0.31 [Cb]	152.47 ± 2.36 [Aa]	152.07 ± 0.72 [Ca]	152.80 ± 0.95 [Ca]
	80	153.73 ± 1.54 [Ba]	153.93 ± 3.62 [Aa]	154.27 ± 0.74 [Ba]	157.20 ± 2.60 [Ba]
	90	153.00 ± 3.85 [Bb]	158.13 ± 1.83 [Aa]	161.67 ± 0.85 [Aa]	161.47 ± 1.15 [Aa]
	100	161.47 ± 3.62 [Aa]	152.13 ± 0.99 [Ab]	147.60 ± 1.00 [Dc]	145.73 ± 1.14 [Dc]
	121	152.33 ± 5.28 [Ba]	151.20 ± 0.47 [Aab]	146.53 ± 0.92 [Dab]	145.00 ± 3.59 [DEc]
oil	25	151.80 ± 0.64 [Ea]	151.80 ± 0.64 [Ea]	151.80 ± 0.64 [Ea]	151.80 ± 0.64 [Ea]
	60	152.87 ± 2.16 [DEa]	154.33 ± 1.90 [Da]	155.40 ± 3.60 [Da]	156.00 ± 1.40 [Da]
	70	154.00 ± 1.87 [Db]	154.53 ± 0.63 [Db]	155.80 ± 2.17 [Dab]	159.87 ± 3.67 [Ca]
	80	159.27 ± 2.16 [Cb]	166.73 ± 3.38 [Aa]	167.40 ± 2.06 [Aa]	168.00 ± 1.56 [Ba]
	90	163.40 ± 0.36 [Bc]	166.20 ± 1.17 [Abc]	167.67 ± 2.33 [Ab]	173.33 ± 2.42 [Aa]
	100	171.33 ± 2.73 [Aa]	162.20 ± 5.46 [Bb]	162.13 ± 4.30 [Bb]	157.07 ± 0.90 [Db]
	121	160.60 ± 2.54 [Ca]	159.07 ± 4.03 [Ca]	159.67 ± 5.49 [Ca]	156.60 ± 1.56 [Da]

3.2.3. Emulsifying Activity (EA) and Emulsion Stability (ES)

EA and ES characterize the ability of protein to adsorb to the oil-water interface and to form a stable emulsion, respectively [68]. In this study, we found that the EA and ES of QPI after hydrothermal treatment were significantly higher than those of the control. When the temperature was less than 90 °C, the EA and ES of QPI increased with the increase in temperature, and reached a maximum of 90 °C for 30 min of hydrothermal treatment, which was significantly higher than those of the control by 84.4% and 27.1% ($p < 0.05$) (Tables 3 and 4). This is similar to the results of the study in which the ES of faba bean protein concentrate heat-treated at 95 °C for 15 min was significantly higher than that of the control [26]. However, when the temperature was 100 °C and 121 °C, the EA and ES of QPI decreased gradually with the extension of hydrothermal treatment time, and the minimum value was reached at 121 °C, 30 min heat treatment; at which time, the EA was lower than the control by 5.95%, while the ES was higher than the control by 10.1% ($p < 0.05$). The reason for this result might be a change in the solubility of QPI [69].

Table 3. Effects of different hydrothermal treatment conditions on the emulsifying activity, $m^2 \cdot g^{-1}$. A–D indicates the significant differences between different temperatures and a–c indicates the significant differences between different times ($p < 0.05$).

Temperature (°C)	Time (min)			
	5	10	20	30
25	6.55 ± 0.38 [Da]	6.55 ± 0.38 [Da]	6.55 ± 0.38 [Ca]	6.55 ± 0.38 [Da]
60	7.65 ± 0.25 [CDb]	7.72 ± 0.39 [CDb]	8.06 ± 0.73 [BCb]	9.17 ± 0.30 [BCa]
70	7.95 ± 0.28 [BCDc]	8.73 ± 0.46 [BCbc]	9.46 ± 0.52 [Bb]	10.57 ± 0.64 [ABa]
80	9.56 ± 0.68 [ABb]	10.19 ± 0.40 [ABb]	11.57 ± 0.71 [Aa]	11.68 ± 0.66 [Aa]
90	11.05 ± 0.38 [Aa]	11.76 ± 0.67 [Aa]	11.82 ± 0.58 [Aa]	12.05 ± 0.38 [Aa]
100	10.31 ± 0.59 [Aa]	9.84 ± 0.80 [Bab]	8.68 ± 0.36 [Bb]	8.64 ± 0.59 [Cb]
121	9.28 ± 0.29 [ABCa]	8.46 ± 0.37 [BCab]	7.72 ± 0.39 [BCb]	6.16 ± 0.56 [Dc]

Table 4. Effects of different hydrothermal treatment conditions on the emulsion stability, %. A–F indicates the significant differences between different temperatures and a–c indicates the significant differences between different times ($p < 0.05$).

Temperature (°C)	Time (min)			
	5	10	20	30
25	56.08 ± 0.59 [Da]	56.08 ± 0.59 [Da]	56.08 ± 0.59 [Ca]	56.08 ± 0.59 [Fa]
60	57.13 ± 0.88 [CDb]	64.37 ± 2.70 [Ca]	65.87 ± 0.68 [Ba]	66.10 ± 2.14 [Ca]
70	58.13 ± 1.73 [Cb]	65.34 ± 2.30 [BCa]	68.51 ± 0.86 [Aa]	68.00 ± 0.41 [Ba]
80	63.57 ± 0.66 [Bb]	68.62 ± 1.42 [Aa]	68.86 ± 1.06 [Aa]	64.21 ± 0.50 [Db]
90	64.15 ± 1.10 [Bb]	69.63 ± 0.39 [Aab]	68.62 ± 1.42 [Aab]	71.25 ± 1.60 [Aa]
100	70.49 ± 1.74 [Aa]	69.27 ± 1.45 [Aa]	67.37 ± 0.74 [ABab]	64.48 ± 1.79 [CDb]
121	70.55 ± 0.45 [Aa]	66.31 ± 2.20 [Bb]	65.80 ± 2.09 [Bb]	61.76 ± 1.27 [Ec]

It was shown that the EA and ES of vicilin-rich proteins isolated from kidney beans after high-temperature treatment were elevated under moderate heating conditions and decreased after excessive heating [70]. The possible reasons for this may be because the moderate heating induced structural changes in the protein in favor of EA and ES, which might be the driving force for improving the EA and ES of the protein [29]. A hydrothermal treatment temperature greater than 90 °C will cause more unfolding of the protein, exposing their internal hydrophobic groups, resulting in a decrease in solubility, which in turn reduces EA and ES [71]. Therefore, we speculate that protein solubility might have an effect on its EA and ES. The above results show that the EA and ES of QPI could be improved by heat treatment below 121 °C, which is similar to the results of Mir et al., (2021) [25]. They found that the EA and ES of QPI increased significantly after water a bath treatment at 80, 90 and 100 °C for 15 and 30 min

4. Conclusions

In this study, the QPI after hydrothermal treatment was studied from the perspective of structure and functional properties. The results indicated that hydrothermal treatment had significant effects on both the structural and functional properties of QPI. Hydrothermal treatment at 60–121 °C for 5–30 min increased the particle size and thermal stability of QPI, and significantly changed its secondary and tertiary structures. In addition, hydrothermal treatment at 60–90 °C for 5–30 min had a positive effect on improving the functional properties of QPI such as WHC, OHC, EA, ES, and solubility, while hydrothermal treatments at 100 and 121 °C damaged these properties of QPI. Overall, the functional properties of the QPI after hydrothermal treatment were all superior to those of the control. Moreover, several other functional properties of QPI appeared to depend on the the its solubility. Insights gained from this study may help improve the functional properties of QPI by adjusting the hydrothermal treatment conditions. Moreover, our findings provide further support for studying the structure and functional properties of QPI after hydrothermal treatment, which is crucial for their application in food. These findings demonstrate that QPI could be added to foods involving thermal processing. Furthermore, based on the abundant nutritional value of QPI and its good functional properties after heat treatment, it can also be added to functional foods to increase the added value of the product.

Supplementary Materials: The following supporting information can be downloaded at: https://www.mdpi.com/article/10.3390/foods11192954/s1, Figure S1: Deconvolution and curve fitting of the Amide I region for QPI with different hydrothermal treatment conditions.

Author Contributions: Data curation, Methodology, Visualization, and Writing—original draft, X.H.; Formal analysis, Software, and Writing—review and editing, B.W. and Y.M.; Project administration, B.Z.; Conceptualization, Y.M.; Resources, and Supervision, J.C.; Funding acquisition, F.Y. All authors have read and agreed to the published version of the manuscript.

Funding: Key Research and Development Project of Gansu Provincial Science and Technology Department.; the funder, F.Y.; the funding number, 18YF1NA076.

Institutional Review Board Statement: Not applicable.

Informed Consent Statement: Not applicable.

Data Availability Statement: The data presented in this study are available on request from the corresponding author.

Acknowledgments: This work was financially supported by the Key Research and Development Project of Gansu Provincial Science and Technology Department (18YF1NA076).

Conflicts of Interest: The authors declare no financial or other conflict of interest in this work.

References

1. Ruiz, G.A.; Xiao, W.; Boekel, M.V.; Minor, M.; Stieger, M. Effect of extraction pH on heat-induced aggregation, gelation and microstructure of protein isolate from quinoa (*Chenopodium quinoa* Willd). *Food Chem.* **2016**, *209*, 203–210. [CrossRef] [PubMed]
2. Mota, C.; Santos, M.; Mauro, R.; Samman, N.; Matos, A.S.; Torres, D. Protein content and amino acids profile of pseudocereals. *Food Chem.* **2016**, *193*, 55. [CrossRef] [PubMed]
3. Dakhili, S.; Abdolalizadeh, L.; Hosseini, S.M.; Shojaee-Aliabadi, S.; Mirmoghtadaie, L. Quinoa protein: Composition, structure and functional properties. *Food Chem.* **2019**, *299*, 125161.1–125161.10. [CrossRef] [PubMed]
4. Brinegar, C.; Goundan, S. Isolation and characterization of chenopodin, the 11S seed storage protein of quinoa (*Chenopodium quinoa*). *J. Agric. Food Chem.* **1993**, *41*, 182–185. [CrossRef]
5. Brinegar, C.; Sine, B.; Nwokocha, L. High-cysteine 2S seed storage proteins from quinoa (*Chenopodium quinoa*). *J. Agric. Food Chem.* **1996**, *44*, 1621–1623. [CrossRef]
6. Mir, N.A.; Riar, C.S.; Singh, S. Effect of pH and holding time on the characteristics of protein isolates from *Chenopodium* seeds and study of their amino acid profile and scoring. *Food Chem.* **2019**, *272*, 165–173. [CrossRef]
7. Elsohaimy, S.; Refaay, T.; Zaytoun, M. Physicochemical and functional properties of quinoa protein isolate. *Ann. Agric. Sci.-Cairo* **2015**, *60*, 297–305. [CrossRef]
8. Chauhan, G.; Cui, W.; Eskin, N. Effect of saponin on the surface properties of quinoa proteins. *Int. J. Food Prop.* **1999**, *2*, 13–22. [CrossRef]
9. Ma, C.Y.; Harwalkar, V.R. Chemical characterization and functionality assessment of oat protein fractions. *J. Agric. Food Chem.* **1984**, *32*, 144–149. [CrossRef]
10. Ashraf, S.; Saeed, S.M.G.; Sayeed, S.A.; Ali, R. Impact of microwave treatment on the functionality of cereals and legumes. *Int. J. Agric. Biol.* **2012**, *14*, 356–370.
11. Li, F.; Kong, X.; Zhang, C.; Hua, Y. Effect of heat treatment on the properties of soy protein-stabilised emulsions. *Int. J. Food Sci. Technol.* **2011**, *46*, 1554–1560. [CrossRef]
12. Jiang, L.; Wang, J.; Li, Y.; Wang, Z.; Liang, J.; Wang, R.; Chen, Y.; Ma, W.; Qi, B.; Zhang, M. Effects of ultrasound on the structure and physical properties of black bean protein isolates. *Food Res. Int.* **2014**, *62*, 595–601. [CrossRef]
13. Cadesky, L.; Walkling-Ribeiro, M.; Kriner, K.T.; Karwe, M.V.; Moraru, C.I. Structural changes induced by high-pressure processing in micellar casein and milk protein concentrates. *Int. J. Dairy Technol.* **2017**, *100*, 7055–7070. [CrossRef] [PubMed]
14. Jiang, J.; Chen, J.; Xiong, Y. Structural and emulsifying properties of soy protein isolate subjected to acid and alkaline pH-shifting processes. *J. Agric. Food Chem.* **2009**, *57*, 7576–7583. [CrossRef] [PubMed]
15. Chen, J.; Mu, T.; Miao, Z.; Goffin, D. Effect of heat treatments on the structure and emulsifying properties of protein isolates from cumin seeds (*Cuminum cyminum*). *Food Sci. Technol. Int.* **2018**, *24*, 673–687. [CrossRef]
16. Zhao, M.; Xiong, W.; Chen, B.; Zhu, J.; Wang, L. Enhancing the solubility and foam ability of rice glutelin by heat treatment at pH 12: Insight into protein structure. *Food Hydrocoll.* **2020**, *103*, 105626. [CrossRef]
17. Zhao, C.; Chu, Z.; Miao, Z.; Liu, J.; Liu, J.; Xu, X.; Wu, Y.; Qi, B.; Yan, J. Ultrasound heat treatment effects on structure and acid-induced cold set gel properties of soybean protein isolate. *Food Biosci.* **2020**, *39*, 100827. [CrossRef]
18. Zhao, X.; Cheng, M.; Zhang, X.; Li, X.; Wang, C. The effect of heat treatment on the microstructure and functional properties of whey protein from goat milk. *Int. J. Dairy Technol.* **2019**, *103*, 1289–1302. [CrossRef]
19. Espinosa, M.; Guevara-Oquendo, V.H.; Newkirk, R.W.; Yu, P. Effect of heat processing methods on the protein molecular structure, physicochemical, and nutritional characteristics of faba bean (low and normal tannin) grown in western Canada. *Anim. Feed Sci. Technol.* **2020**, *269*, 114681. [CrossRef]
20. Yu, N.; Jiang, C.; Ning, F.; Hu, Z.; Shao, S.; Zou, X.; Meng, X.; Xiong, H. Protein isolate from *Stauntonia brachyanthera* seed: Chemical characterization, functional properties, and emulsifying performance after heat treatment. *Food Chem.* **2020**, *345*, 128542. [CrossRef]
21. Malik, M.A.; Saini, C.S. Improvement of functional properties of sunflower protein isolates near isoelectric point: Application of heat treatment. *LWT-Food Sci. Technol.* **2018**, *98*, 411–417. [CrossRef]

22. Wang, L.; Dong, J.; Zhu, Y.; Shen, R.; Wu, L.; Zhang, K. Effects of microwave heating, steaming, boiling and baking on the structure and functional properties of quinoa (*Chenopodium quinoa* Willd.) protein isolates. *Int. J. Food Sci. Technol.* **2020**, *56*, 14706. [CrossRef]
23. Vondel, J.; Lambrecht, M.A.; Housmans, J.; Rousseau, F.; Delcour, J.A. Impact of hydrothermal treatment on denaturation and aggregation of water-extractable quinoa (*Chenopodium quinoa* Willd.) protein. *Food Hydrocoll.* **2021**, *115*, 106611. [CrossRef]
24. Cerdán-Leal, M.A.; López-Alarcón, C.A.; Ortiz-Basurto, R.I.; Luna-Solano, G.; Jiménez-Fernández, M. Influence of heat denaturation and freezing-lyophilization on physicochemical and functional properties of quinoa protein isolate. *Cereal Chem.* **2019**, *97*, 373–381. [CrossRef]
25. Mir, N.A.; Riar, C.S.; Singh, S. Improvement in the functional properties of quinoa (*Chenopodium quinoa*) protein isolates after the application of controlled heat-treatment: Effect on structural properties. *Food Struct.* **2021**, *28*, 100189. [CrossRef]
26. Mir, N.A.; Riar, C.S.; Singh, S. Structural modification of quinoa seed protein isolates (QPIs) by variable time sonification for improving its physicochemical and functional characteristics. *Ultrason. Sonochem.* **2019**, *58*, 104700. [CrossRef]
27. Hall, A.E.; Moraru, C.I. Structure and function of pea, lentil and faba bean proteins treated by high pressure processing and heat treatment. *LWT-Food Sci. Technol.* **2021**, *152*, 112349. [CrossRef]
28. Zhu, Q.; Li, Y.; Li, S.; Wang, W. Fabrication and characterization of acid soluble collagen stabilized Pickering emulsions. *Food Hydrocoll.* **2020**, *106*, 105875. [CrossRef]
29. Nawrocka, A.; Szymanska-Chargot, M.; Mis, A.; Wilczewska, A.Z.; Markiewicz, K.H. Effect of dietary fibre polysaccharides on structure and thermal properties of gluten proteins—A study on gluten dough with application of FT-Raman spectroscopy, TGA and DSC. *Food Hydrocoll.* **2017**, *69*, 410–426. [CrossRef]
30. Guo, L.; Fang, Y.; Shao, Z.P.; Fang, S.; Li, Y.; Chen, J.; Meng, Y. pH-induced structural transition during complexation and precipitation of sodium caseinate and ε -poly-L-lysine. *Int. J. Biol. Macromol.* **2020**, *154*, 644–653. [CrossRef]
31. Vera, A.; Valenzuela, M.A.; Yazdani-Pedram, M.; Tapia, C.; Abugoch, L. Conformational and physicochemical properties of quinoa proteins affected by different conditions of high-intensity ultrasound treatments. *Ultrason. Sonochem.* **2019**, *51*, 186–196. [CrossRef] [PubMed]
32. Wang, X.; Zhao, R.; Yuan, W. Composition and secondary structure of proteins isolated from six different quinoa varieties from china. *J. Cereal Sci.* **2020**, *95*, 103036. [CrossRef]
33. Wang, S.; Wang, T.; Sun, Y.; Cui, Y.; Yu, G.; Jiang, L. Effects of high hydrostatic pressure pretreatment on the functional and structural properties of rice bran protein hydrolysates. *Foods* **2022**, *11*, 29. [CrossRef] [PubMed]
34. Bradford, M.M. A rapid and sensitive method for the quantitation of microgram quantities of protein utilizing the principle of protein-dye binding. *Anal. Biochem.* **1976**, *72*, 248–254. [CrossRef]
35. Deng, Y.; Huang, L.; Zhang, C.; Xie, P.; Cheng, J.; Wang, X.; Li, S. Physicochemical and functional properties of Chinese quince seed protein isolate. *Food Chem.* **2019**, *283*, 539–548. [CrossRef]
36. Lawal, O.S.; Adebowale, K.O.; Adebowale, Y.A. Functional properties of native and chemically modified protein concentrates from bambarra groundnut. *Food Res. Int.* **2007**, *40*, 1003–1011. [CrossRef]
37. Zhu, Z.; Zhu, W.; Yi, J.; Liu, N.; Cao, Y.; Lu, J.; Decker, E.A.; McClements, D.J. Effects of sonication on the physicochemical and functional properties of walnut protein isolate. *Food Res. Int.* **2018**, *106*, 853–861. [CrossRef]
38. Jia, X.; Wang, J.; Lu, X.; Zheng, B.; Guo, Z. Structure and dilatational rheological behavior of heat-treated lotus (*Nelumbo nucifera* Gaertn.) seed protein. *LWT-Food Sci. Technol.* **2019**, *116*, 108579. [CrossRef]
39. Wang, Y.; Yang, Q.; Fan, J.; Zhang, B.; Chen, H. The effects of phosphorylation modification on the structure, interactions and rheological properties of rice glutelin during heat treatment. *Food Chem.* **2019**, *297*, 124978. [CrossRef]
40. Zhao, X.; Hou, C.; Tian, M.; Zhou, Y.; Yang, R.; Wang, X.; Gu, Z.; Wang, P. Effect of water-extractable arabinoxylan with different molecular weight on the heat-induced aggregation behavior of gluten. *Food Hydrocoll.* **2020**, *99*, 105318. [CrossRef]
41. Ogungbenle, H.N. Nutritional evaluation and functional properties of quinoa (*Chenopodium quinoa*) flour. *Int. J. Food Sci. Nutr.* **2009**, *54*, 153–158. [CrossRef] [PubMed]
42. Eugenia, S.M.; Paula, V.; Eduardo, M.S.R.; Ritva, R.C.; Alberto, L.E.; Gabriela, P.T. Physico-chemical and functional characterization of protein isolated from different quinoa varieties (*Chenopodium quinoa* willd). *Cereal Chem. J.* **2015**, *93*, 275–281.
43. Lqari, H.; Vioque, J.; Pedroche, J.; Millán, F. Lupinus angustifolius protein isolates: Chemical composition, functional properties and protein characterization. *Food Chem.* **2002**, *76*, 349–356. [CrossRef]
44. Yu, L.; Yang, W.; Sun, J.; Zhang, C.; Bi, J.; Yang, Q. Preparation, characterisation and physicochemical properties of the phosphate modified peanut protein obtained from *Arachin Conarachin* L. *Food Chem.* **2015**, *170*, 169–179. [CrossRef] [PubMed]
45. Kumar, K.S.; Ganesan, K.; Selvaraj, K.; Rao, P. Studies on the functional properties of protein concentrate of *kappaphycus alvarezii* (Doty) Doty–An edible seaweed. *Food Chem.* **2014**, *153*, 353–360. [CrossRef] [PubMed]
46. Malik, M.A.; Saini, C.S. Heat treatment of sunflower protein isolates near isoelectric point: Effect on rheological and structural properties. *Food Chem.* **2019**, *276*, 554–561. [CrossRef]
47. Zhang, S.; Zheng, L.; Zheng, X.; Ai, B.; Yang, Y.; Pan, Y.; Sheng, Z. Effect of steam explosion treatments on the functional properties and structure of camellia (*Camellia oleifera* Abel.) seed cake protein. *Food Hydrocoll.* **2019**, *93*, 189–197. [CrossRef]
48. Chao, D.; Aluko, R.E. Modification of the structural, emulsifying, and foaming properties of an isolated pea protein by thermal pretreatment. *CyTA-J. Food* **2018**, *16*, 357–366. [CrossRef]

49. Zhong, L.; Ma, N.; Wu, Y.; Zhao, L.; Ma, G.; Pei, F.; Hu, Q. Characterization and functional evaluation of oat protein isolate-Pleurotus ostreatus β-glucan conjugates formed via Maillard reaction. *Food Hydrocoll.* **2019**, *87*, 459–469. [CrossRef]
50. Zhang, F.; Jiang, S.; Feng, X.; Wang, R.; Zeng, M.; Zhao, Y. Effect of heat treatment on physicochemical state and in vitro digestion of salt-soluble protein from pacific oyster (*Crassostrea gigas*). *LWT-Food Sci. Technol.* **2020**, *134*, 110126. [CrossRef]
51. Yao, F.; Wu, Q.; Yong, L.; Guo, W.; Xu, Y. Thermal decomposition kinetics of natural fibers: Activation energy with dynamic thermogravimetric analysis. *Polym. Degrad. Stab.* **2008**, *93*, 90–98. [CrossRef]
52. Zhao, X.; Chen, F.; Xue, W.; Lee, L. FTIR spectra studies on the secondary structures of 7s and 11s globulins from soybean proteins using AOT reverse micellar extraction. *Food Hydrocoll.* **2008**, *22*, 568–575. [CrossRef]
53. He, R.; He, H.Y.; Chao, D.; Ju, X.; Aluko, R. Effects of high pressure and heat treatments on physicochemical and gelation properties of rapeseed protein isolate. *Food Bioprocess Technol.* **2014**, *7*, 1344–1353. [CrossRef]
54. Keerati-U-Rai, M.; Miriani, M.; Iametti, S.; Bonomi, F.; Corredig, M. Structural changes of soy proteins at the oil–water interface studied by fluorescence spectroscopy. *Colloids Surf. B* **2012**, *93*, 41–48. [CrossRef]
55. Peng, Q.; Khan, N.A.; Wang, Z.; Yu, P. Moist and dry heating-induced changes in protein molecular structure, protein subfractions, and nutrient profiles in camelina seeds. *J. Dairy Sci.* **2013**, *97*, 446–457. [CrossRef]
56. Meziani, S.; Jasniewski, J.; Ribotta, P.; Arab-Tehrany, E.; Muller, J.M.; Ghoul, M.; Desobry, S. Influence of yeast and frozen storage on rheological, structural and microbial quality of frozen sweet dough. *J. Food Eng.* **2012**, *109*, 538–544. [CrossRef]
57. Shilpashree, B.G.; Arora, S.; Chawla, P.; Tomar, S.K. Effect of succinylation on physicochemical and functional properties of milk protein concentrate. *Food Res. Int.* **2015**, *72*, 223–230. [CrossRef]
58. Liu, G.; Li, J.; Shi, K.; Wang, S.; Chen, J.; Liu, Y.; Huang, Q. Composition, secondary structure, and self-assembly of oat protein isolate. *J. Agric. Food Chem.* **2009**, *57*, 4552–4558. [CrossRef]
59. Shima, M.; Maryam, S.; Farhad, A.; Zahra, E.D.; Elnaz, H.; Nader, S.; Ali, A.M.M. Effect of dry heating on physico-chemical, functional properties and digestibility of camel whey protein. *Int. Dairy J.* **2018**, *86*, 9–20.
60. Shao, Y.; Lin, K.; Kao, Y. Modification of foaming properties of commercial soy protein isolates and concentrates by heat treatments. *J. Food Qual.* **2016**, *39*, 695–706. [CrossRef]
61. Beck, S.M.; Knoerzer, K.; Sellahewa, J.; Emin, M.A.; Arcot, J. Effect of different heat-treatment times and applied shear on secondary structure, molecular weight distribution, solubility and rheological properties of pea protein isolate as investigated by capillary rheometry. *J. Food Eng.* **2017**, *208*, 66–76. [CrossRef]
62. Lv, S.; Sun, L.; Zhao, S.; Bao, Y. Effect of dry heat stabilisation on the functional properties of rice bran proteins. *Int. J. Food Sci. Technol.* **2017**, *52*, 1836–1843. [CrossRef]
63. Yu, P.; Kyriakopoulou, K.; Rahmani, A.; Venema, P.; Goot, A. Isochoric moisture heating as a tool to control the functionality of soy protein. *LWT-Food Sci. Technol.* **2021**, *150*, 111979.
64. Khan, S.H.; Butt, M.S.; Sharif, M.K.; Sameen, A.; Mumtaz, S.; Sultan, M.T. Functional properties of protein isolates extracted from stabilized rice bran by microwave, dry heat, and parboiling. *J. Agric. Food Chem.* **2011**, *59*, 2416–2420. [CrossRef] [PubMed]
65. Li, P.; Wen, J.; Ma, X.; Lin, F.; Zhuo, J.; Bing, D. Structural, functional properties and immunomodulatory activity of isolated Inca peanut (*Plukenetia volubilis* L.) seed albumin fraction. *Int. J. Biol. Macromol.* **2018**, *118*, 1931–1941. [CrossRef]
66. Hu, H.; Li-Chan, E.C.Y.; Wan, L.; Tian, M.; Pan, S. The effect of high intensity ultrasonic pre-treatment on the properties of soybean protein isolate gel induced by calcium sulfate. *Food Hydrocoll.* **2013**, *32*, 303–311. [CrossRef]
67. Arzeni, C.; Martínez, K.; Zema, P.; Arias, A.; Pérez, O.E.; Pilosof, A.M.R. Comparative study of high intensity ultrasound effects on food proteins functionality. *J. Food Eng.* **2012**, *108*, 463–472. [CrossRef]
68. Du, Y.; Jiang, Y.; Zhu, X.; Xiong, H.; Shi, S.; Hu, J.; Peng, H.; Zhou, Q.; Sun, W. Physicochemical and functional properties of the protein isolate and major fractions prepared from *Akebia trifoliata var. australis* seed. *Food Chem.* **2012**, *133*, 923–929. [CrossRef]
69. Nidhina, N.; Muthukumar, S.P. Antinutritional factors and functionality of protein-rich fractions of industrial guar meal as affected by heat processing. *Food Chem.* **2015**, *173*, 920–926. [CrossRef]
70. Tang, C.; Ma, C. Heat-induced modifications in the functional and structural properties of vicilin-rich protein isolate from kidney (*Phaseolus vulgaris* L.) bean. *Food Chem.* **2009**, *115*, 859–866. [CrossRef]
71. Mir, N.A.; Riar, C.S.; Singh, S. Structural modification in album (*Chenopodium album*) protein isolates due to controlled thermal modification and its relationship with protein digestibility and functionality. *Food Hydrocoll.* **2020**, *103*, 105708. [CrossRef]

MDPI AG
Grosspeteranlage 5
4052 Basel
Switzerland
Tel.: +41 61 683 77 34

Foods Editorial Office
E-mail: foods@mdpi.com
www.mdpi.com/journal/foods

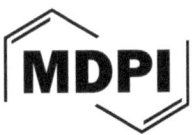

Disclaimer/Publisher's Note: The title and front matter of this reprint are at the discretion of the Guest Editors. The publisher is not responsible for their content or any associated concerns. The statements, opinions and data contained in all individual articles are solely those of the individual Editors and contributors and not of MDPI. MDPI disclaims responsibility for any injury to people or property resulting from any ideas, methods, instructions or products referred to in the content.

www.ingramcontent.com/pod-product-compliance
Lightning Source LLC
LaVergne TN
LVHW072329090526
838202LV00019B/2383